THE LIBRARY
THE LEARNING AND DEVELOPMENT CENTRE
THE CALDERDALE ROYAL HOSPITAL
HALIFAX HX3 0PW

Property of:-   The Library

£78.84.

D1433856

Calde

B59499

THE LIBRARY
THE LEARNING AND DEVELOPMENT CENTRE
THE CALDERDALE ROYAL HOSPITAL
HALIFAX HX3 0PW

Retina and Vitreous Surgery

Surgical Techniques in Ophthalmology

Series Editors

F Hampton Roy MD FACS **and Larry Benjamin** FRCS FRCOphth DO

Strabismus Surgery
ISBN 978 1 4160 3020 1

Cataract Surgery
ISBN 978 1 4160 2969 4

Glaucoma Surgery
ISBN 978 1 4160 3020 8

Refractive Surgery
ISBN 978 1 4160 3022 5

Retina and Vitreous Surgery
ISBN 978 1 4160 4206 8

Oculoplastic Surgery
ISBN 978 1 4160 3286 1

Retina and Vitreous Surgery

Edited by

Abdhish R. Bhavsar MD

Director, Clinical Research, Retina Center, PA;
Attending Surgeon, Phillips Eye Institute
Adjunct Assistant Professor
University of Minnesota
Minneapolis, MN, USA

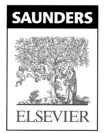

SAUNDERS

ELSEVIER

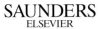

© 2009, Elsevier Inc. All rights reserved.

First published 2009

No part of this publication may be reproduced or transmitted in any form or by any means, electronic or mechanical, including photocopying, recording, or any information storage and retrieval system, without permission in writing from the publisher. Permissions may be sought directly from Elsevier's Rights Department: phone: (+1) 215 239 3804 (US) or (+44) 1865 843830 (UK); fax: (+44) 1865 853333; e-mail: healthpermissions@ elsevier.com. You may also complete your request on-line via the Elsevier website at http://www.elsevier. com/permissions.

ISBN 978 1 4160 4206 8

British Library Cataloguing in Publication Data
A catalogue record for this book is available from the British Library

Library of Congress Cataloging in Publication Data
A catalog record for this book is available from the Library of Congress

Notice
Medical knowledge is constantly changing. Standard safety precautions must be followed, but as new research and clinical experience broaden our knowledge, changes in treatment and drug therapy may become necessary or appropriate. Readers are advised to check the most current product information provided by the manufacturer of each drug to be administered to verify the recommended dose, the method and duration of administration, and contraindications. It is the responsibility of the practitioner, relying on experience and knowledge of the patient, to determine dosages and the best treatment for each individual patient. Neither the Publisher nor the author assumes any liability for any injury and/or damage to persons or property arising from this publication.
The Publisher

Printed in China
Last digit is the print number: 9 8 7 6 5 4 3 2 1

Working together to grow
libraries in developing countries

www.elsevier.com | www.bookaid.org | www.sabre.org

ELSEVIER   BOOK AID International   Sabre Foundation

Commissioning Editor: Russell Gabbedy
Development Editor: Joanne Scott
Project Manager: Rory MacDonald
Design Manager: Judith Wright
Illustration Manager: Kirsteen Wright
Illustrator: Danny Pyne
Marketing Managers: Bill Veltre (USA)/John Canelon (UK)

Contents

Contributors

Everett Ai MD
Director, Retina Unit
California Pacific Medical Center
West Coast Retina Medical Group
San Francisco, CA, USA

Marcus L. Allen MD
Physician/Associate
Retina Institute of Texas, PA
Dallas, TX, USA

Pawan Bhatnagar MD
Vitreoretinal Surgery Fellow
LuEsther T. Mertz Retinal Research Center
Department of Ophthalmology
Manhattan Eye, Ear and Throat Hospital
New York, NY, USA

Abdhish R. Bhavsar MD
Director, Clinical Research, Retina Center, PA;
Attending Surgeon, Phillips Eye Institute
Adjunct Assistant Professor
University of Minnesota
Minneapolis, MN, USA

Alex Bui MD
Vitreoretinal Surgery Fellow
California Pacific Medical Center
West Coast Retina Medical Group
San Francisco, CA, USA

Antonio Capone Jr MD
Clinical Associate Professor of Biomedical
Sciences
Eye Research Institute
Oakland University, Royal Oak, MI;
Director, Fellowship of Vitreoretinal Diseases
and Surgery
Associated Retinal Consultants PC
St Clair Shores, MI, USA

Steve Charles MD
Clinical Professor of Ophthalmology
University of Tennessee College of Medicine
Department of Ophthalmology
Memphis, TN, USA

Bertil E. Damato MD PhD FRCOphth
Professor of Ophthalmology
Ocular Oncology Service
Royal Liverpool University Hospital
Liverpool, UK

Kimberly Drenser MD PhD
Director of Research and Viteroretinal Surgeon
Associated Retinal Consultants;
Assistant Professor, Oakland Unit
Associated Retinal Consultants
Royal Oak, MI, USA

Howard F. Fine MD MHSc
Medical Director, Gerstner Clinical Research
Center
Edward S. Harkness Eye Institute
Columbia University Medical Center
New York, NY, USA

Carl Groenewald MD
Consultant Vitreoretinal Surgeon
St Paul's Eye Unit
Royal Liverpool University Hospital
Liverpool, UK

Anurag Gupta MD
Assistant Professor of Ophthalmology, Director
David Geffen School of Medicine at UCLA
International Vitreoretinal Surgery Fellowship
Jules Stein Eye Institute
Los Angeles, CA, USA

Mark E. Hammer MD
Clinical Associate Professor of Ophthalmology,
University of South Florida
Retina Associates of Florida
Tampa, FL, USA

Robert G. Josephberg MD
Chief of Retina and Vitreous, Westchester
Medical Center
Assistant Clinical Professor, New York Medical
College, Valhalla, New York,
and University of Medicine and Dentistry
Newark, NJ, USA

J. Michael Jumper MD
Chief, Retina Section
California Pacific Medical Center
Assistant Clinical Professor
University of California San Francisco
West Coast Retina Medical Group
San Francisco, CA, USA

Neil E. Kelly MD
Retired, formerly with Retina Consultants
Sacrament
Eye Life Institute
Sacaramento, CA, USA

Gregory F. Kozielec
Physician/Partner
Retina Institute of Texas, PA
Dallas, TX, USA

Allan E. Kreiger MD
Professor of Ophthalmology
Jules Stein Eye Institute
UCLA School of Medicine
Los Angeles, CA, USA

William F. Mieler MD
Professor and Chairman
University of Chicago
Department of Ophthalmology and Visual
Sciences
Chicago, IL, USA

Sachin Mudvari MD
Resident
Department of Ophthalmology
California Pacific Medical Center
San Francisco, CA, USA

Michael P. Rubin MD
Retina Fellow
Harvard Medical School
Massachusetts Eye and Ear Infirmary
Boston, MA, USA

W. Sanderson Grizzard MD
Clinical Professor of Ophthalmology
University of South Florida
Retina Associates of Florida
Tampa, FL, USA

Steven D. Schwartz MD
Chief
Retina Divsion
Jules Stein Eye Institute, UCLA
Los Angeles, CA, USA

Kent W. Small MD
President
Molecular Insight LLC
Los Angeles, CA, USA

Richard F. Spaide MD
Associate Clinical Professor of Ophthalmology
Manhattan Eye, Ear, and Throat Hospital
Vitreous, Retina, Macula Consultants of New
York & the LuEsther T. Mertz Retina Research
Laboratory
New York, NY, USA

Maurice G. Syrquin MD
Physician/Partner Retina Institute of Texas
Dallas, TX, USA

Khaled A. Tawansy MD
Director, Children's Retina Institute of California
Assistant Professor of Ophthalmology and
Pediatrics
Children's Hospital Los Angeles
Los Angeles, CA, USA

Bruce C. Taylor MD
Retired, formerly Physician/Partner
Retina Institute of Texas
Dallas, TX, USA

Edgar L. Thomas MD (Deceased)
Retina-Vitreous Associates
Los Angeles, CA, USA

Michael T. Trese MD
Clinical Professor of Biomedical Sciences
Eye Research Institute, Oakland University
Royal Oak, MI;
Associated Retinal Consultants PC
St Clair Shores, MI, USA

Anand Vinekar MD FRCS
Chief, Pediatric Vitreo-Retina and Rehabilitation
Service
Narayana Nethralaya Postgraduate Institute
Bangalore, India;
International Fellow
Associated Retinal Consultants
Royal Oak, MI, USA

Charles P. Wilkinson MD
Chairman, Department of Ophthalmology
Greater Baltimore Medical Center;
Professor, Department of Ophthalmology
Johns Hopkins University
Baltimore, MD, USA

George A. Williams MD
Chief, Department of Ophthalmology
Director, Beaumont Eye Institute
Royal Oak, MI, USA

Richard L. Winslow MD
Formerly Physician/Partner
Retina Institute of Texas
Dallas, TX, USA

Keye L. Wong MD
Associate Clinical Professor
University of South Florida;
Retina Associates of Sarasota
Sarasota, FL USA

Additional Video Contributors

Haris I. Amin MD
President
Ocean County Retina, PC
Toms River, NJ, USA

Subhadra Jalali MD
Retina Consultant
L.V.Prasad Eye Institute
Hyderabad, India

Virgilio Morales-Canton MD
Attending Physician, Retina Service
Asociacion para Evitar la Ceguera en México
Mexico City, Mexico

Series Preface

Modern ophthalmic surgery is a combination of dexterity, knowledge, judgement and experience which is gained over many years. Properly applied it can produce results which can be life changing for the patient and tremendously rewarding for the team looking after the patient. Complications arising from the surgery can be just as life altering, more so perhaps than in many other branches of surgery because of the emotive implications of loss of sight.

Training in ophthalmology is becoming shorter and more intense on both sides of the Atlantic and the trainee surgeon needs clear, structured tuition on which to base their practical surgical experience. Theoretical learning of surgery must always be supported by a positive practical learning environment and this series of books aims to help with the theoretical aspects of techniques but also gives good, practical guidance for the time spent in the operating theatre.

Adaptability is the key to successful surgery. Being able to change a surgical plan part of the way through a procedure, implement that change whilst taking the whole team with you and achieving a good outcome while still making the whole process a positive experience for the patient requires skill and judgement. Learning different approaches to a surgical procedure enables that adaptability whereas a surgeon stuck with a single technique will at some point be unable to complete the operation successfully.

This surgical series is written by an international selection of surgeons with many combined years of surgical practice and teaching. Each volume is written in a clear, structured format with many pictures and diagrams and is also coupled with high quality surgical video footage where these help to illustrate an important surgical concept. Whilst no surgical text can be completely comprehensive, the techniques described in the various volumes are all tried and tested by the authors.

It is hoped that these six volumes will help to enable surgical adaptability.

F. Hampton Roy
Larry Benjamin

Preface

The concept of a textbook on retina and vitreous surgery that centers on the basics of surgical techniques has been in my thoughts every since I was a fellow at the Jules Stein Eye Institute at UCLA over 10 years ago. When I was approached by Elsevier to author and edit a retina volume in this present series of ophthalmology texts, it was received with both pleasure and anticipation.

The basic design of this series and of this volume, *Retina and Vitreous Surgery*, encompasses the essential elements of the surgical approach to ophthalmic diseases. The basic surgical principles involved in each surgical procedure are of paramount importance. This text presents these basic surgical principles in illustrated format for each disease/surgical approach. The precise instruments and equipment required are specified in each chapter, along with the indications and contraindications, description of the step-by-step surgical approach, potential complications and postoperative care.

The main idea of this text is to provide a practical resource for all retina and vitreous surgeons. The text is complimented by a DVD which provides visual and audio support to enable the reader to see the surgical procedure through the eyes of the authoring surgeon(s).

This is a wonderful text for new retina surgeons and it can also be helpful for quite experienced retinal surgeons as well. This is particularly the case for those surgical procedures that are not in one's typical or daily armamentarium. It can be quite helpful, for example to review the chapter covering the principles of the surgical management of tumors if you have not performed such a case in a while.

Furthermore, if you would just like to see how someone else does a particular, even routine, surgical procedure, you can take a look at that chapter and then view the corresponding DVD clip. In many chapters, the authors have described a number of pearls that they have found helpful and these can potentially help you with your surgery every day.

The main distinguishing factor between this text and others is that this is meant for daily consumption, with less emphasis on exhaustive literature reviews and more emphasis on the daily care of patients and on the daily practice of retina and vitreous surgery.

My hope is that you enjoy this text and that it positively impacts the care of your patients with retinal and vitreous diseases every day.

Abdhish R. Bhavsar MD

Dedication

This textbook is dedicated to my children, Nirayudh, Niharika and Atreyus, from whom I have borrowed the time to produce this text, but to whom I will never be able to repay that time.

I owe the creative spirit responsible for this production to my parents Raman N. Bhavsar, MD and Bhartibala (Meena) R. Bhavsar, who taught me the value of perseverance, hard work and self-confidence even in the face of defeat. My father always taught me that the human mind has tremendous capacity, and that being kind and compassionate to everyone while having a "Teflon coating" for protection is essential for dealing with great adversity and even failure.

I owe to my teachers the fostering of internal values and excellence in retina medical and surgical care that I provide to patients every day: Normal P. Blair, MD at the University of Illinois Eye and Ear Infirmary, Allan E. Kreiger, MD, Marc O. Yoshizumi, MD, Kent W. Small, MD, John R. Heckenlively, MD, Steven D. Schwartz, MD, Bradley R. Straatsma, MD, JD, and of course to my senior retina fellow at the Jules Stein Eye Institute at UCLA, Maurice G. Syrquin, MD.

If I were to select one retina surgeon whose example I have tried to model my life after, it would be Edgar (Garee) L. Thomas, MD. Garee has taught me: the value of always carrying oneself as a gentleman, even in the face of blatant mistreatment by others; the value of always being gracious when younger folk ask for your help; the value of persevering in caring for patients, keeping one's word and completing promised projects and book chapters, even in the face of devastating cancer and imminent death.

I owe to my spouse, Mary A. Bhavsar, MD, the time that she has allowed me to take from my responsibilities to our family, while absorbing those responsibilities herself; and for insisting that I should constantly push the envelope for self-improvement and accomplishment ever since we were fellows together at the Jules Stein Eye Institute at UCLA many years ago.

I express my sincere gratitude to all the dedicated retina surgeons and authors who have made this text possible.

ELSEVIER DVD-ROM LICENSE AGREEMENT

PLEASE READ THE FOLLOWING AGREEMENT CAREFULLY BEFORE USING THIS DVD-ROM PRODUCT. THIS DVD-ROM PRODUCT IS LICENSED UNDER THE TERMS CONTAINED IN THIS DVD-ROM LICENSE AGREEMENT ("Agreement"). BY USING THIS DVD-ROM PRODUCT, YOU, AN INDIVIDUAL OR ENTITY INCLUDING EMPLOYEES, AGENTS AND REPRE-SENTATIVES ("You" or "Your"), ACKNOWLEDGE THAT YOU HAVE READ THIS AGREEMENT, THAT YOU UNDERSTAND IT, AND THAT YOU AGREE TO BE BOUND BY THE TERMS AND CONDITIONS OF THIS AGREEMENT. ELSEVIER INC. ("Elsevier") EXPRESSLY DOES NOT AGREE TO LICENSE THIS DVD-ROM PRODUCT TO YOU UNLESS YOU ASSENT TO THIS AGREEMENT. IF YOU DO NOT AGREE WITH ANY OF THE FOLLOWING TERMS, YOU MAY, WITHIN THIRTY (30) DAYS AFTER YOUR RECEIPT OF THIS DVD-ROM PRODUCT RETURN THE UNUSED, PIN NUMBER PROTECTED, DVD-ROM PRODUCT, ALL ACCOMPANYING DOCUMENTATION TO ELSEVIER FOR A FULL REFUND.

DEFINITIONS As used in this Agreement, these terms shall have the following meanings:

"Proprietary Material" means the valuable and proprietary information content of this DVD-ROM Product including all indexes and graphic materials and software used to access, index, search and retrieve the information content from this DVD-ROM Product developed or licensed by Elsevier and/or its affiliates, suppliers and licensors.

"DVD-ROM Product" means the copy of the Proprietary Material and any other material delivered on DVD-ROM and any other human-readable or machine-readable materials enclosed with this DVD-ROM Product, including without limitation documentation relating to the same.

OWNERSHIP This DVD-ROM Product has been supplied by and is proprietary to Elsevier and/or its affiliates, suppliers and licensors. The copyright in the DVD-ROM Product belongs to Elsevier and/or its affiliates, suppliers and licensors and is protected by the national and state copyright, trademark, trade secret and other intellectual property laws of the United States and international treaty provisions, including without limitation the Universal Copyright Convention and the Berne Copyright Convention. You have no ownership rights in this DVD-ROM Product. Except as expressly set forth herein, no part of this DVD-ROM Product, including without limitation the Proprietary Material, may be modified, copied or distributed in hardcopy or machine-readable form without prior written consent from Elsevier. All rights not expressly granted to You herein are expressly reserved. Any other use of this DVD-ROM Product by any person or entity is strictly prohibited and a violation of this Agreement.

SCOPE OF RIGHTS LICENSED (PERMITTED USES) Elsevier is granting to You a limited, non-exclusive, non-transferable license to use this DVD-ROM Product in accordance with the terms of this Agreement. You may use or provide access to this DVD-ROM Product on a single computer or terminal physically located at Your premises and in a secure network or move this DVD-ROM Product to and use it on another single computer or terminal at the same location for personal use only, but under no circumstances may You use or provide access to any part or parts of this DVD-ROM Product on more than one computer or terminal simultaneously.

You shall not (a) copy, download, or otherwise reproduce the DVD-ROM Product in any medium, including, without limitation, online transmissions, local area networks, wide area networks, intranets, extranets and the Internet, or in any way, in whole or in part, except for printing out or downloading nonsubstantial portions of the text and images in the DVD-ROM Product for Your own personal use; (b) alter, modify, or adapt the DVD-ROM Product, including but not limited to decompiling, disassembling, reverse engineering, or creating derivative works, without the prior written approval of Elsevier; (c) sell, license or otherwise distribute to third parties the DVD-ROM Product or any part or parts thereof; or (d) alter, remove, obscure or obstruct the display of any copyright, trademark or other proprietary notice on or in the DVD-ROM Product or on any printout or download of portions of the Proprietary Materials.

RESTRICTIONS ON TRANSFER This License is personal to You, and neither Your rights hereunder nor the tangible embodiments of this DVD-ROM Product, including without limitation the Proprietary Material, may be sold, assigned, transferred or sublicensed to any other person, including without limitation by operation of law, without the prior written consent of Elsevier. Any purported sale, assignment, transfer or sublicense without the prior written consent of Elsevier will be void and will automatically terminate the License granted hereunder.

TERM This Agreement will remain in effect until terminated pursuant to the terms of this Agreement. You may terminate this Agreement at any time by removing from Your system and destroying the DVD-ROM Product. Unauthorized copying of the DVD-ROM Product, including without limitation, the Proprietary Material and documentation, or otherwise failing to comply with the terms and conditions of this Agreement shall result in automatic termination of this license and will make available to Elsevier legal remedies. Upon termination of this Agreement, the license granted herein will ter-minate and You must immediately destroy the DVD-ROM Product and accompanying documentation. All provisions relating to proprietary rights shall survive termination of this Agreement.

LIMITED WARRANTY AND LIMITATION OF LIABILITY NEITHER ELSEVIER NOR ITS LICENSORS REPRESENT OR WARRANT THAT THE DVD-ROM PRODUCT WILL MEET YOUR REQUIREMENTS OR THAT ITS OPERATION WILL BE UNINTERRUPTED OR ERROR-FREE. WE EXCLUDE AND EXPRESSLY DISCLAIM ALL EXPRESS AND IMPLIED WARRANTIES NOT STATED HEREIN, INCLUDING THE IMPLIED WARRANTIES OF MERCHANTABILITY AND FITNESS FOR A PARTICULAR PURPOSE. IN ADDITION, NEITHER ELSEVIER NOR ITS LICENSORS MAKE ANY REPRESENTATIONS OR WARRANTIES, EITHER EXPRESS OR IMPLIED, REGARDING THE PERFORMANCE OF YOUR NETWORK OR COMPUTER SYSTEM WHEN USED IN CONJUNCTION WITH THE DVD-ROM PRODUCT. WE SHALL NOT BE LIABLE FOR ANY DAMAGE OR LOSS OF ANY KIND ARISING OUT OF OR RESULTING FROM YOUR POSSESSION OR USE OF THE SOFTWARE PRODUCT CAUSED BY ERRORS OR OMISSIONS, DATA LOSS OR CORRUPTION, ERRORS OR OMISSIONS IN THE PROPRIETARY MATERIAL, REGARDLESS OF WHETHER SUCH LIABILITY IS BASED IN TORT, CONTRACT OR OTHERWISE AND INCLUDING, BUT NOT LIMITED TO, ACTUAL, SPECIAL, INDIRECT, INCIDENTAL OR CONSEQUENTIAL DAMAGES. IF THE FOREGOING LIMITATION IS HELD TO BE UNENFORCEABLE, OUR MAXIMUM LIABILITY TO YOU SHALL NOT EXCEED THE AMOUNT OF THE LICENSE FEE PAID BY YOU FOR THE SOFTWARE PRODUCT. THE REMEDIES AVAILABLE TO YOU AGAINST US AND THE LICENSORS OF MATERIALS INCLUDED IN THE SOFTWARE PRODUCT ARE EXCLUSIVE.

If this DVD-ROM Product is defective, Elsevier will replace it at no charge if the defective DVD-ROM Product is returned to Elsevier within sixty (60) days (or the greatest period allowable by applicable law) from the date of shipment.

Elsevier warrants that the software embodied in this DVD-ROM Product will perform in substantial compliance with the documentation supplied in this DVD-ROM Product. If You report a significant defect in performance in writing to Elsevier, and Elsevier is not able to correct same within sixty (60) days after its receipt of Your notification, You may return this DVD-ROM Product, including all copies and documentation, to Elsevier and Elsevier will refund Your money.

YOU UNDERSTAND THAT, EXCEPT FOR THE 60-DAY LIMITED WARRANTY RECITED ABOVE, ELSEVIER, ITS AFFILIATES, LICENSORS, SUPPLIERS AND AGENTS, MAKE NO WARRANTIES, EXPRESSED OR IMPLIED, WITH RESPECT TO THE DVD-ROM PRODUCT, INCLUDING, WITHOUT LIMITATION THE PROPRIETARY MATERIAL, AND SPECIFICALLY DISCLAIM ANY WARRANTY OF MERCHANTABILITY OR FITNESS FOR A PARTICULAR PURPOSE.

If the information provided on this DVD-ROM Product contains medical or health sciences information, it is intended for professional use within the medical field. Information about medical treatment or drug dosages is intended strictly for professional use, and because of rapid advances in the medical sciences, independent verification of diagnosis and drug dosages should be made.

IN NO EVENT WILL ELSEVIER, ITS AFFILIATES, LICENSORS, SUPPLIERS OR AGENTS, BE LIABLE TO YOU FOR ANY DAMAGES, INCLUDING, WITHOUT LIMITA-TION, ANY LOST PROFITS, LOST SAVINGS OR OTHER INCIDENTAL OR CONSEQUENTIAL DAMAGES, ARISING OUT OF YOUR USE OR INABILITY TO USE THE DVD-ROM PRODUCT REGARDLESS OF WHETHER SUCH DAMAGES ARE FORESEEABLE OR WHETHER SUCH DAMAGES ARE DEEMED TO RESULT FROM THE FAILURE OR INADEQUACY OF ANY EXCLUSIVE OR OTHER REMEDY.

U.S. GOVERNMENT RESTRICTED RIGHTS The DVD-ROM Product and documentation are provided with restricted rights. Use, duplication or disclosure by the U.S. Government is subject to restrictions as set forth in subparagraphs (a) through (d) of the Commercial Computer Restricted Rights clause at FAR 52.22719 or in subparagraph (c)(1)(ii) of the Rights in Technical Data and Computer Software clause at DFARS 252.2277013, or at 252.2117015, as applicable. Contractor/Manufacturer is Elsevier Inc., 360 Park Avenue South, New York, NY 10010 USA.

GOVERNING LAW This Agreement shall be governed by the laws of the State of New York, USA. In any dispute arising out of this Agreement, You and Elsevier each consent to the exclusive personal jurisdiction and venue in the state and federal courts within New York County, New York, USA.

1

Scleral buckling surgery

Charles P. Wilkinson and Abdhish R. Bhavsar

Rhegmatogenous retinal detachments are repaired by preventing access of intravitreal (vitreous) fluid to the subretinal space via retinal breaks. By the early 1950s, scleral buckling techniques were employed by most vitreoretinal surgeons to repair the vast majority of retinal detachments. The introduction of pneumatic retinopexy for selected cases in 1984 and the increasing popularity of vitrectomy for relatively routine cases have resulted in scleral buckling losing its role as the procedure of choice for most detachment cases.[1,2] Still, the specific indications for the use of a single technique or combination of techniques are controversial and a matter of surgeon preference in most instances, and scleral buckling remains an important component in the arsenal of the contemporary vitreoretinal surgeon.

This chapter will describe and illustrate personally favored scleral buckling techniques that can be employed in the management of most types of uncomplicated primary rhegmatogenous retinal detachments.

INSTRUMENTS AND DEVICES

The most important skill required in surgery for retinal detachment is the ability to detect all retinal breaks and additional areas of vitreoretinal pathology. The only indispensable pieces of equipment for scleral buckling are an indirect ophthalmoscope and a condensing lens. Many excellent models of the former are available, and we favor a 20-diopter lens. (Microscopic scleral buckling techniques have been described, and these may be reasonable if placement of an encircling band at the time of vitrectomy is planned, but we avoid the microscope in routine buckling cases.) Magnifying loupes are recommended for suture placement and drainage, and the authors use old Zeiss loupes that do not require removal when the indirect ophthalmoscope is employed. A cryotherapy unit is used to create a chorioretinal adhesion in the vast majority of cases managed by the authors. Virtually all additional instruments listed below are personal choices, and similar but different equipment can be successfully employed.[3] These will be listed in the order in which they are usually used during a typical case (see Box 1.1).

INDICATIONS AND CONTRAINDICATIONS

At the present time, there is considerable debate among vitreoretinal surgeons in regard to the appropriate role of scleral buckling. Phakic cases that are not ideal for pneumatic retinopexy, which is described in Chapter 12, are usually indications for scleral buckling. In phakic eyes, as the sizes of the breaks become larger, the distances of the retinal breaks become more posterior, and the numbers of such breaks become greater, scleral buckling becomes both more difficult for the surgeon and more painful for the patient, and there is a trend for increasing use of vitrectomy techniques instead of buckles. In pseudophakic cases, there is clearly a worldwide trend for increasing use of vitrectomy techniques, either alone or in conjunction with buckles (see Ch. 2).

Currently, the most common literal contraindication for buckling is vitreous opacification associated with vitreous hemorrhage, and the most common clear media problem is scleral ectasia, but we commonly employ non-buckling techniques instead of buckles,

Box 1.1 Equipment

Exposure

- Lid speculum of choice
- Westcott blunt scissors
- Castroviejo toothed forceps
- Muscle hooks with fenestrated ends
- Large silk suture or umbilical tape to be placed around rectus muscles
- Cotton-tipped applicators, short
- Balanced salt solution to irrigate the cornea

Localization

- A blunt diathermy probe is preferred because it marks internally the edge of the break(s).
- A Gass or other pressure-localizing device can also be used.
- Marking pencil to permanently mark the spots created with the localizer.

Buckling[a]

- Double-armed 5-0 Mersilene suture attached to spatula needles
- Silicone buckling materials
    - Silicone sponge (round 3-mm, 5-mm; ovoid 5 × 7.5 mm) for segmental buckles
    - Hard silicone bands for encircling cases (no. 240, 41 with or without tires or 42 without)
    - Hard silicone tires to provide added height and width of different lengths (no. 287, 289 with 240 band, and 287WG with 41 band)
    - Hard silicone pieces to provide focal augmentation without sutures (no. 103, no. 106)
    - Watzke silicone sleeve to join ends of an encircling band
    - Tennessee blunt forceps to maneuver silicone pieces
- Broad-spectrum antibiotic solution in which to soak buckling element(s)
- Strong straight scissors to trim silicone buckling material

Drainage

- Black tapered penetrating diathermy pin
- Suture needle is a suitable alternative
- Diathermy with blunt probe to treat lightly the exposed choroids

Closure

- 5-0 plain catgut suture
- Use antibiotic solution mentioned above to lavage sub-Tenon's space
- 0.2–0.4 cc of dexamethasone for subconjunctival injection

Accessory products

- 3- to 5-cc syringes with 30-gauge needles
- Available gasses other than air
    - Sulfur hexafluoride (SF_6)
    - Perfluoropropane (C_3F_8)
- Millipore filter
- Balanced salt solution mentioned above can be injected to increase intraocular pressure

[a]*Buckling almost always follows cryotherapy of the retinal break(s).*

primarily to avoid complications of buckling or because the alternative choices appear to be wiser.

SURGICAL TECHNIQUE

A typical scleral buckling procedure involves a sequence of steps that include exposure, localization of breaks, treatment of breaks, suturing of buckling material, management of subretinal fluid, adjustment of the buckle, accessory manipulations, and closure.

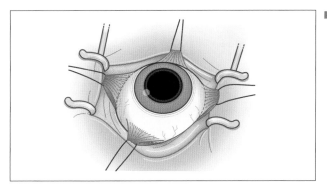

FIGURE 1.1 360-degree circumferential peritomy with isolation of two rectus muscles on large silk sutures.

Exposure

A peritomy is created circumferentially at the limbus or 3–4 mm posteriorly. Although a 360° peritomy is frequently employed, a partial peritomy is sufficient for a limited detachment. Relaxing incisions perpendicular to the limbus can be added. Traction sutures (2-0) or umbilical tapes (or Steristrips) are placed beneath the insertions of the exposed rectus muscles to facilitate positioning the globe (Fig. 1.1). After the appropriate number of rectus muscles is secured with traction sutures, the sclera should be examined for areas of thinning.

1.1
1.2
1.3
1.4

Localization of breaks

After examination of the sclera, the fundus is carefully reevaluated. Most routine tears are marked with a flat diathermy probe or a pressure localization device (e.g. Gass or O'Connor localizer) placed in the center of their anterior edges. This location is preferred because:

1.5
1.6
1.7

- the anterior edge is the usual site of persistent vitreoretinal traction,
- the anterior edge is easier to mark than the posterior border,
- a buckling effect extending from the anterior edge into the area of the vitreous base is desirable, and
- it is relatively easy to estimate the amount of buckling effect required more posteriorly to support the posterior margins of the break(s).

The localization site is immediately touched with a marking pencil (or pen), because the visible initial mark usually disappears quickly. If a break is large, marks should be placed at the posterior, anterior, and lateral margins.

Treatment of breaks

All retinal breaks and most areas of lattice degeneration are treated with transscleral cryotherapy applied under direct visualization. Scleral depression sufficient to approximate the pigment epithelium to the retina is attempted, and treatment is begun anteriorly, where this is easiest. A single row of confluent burns is created around the break(s) and areas of vitreoretinal degeneration, although more than one row may be required anteriorly to extend the future adhesion into the vitreous base (Fig. 1.2). Freezing is promptly terminated as the ice ball just begins to involve the retina. The time required for this effect varies as a function of the cryotherapy equipment, the thickness of the sclera, the choroid and subretinal fluid, and the amount of fluid and episcleral tissue on the scleral surface. The cryotherapy probe must be allowed to thaw after each application before it is moved along the scleral surface.

1.8

A major deficiency in the use of cryotherapy is the inability to visualize treated retina for many minutes following thawing. This can lead to over-treatment by treating the same area twice. Alternatively, an inadequate adhesion will be produced if the burns are not

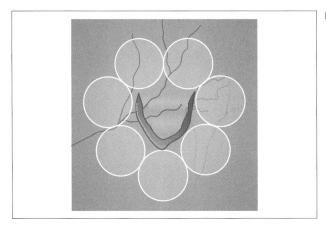

■ **FIGURE 1.2** Cryotherapy should be applied around retinal breaks and into the vitreous base anterior to the break. Treatment of bare pigment epithelium is avoided to reduce dispersion of retinal pigment epithelial cells.

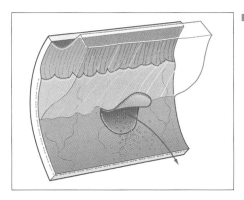

■ **FIGURE 1.3** Dispersion of pigment epithelial cells into the vitreous cavity as a result of cryotherapy. Additional dispersion is caused by retreatment or repeat scleral depression.

contiguous in appropriate areas. Therefore the surgeon must form an optimal visual image of the precise limits of applications of cryotherapy.

Cryotherapy burns should extend only to the edges of medium and large retinal breaks. If the pigment epithelium lying beneath the break is included in the cryotherapy burn, an intravitreal dispersion of pigmented cells capable of proliferation will occur (Fig. 1.3). For the same reason, scleral depression of a treated area at the edge of a break should not be repeated after the treatment, and localization of retinal breaks should always precede cryotherapy.

The development of indirect laser delivery systems has made it possible to treat retinal breaks with photocoagulation, but we do not use this modality except in very unusual circumstances, when breaks in reattached retina are treated postoperatively through a gas bubble.

Suturing of scleral buckling material

1.9
1.10
1.11

Silicone exoplants are secured to the sclera with 5-0 non-absorbable synthetic mattress sutures (e.g. nylon, Mersilene, or silk) attached to spatula needles. One-half to two-thirds thickness intrascleral passes at least 6 mm long are usually attempted for sponges and broad exoplants, whereas shorter intrascleral passes can be used to support encircling bands. The eye is immobilized with the traction sutures held by the assistant. The surgeon applies focal pressure with a cotton applicator near the intended suture site to prevent buckling of the sclera in front of the needle as it is passed through the sclera. Alternatively, a nearby muscle insertion can be grasped with a forceps to provide increased stability and to elevate intraocular pressure (IOP). The needle tip should be visualized at all times during its passage through the sclera.

Buckle configuration generalities

Placement of sutures for buckling initially requires a consideration of buckle configuration. The location, number, size, and types of retinal breaks are important variables affecting the selection of a specific buckling technique. Similarly, zones of vitreoretinal degeneration, with or without retinal breaks, and regions of significant vitreoretinal traction unassociated with retinal breaks should be considered in the preoperative assessment. The most important variable affecting the choice of a scleral buckling technique is the extent of significant vitreoretinal pathology (see Table 1.1). If retinal breaks, vitreoretinal degenerative disorders, and significant vitreoretinal traction are present in multiple quadrants, a procedure with a relatively extensive circumferential component is favored. A single retinal break unassociated with additional significant problems is usually managed with an isolated radial segmental buckle.

Internal morphologic changes caused by scleral buckling are determined by the size, shape, and consistency of the buckling material; the width of the suture bites placed to attach the silicone to the sclera; and the tightness of the tied sutures. In addition, a significant shortening of an encircling band, sponge, or tire will cause a major reduction in the circumference of the eye wall, and a high buckling effect will result. The placement of a scleral buckle is associated with a significant displacement of intraocular fluid volume, and the amount depends on the total volume of the buckling effect. Therefore the need for a relatively extensive buckling of sclera usually requires drainage of subretinal fluid or a paracentesis.

Typical scleral buckle configurations

Localized scleral buckles may be radially or circumferentially oriented, and a combination of the two may be considered if more extensive buckling is required. Radial scleral buckles provide localized support for a retinal tear and minimize the development of radial retinal folds commonly associated with circumferential buckles, which shorten the circumference of the eye wall but not the circumference of the retina. Circumferential buckles provide a zone of support oriented parallel to the region where vitreous traction is usually most severe, and they are an efficient means of supporting multiple areas of vitreoretinal pathology. If the area to be buckled is less than 160°, a segmental buckle is usually employed, and buckles greater than 180° are usually created with an encircling component.

For segmental buckles, the piece of silicone sponge is reduced in thickness by 50–70%, and the convex side is placed against the sclera to reduce chances of later extrusion (Fig. 1.4). The width of the sponge depends on the size of the breaks that are to be supported.

TABLE 1.1 The circumferential extent of vitreoretinal pathology dictates the configuration of the scleral buckle

Strategy	Extent (°)	Buckle
Radial sponge	10–30	Silicone sponge: 3 mm, 5 mm, 5 × 7.5 mm
Circumferential sponge	20–160	Silicone sponge: 3 mm, 5 mm, 5 × 7.5 mm
360° encircling buckle	360	Bands: 240, 41, 42 Tires: 287, 289, 276 Pieces: 103, 106

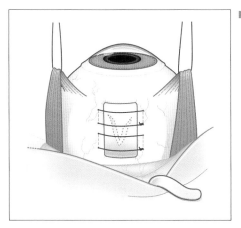

■ **FIGURE 1.4** Radial segmental buckle. Silicone sponges are split lengthwise to reduce their volume. The convex surface is placed against the sclera, and sutures are tied over the cut flat external surface. Mattress sutures are placed so that the knots are tied posteriorly.

Sutures are placed beneath significant areas of pathology and also sufficiently close to the ends of the sponge to keep them flat against the sclera.

A circumferential buckle of 180° or more is usually created with an encircling silicone band with or without a piece of grooved silicone tire placed beneath an encircling band in areas needing additional support of retinal breaks or vitreoretinal traction. The addition of the band ensures a permanent buckling effect and provides some degree of support for 360°.

Segmental buckles

When a radially oriented segmental buckle is needed, intrascleral suture limbs are placed perpendicular to the ora straddling the meridian of the retinal break and equidistant from its edges; the needle is passed so that the mattress suture knot can be tied posteriorly (Fig. 1.4). The size and type of the retinal break usually dictate the width and length of the exoplant, as well as the distance between suture bites. In general, the width of the silicone element should be at least as wide as the edges of the break marked on the sclera, and the buckle length should support both the posterior end of the break and the vitreous base immediately anterior to the break and posterior to the ora serrata. The further apart the suture bites are placed and the tighter they are tied, the greater will be the internal indentation.

If a circumferentially oriented segmental buckle is required, suture limbs are placed parallel to the limbus. The anterior bite is usually placed just anterior to the posterior margin of the vitreous base, a location estimated as lying about 2–3 mm posterior to an imaginary line drawn between the muscle insertions (and forming a portion of the spiral of Tillaux). A silicone element of sufficient width to support both the anterior and posterior edges of the retinal break(s) or other pathology is used, and the posterior suture bite is placed in a position that will produce an optimal buckling effect.

Encircling buckles

1.12

If a 360° encircling circumferential buckle of modest width and height is needed, an encircling no. 240, 41, or 42 silicone band is passed around the circumference of the globe and beneath the rectus muscles. The band is anchored with a single mattress suture with bites parallel to the limbus placed in the center of each quadrant (Fig. 1.5). Although they are an elegant and effective means of securing a band, scleral tunnels are usually not employed. Suture bites that straddle a silicone band should

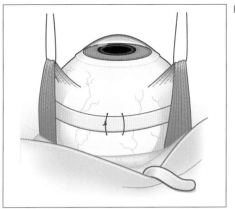

■ **FIGURE 1.5** Encircling silicone band. Mattress sutures are placed in the center of each quadrant, and their width should allow the band to slide beneath them but not move anteriorly when the suture is knotted.

be placed just far enough apart to allow the band to move freely beneath the suture, and this distance equals the width of the band plus its thickness. Narrower bites inhibit circumferential movement of the band, particularly if the sutures are pulled tight. Wider bites will allow the band to move anterior to its desired location when its ends are joined. In its proper position, the band is usually intended to support breaks in the region of the posterior edge of the vitreous base, and these are marked and treated before suture placement. In quadrants without retinal breaks, the vitreous base margin can be marked, or its location can be estimated and the anterior suture bite placed about 3 mm posterior to the imaginary line mentioned above.

When using segmental scleral buckles produced by circumferentially oriented silicone materials, suture bites are always placed in the location overlying the responsible retinal break(s), because the maximum buckle height is produced in this spot. However, sutures placed to anchor encircling silicone bands are usually not placed beneath retinal breaks, so that any subsequent augmentation of the buckling effect can be obtained by simply placing a hard silicone element beneath the band without sutures. If the increased buckling effect is needed in only a small area, a radially oriented piece is used in this situation. If a grooved segment of silicone tire is required because of a need for more extensive circumferential augmentation of the buckle, additional sutures may or may not be required, depending on the characteristics of the specific case.

If a high broad 360° encircling scleral buckle is required, two broad mattress sutures are placed in each quadrant to accommodate a silicone tire of at least 7-mm width and its overlying silicone band (Fig. 1.6). The anterior suture bite is placed at the estimated location of the ora, and the posterior bite is placed far posteriorly, at a spot dictated by the specifics of the case. Frequently, this distance is equal to twice the distance from the anterior bite to the marked posterior edge of the retinal break(s).

The ends of an encircling band are always joined with a silicone Watzke sleeve. Tantalum clips and suture clove hitch techniques are not used, primarily because of the extra time required for their use, particularly if later adjustment of the length of the band is required. Some degree of twisting of the band near the elastic sleeve can occur when the band is tightened, and this should be avoided. Because

1.13

even minimal twisting of the sleeve can affect the inner morphology of the buckling effect, the sleeve should be located in a quadrant relatively free of significant vitreoretinal pathology.

Management of subretinal fluid

Decisions regarding the drainage of subretinal fluid are among the most difficult associated with scleral buckling procedures, and considerable differences in opinion exist regarding

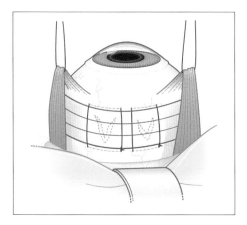

■ **FIGURE 1.6** If a broad and high buckling effect is desired, two broad mattress sutures are placed in each quadrant to accommodate the tire and overlying band.

many types of cases. Drainage is almost never performed if responsible breaks can be easily and nearly completely closed with a non-drainage technique. Drainage is always performed if a high and broad encircling scleral buckle is required. However, in most cases the criteria for drainage or non-drainage are less obvious. In eyes in which drainage was considered to be neither mandatory nor contraindicated, a small randomized trial demonstrated comparable results with both techniques.[4]

Most non-drainage procedures are effective if the crest of the buckle is within approximately 3 mm of the respective retinal break. Although this may be relatively easy to accomplish when buckling a single break, the need for more extensive buckling of multiple breaks makes this a more difficult goal and favors a drainage procedure, in which all breaks are usually efficiently placed on the crest of the buckle. Because of complications associated with this maneuver, drainage of subretinal fluid is avoided unless it is considered to be necessary for surgical success. Nevertheless, most surgeons perform transscleral drainage of subretinal fluid in approximately 75% of retinal detachment cases managed with scleral buckling.[5] Still, both techniques play a major role in the management of a routine series of cases, and familiarity with both non-drainage and drainage techniques is essential.

Non-drainage technique

The most common indication for a non-drainage technique is a retinal detachment caused by a single superior break that can be approximated close to the pigment epithelium during the scleral depression associated with placing cryotherapy. Following the placement of appropriate sutures, the scleral buckle is elevated to the desired height, and the relation of the retinal break to the surface of the buckle is reevaluated. If the break is not perfectly positioned, the scleral buckle must be adjusted. The length of the buckling effect can be extended with additional sutures placed anterior or posterior to those already holding the buckle. If the break is not positioned on the center of the buckle crest, at least one arm of the mattress suture must be repositioned.

Perfusion of the optic nerve must be documented each time that sutures over any portion of the scleral buckle are tightened further, and this is particularly important in eyes with reduced outflow facilities. Frequently, pulsations of the central retinal artery are observed. If pulsations are not visualized and perfusion is questioned, additional digital pressure should be applied to the globe to elicit pulsations. If these do not occur, the arterial flow into the eye has probably ceased, and the sutures should be relaxed if pulsations do not begin to occur within 1–2 min.

Drainage technique

Drainage of subretinal fluid is performed at the most optimal site available, and this is determined by the configuration of the retinal detachment. A number of factors are important in selecting a location at which sufficient subretinal fluid allows safe drainage, and these include:

- the distribution of subretinal fluid when the eye is in a position at which drainage will be performed,
- the location of the retinal break(s),
- the location and configuration of the buckle,
- features of vitreoretinal and epiretinal membrane traction, and
- the ease of exposure of the proposed drainage site.

The optimal locations for drainage are just above or below the lateral rectus muscle, because major choroidal vessels are avoided, and exposure of sclera is ideal. Major choroidal vessels are also avoided by draining on either side of the three remaining rectus muscles, but exposure is frequently more difficult. If possible, drainage is usually performed some distance from retinal breaks, so that passage of fluid through the break(s) and out of the eye can be minimized by the scleral depression effect provided by the buckle or a cotton-tipped applicator. (In unusual situations in which a large buckling effect is required and very little subretinal fluid exists, drainage can be performed immediately beneath a large tear to allow both subretinal and intravitreal fluids to exit the globe.)

1.14

Drainage is usually performed at or slightly anterior to the equator, and a site that will ultimately be closed by the exoplant is preferred. This avoids the need for a preplaced suture at the sclerotomy site, and it facilitates subsequent management of drainage complications. In the unusual situation in which drainage cannot be performed optimally at a 'covered' site, a preplaced non-absorbable suture is employed to close the scleral incision following drainage.

1.16

A 3- to 4-mm radial incision through sclera is performed. (Drainage with a small needle with ophthalmoscopic visualization[6] appears to be becoming more popular, and drainage with a 20-diopter lens and indirect laser has been described,[7,8] but we have little experience with these techniques.) All scleral fibers are divided until subtle prolapse of uveal tissue is observed. The choroid is then closely inspected for prominent choroidal vessels using loupes and/or the 20-diopter condensing lens and indirect ophthalmoscope. If large visible vessels cannot be avoided during penetration, a second site nearby is selected, and another scleral incision is performed. If the area of exposed choroid is free of prominent vessels, it is lightly treated with a flat diathermy probe. This causes minimal retraction of the edges of the sclera to improve visualization, and it may reduce the chances of hemorrhage.

1.15

All significant traction on the eye is then eliminated to reduce IOP. The subretinal space is then entered with a sharp-tipped conical penetrating diathermy electrode. Modest pressure is used to insert the device perpendicular to the surface of the sclera until the subretinal space is entered. This event is usually heralded by a sudden subtle pop that is usually perceived by touch or observation. Because of the tapered shape of the electrode, significant amounts of subretinal fluid do not exit the eye until this device is very slowly withdrawn from the eye.

Although an oblique or tangential path of penetration is recommended by some authors to avoid perforating the retina, this can result in a flap valve that can limit drainage. If a proper drainage site has been selected, penetration of the retina with the tapered diathermy pin is exceptionally rare, because it is removed prior to the release of significant amounts of subretinal fluid.

1.17

As the globe softens during drainage, IOP is very slowly increased to encourage further drainage and to avoid complications associated with hypotony. If a large tear is present, the sclera or the buckle and sclera overlying the break are indented with a cotton applicator. This maintains IOP and inhibits passage of intravitreal fluid to the subretinal space. Pressure can also be increased by placing applicators on either side of the sclerotomy site and gently pushing both toward the center of the eye, and these maneuvers also tend to keep the sclerotomy open. Relatively normal IOP can also be maintained by indenting the sclera at a location far from the sclerotomy site with numbers of cotton applicators.

The drainage site is not touched as long as fluid flows through it. Sudden and significant increases in IOP are avoided to reduce chances of retinal incarceration. The appearance of pigment granules suspended in the subretinal fluid usually indicates that the last of the subretinal fluid is exiting the eye. When drainage ceases, the sclerotomy site is closed by temporarily tying the sutures over an exoplant or by pulling together the ends of an encircling band. If the buckling material does not adequately close the sclerotomy, the scleral incision is closed with a suture.

The eye is quickly inspected following closure of the sclerotomy site and a preliminary adjustment of the scleral buckle. The site of drainage is first evaluated for signs of subretinal bleeding, retinal incarceration, and iatrogenic hole formation. The amount of persistent subretinal fluid is then determined, and the need for further drainage is considered. Significant amounts of subretinal fluid are allowed to persist if an effective buckling effect has been produced. If drainage of additional subretinal fluid is required, the sclerotomy site must be closely evaluated with mobile scleral depression. If the pigment epithelium is clearly not in contact with the retina, the sclerotomy site can be reopened by reducing IOP and/or removing the portion of the exoplant that covers the scleral incision. Additional drainage usually occurs spontaneously, or it can be initiated by gently manipulating the edges of the sclerotomy with applicators or a forceps. In some cases, particularly those with exceptionally viscous subretinal fluid, the retina may flatten completely at the site of the sclerotomy while large amounts of subretinal fluid persist elsewhere. In this situation, additional sclerotomies must be performed if additional drainage is required to produce an adequate buckling effect.

Adjustment of scleral buckle

1.19

Following drainage of appropriate amounts of subretinal fluid, an optimal scleral buckling effect is created by adjusting the scleral sutures and the length of the encircling band. Broad sutures over the portion of the buckle supporting large retinal breaks are first temporarily tied in a manner intended to provide optimal width and height. If IOP remains low and the breaks are in optimal position, the sutures are permanently tied. The height of the buckle is adjusted if it is inadequate or excessive. If a circumferential fold of retina continues to communicate with an open retinal break ('fish mouth' phenomenon) following buckle adjustment, a gas injection is used to solve the dilemma.

If an encircling band has been employed in combination with a wider circumferential buckle of hard silicone, its ends are adjusted to provide a modest buckling component supporting the posterior edge of the vitreous base in areas not occupied by the tire. If the encircling band is intended to provide all of the buckling effect, it is adjusted to create an indentation of somewhat greater height. The degree to which the band should be tightened depends on the IOP, the nature and extent of vitreoretinal pathology, and the necessity of a subsequent intravitreal gas injection. If the IOP remains quite soft following appropriate adjustment of the scleral buckle and retinal breaks are flat, balanced salt solution should be injected into the vitreous cavity via the pars plana. Attempts to restore normal pressure with further increases in buckle height can lead to a number of postoperative problems.

The need to replace buckling materials or sutures is quite unusual if appropriate localization of retinal breaks has been performed. However, augmentation of the buckle in certain areas is frequently desired. This can be accomplished with suture adjustments if wide elements are already in place. If an encircling band has been used, and an augmentation of the buckle is needed in an area supported only by the band, hard silicone pieces of an appropriate size are placed beneath the band, as noted earlier.

Accessory techniques

Although scleral buckles are successful in producing a functional closure of retinal breaks in most cases, their effectiveness can be enhanced with accessory techniques, the most important of which is intravitreal gas injection.

Intravitreal gas injection

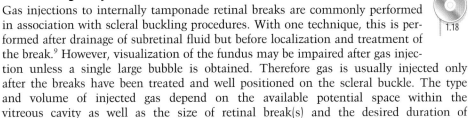

1.18

Gas injections to internally tamponade retinal breaks are commonly performed in association with scleral buckling procedures. With one technique, this is performed after drainage of subretinal fluid but before localization and treatment of the break.[9] However, visualization of the fundus may be impaired after gas injection unless a single large bubble is obtained. Therefore gas is usually injected only after the breaks have been treated and well positioned on the scleral buckle. The type and volume of injected gas depend on the available potential space within the vitreous cavity as well as the size of retinal break(s) and the desired duration of tamponade.

A 0.30-mL bubble will maintain contact with a 45° arc of the retina, and a 1.0-mL bubble of room air will cover approximately 80° and is not absorbed for 3–4 days. However, injection of even 0.5 mL of gas into an eye with normal IOP will usually cause a transient occlusion of the central retinal artery. Therefore the eye must be quite soft prior to an injection of a large gas bubble, or a smaller volume of an expanding gas is employed. Choices regarding the amount of gas injected and the type and concentration of the tamponade depend on the specifics of the case and the opinions of the surgeon.

Numerous techniques of gas injection have been described. A simple method is to grasp a muscle insertion to fixate the eye and to penetrate the globe with a 30-gauge needle attached to a tuberculin syringe containing the desired concentration of gas. The injection is performed 4 mm posterior to the limbus in a phakic eye and 1 mm closer to the limbus in an aphakic case. The best quadrant is the most superior one. Using indirect ophthalmoscopy, passage of the needle tip through the pars plana epithelium must be documented. The needle is then withdrawn a short distance and a predetermined volume of gas is rapidly injected. The optic nerve is immediately inspected to document perfusion of the retinal vessels. If pulsations are visualized in a patient with normal blood pressure, no tension-lowering manipulations are performed. If pulsations are not observed and cannot be produced with digital pressure, the IOP is lowered with a paracentesis or reduction in buckle height if pulsations have not resumed after 1–2 min.

Intravitreal balanced salt injection

Balanced salt solution is occasionally injected in a location similar to gas to restore normal volume after the buckle has been adjusted.

Closure

Sutures of 5-0 or 6-0 catgut are used to close the peritomy. This can be running or interrupted, and it is useful to place some of the central bites through episclera to ensure that retraction of the posterior margin does not occur. Between 0.2 and 0.4 cc of dexamethasone is usually injected in the subconjunctival space.

OUTCOMES

During the past 80 years, retinal reattachment surgery has evolved from being virtually hopeless to being successful in almost all cases in which proliferative vitreoretinopathy (PVR) does not develop. In contrast to anatomic outcomes, visual results remain relatively poor, and there is little unequivocal evidence that they have improved significantly over the past 40 years. This is because of the significant percentage of cases that have permanent macular damage due to preoperative detachment of the central retina. Anatomic success will improve central visual acuity but not restore it to normal. Barring surgical complications, visual results are primarily a function of macular damage sustained prior to reattachment.[10] Most complications of scleral buckling do not impact anatomic or visual success.

Anatomic results

Case selection is a critical factor in any discussion of surgical results, and this is particularly true if certain cases are removed from 'consecutive' series because of preoperative findings that are associated with a relatively poor prognosis. Currently, approximately 90% of retinal detachments that are selected for scleral buckling can be repaired with a single operation.[5,10,11] If the cause of primary failure is an inadequate buckling effect or missed or new retinal breaks in the absence of PVR, reoperations are usually successful. If PVR causes failure of the initial operation, scleral buckling alone is usually not successful, and vitrectomy techniques are traditionally performed.

Good preoperative visual acuity is perhaps surprisingly the most important predictor of both anatomic and visual success.[12] Macula-on detachments have a significantly better anatomic prognosis than macula-off cases, and eyes in the latter group with relatively poor preoperative visual acuity are less likely to be successfully repaired than are those with relatively good preoperative vision.

Visual results

Postoperative visual acuity results are closely related to both anatomic success and preoperative visual acuity. Ultimate anatomic failure is associated with blindness. Successful surgery usually results in stable or improved visual acuity. Approximately 90% of macula-on patients maintain preoperative vision following surgery.[13] Macula-off retinal detachments are almost always associated with damage to the central retina and reduced pre- and postoperative visual acuity.[12]

The best predictor of postoperative visual acuity is preoperative visual acuity,[12] and evaluating preoperative macular function with a potential acuity meter may provide a more precise estimate of potential postoperative visual acuity.[14] The duration and height of macular detachment are also related to postoperative vision, but these are also reflected in preoperative visual acuity.

The relationship between pre- and postoperative visual acuities is of particular importance in any comparison of results following alternative types of reattachment surgery, and valid studies should document vision before and after surgery in all eyes.

COMMON POSTOPERATIVE COMPLICATIONS OF SCLERAL BUCKLING

These are not uncommon, and some, such as altered refractive error, are actually side effects. The most common do not affect anatomic or visual results.

Altered refractive error

The refractive error usually changes following scleral buckling because of alterations in the axial length of the eye.[15] Scleral buckling techniques with an encircling component cause a myopic change in the refractive error. An average increase in axial length of approximately 1 mm induces an average myopic shift of approximately −2.75 diopters.

The effect of radial scleral buckles is usually less significant. Significant astigmatic changes are very unusual unless the buckles are quite anterior, but some degree of astigmatism is occasionally caused by indenting the sclera near the ora serrata.

Although changes in refractive error may be relatively unimportant in eyes with poor postoperative visual acuity, the induction of significant anisometropia can be devastating to some patients, particularly those with excellent postoperative visual acuity and an emmetropic fellow eye. Avoiding anisometropia is an important goal of some alternatives to scleral buckling.

Strabismus

Some degree of extraocular muscle imbalance can occur in up to 50% of patients undergoing scleral buckling procedure.[16] Many of these abnormalities are temporary and caused by intraoperative muscle damage. Nevertheless, permanent muscle imbalance is observed disappointingly frequently.

Causes of strabismus include the following:

- abnormal adhesions between the muscle and the sclera or Tenon's capsule,
- injury to the muscle from surgical trauma,
- mechanical disturbances caused by the location and shape of buckling materials,
- problems associated with disinsertion or reposition of a muscle, and
- possible toxicity of local anesthetic agents.

Factors associated with postoperative muscle imbalance include placement of a buckle beneath a muscle, size of buckling material beneath a muscle, and reoperations.

Cystoid macular edema

Cystoid macular edema is a common complication of ocular inflammatory diseases and surgery. There is no strong relationship between the incidence of CME and macular involvement, drainage of subretinal fluid, and the type of scleral buckle.[17]

The effect of CME on final visual acuity is uncertain, primarily because of a lack of studies correlating preoperative vision with a variety of additional variables associated with scleral buckling procedures. Nevertheless, CME contributes to a loss of visual acuity in eyes without macular involvement, and it probably limits recovery of vision in eyes in which the macula was detached.

Epimacular proliferation

Epiretinal membranes that distort or cover the macula are a relatively common cause of disappointing visual acuity following successful scleral buckling surgery. The reported incidence of this problem varies considerably because of the criteria employed for its diagnosis. Macular puckers have been reported in from 2 to 17% of successfully buckled cases.[18]

Removal of epiretinal membranes with vitrectomy techniques is the only effective means of treating macular puckers.

Proliferative vitreoretinopathy

Proliferative vitreoretinopathy is the only common cause of ultimate failure following retinal reattachment surgery. This cell-mediated process is associated with the production of fibrocellular membranes on the posterior vitreous surface and on both surfaces of the retina. Factors that cause a significant breakdown in the blood–aqueous barrier and that allow an increased number of pigment epithelial cells to enter the vitreous cavity are also associated with an increased incidence of PVR.[19]

Recurrent retinal detachment

Recurrent or persistent retinal detachment is the most significant complication of scleral buckling, and the severity of this problem is related to its cause. Retinal detachment following scleral buckling surgery occurs in from 9 to 25% of primary operations, and the vast majority are associated with open retinal breaks.[20]

If the postoperative retinal detachment is caused by a new tear or an inadequate buckling effect unassociated with PVR, modification of the scleral buckle and creation of a chorioretinal adhesion will usually reattach the retina. If extensive PVR is responsible for the surgical failure, vitrectomy techniques are usually required for a successful repair.

REFERENCES

1. Benson WE, Chan P, Sharma S, et al. Current popularity of pneumatic retinopexy. Retina 1999; 19:238–241.
2. Minihan M, Tanner V, Williamson TH. Primary rhegmatogenous retinal detachment: 20 years of change. Br J Ophthalmol 2001; 85:546–548.
3. Williams GA, Aaberg TM Jr. Techniques of scleral buckling. In: Ryan SJ et al., eds. Retina, 4th edn. Philadelphia: Mosby; 2006:2035–2070.
4. Hilton GF, Grizzard WS. The drainage of subretinal fluid: a randomized controlled clinical trial. Retina 1981; 1:271–280.
5. Wilkinson CP, Bradford RH. Complications of draining subretinal fluid. Retina 1984; 4:1–4.
6. Jaffe GJ, Brownlow R, Hines J. Modified external needle drainage procedure for rhegmatogenous retinal detachment. Retina 2003; 23:80–85.
7. Pitts JF, Schwartz SD, Wells J, et al. Indirect argon laser drainage of subretinal fluid. Eye 1996; 10(part 4):465–468.
8. Challa JK, Hunyor AB, Playfair TJ, et al. External argon laser choroidotomy for subretinal fluid drainage. Aust NZ J Ophthalmol 1998; 26(1):37–40.
9. Gilbert C, McLeod D. D-ACE surgical sequence for selected bullous retinal detachments. Br J Ophthalmol 1985; 69:733–736.
10. Michels RG, Wilkinson CP, Rice TA. Retinal detachment. St Louis: Mosby; 1990:917–958.
11. Hilton GF, McLean EB, Brinton DA. Retinal detachment. Principles and practice, 2nd edn. San Francisco: American Academy of Ophthalmology; 1995:120–128.
12. Tani P, Robertson DM, Langworthy A. Prognosis for central vision and anatomic reattachment in rhegmatogenous retinal detachment with macula detached. Am J Ophthalmol 1981; 92:611–620.
13. Tani P, Robertson DM, Langworthy A. Rhegmatogenous retinal detachment without macular involvement treated with scleral buckling. Am J Ophthalmol 1980; 90:503–508.
14. Friberg TR, Eller AW. Prediction of visual recovery after scleral buckling of macula-off retinal detachments. Am J Ophthalmol 1992; 114:715–722.
15. Smiddy WE, Loupe DN, Michels RG, et al. Refractive changes after scleral buckling surgery. Arch Ophthalmol 1989; 107:1469–1471.
16. Smiddy WE, Loupe DN, Michels RG, et al. Extraocular muscle imbalance after scleral buckling surgery. Ophthalmology 1989; 96:1485–1490.
17. Meredith TA, Reeser FH, Topping TM, et al. Cystoid macular edema after retinal detachment surgery. Ophthalmology 1980; 87:1090–1095.
18. Lobes LA Jr, Burton TC. The incidence of macular pucker after retinal detachment surgery. Am J Ophthalmol 1978; 85:72–77.
19. Sharma T, Challa J, Ravishankar KV, et al. Scleral buckling for retinal detachment: predictors of failure. Retina 1994; 14:338–343.
20. Grizzard WS, Hilton GF, Hammer ME, et al. A multivariate analysis of anatomic success of retinal detachments treated with scleral buckling. Graefes Arch Clin Exp Ophthalmol 1994; 232:1–7.

2 Vitrectomy surgery

Abdhish R. Bhavsar

INSTRUMENTATION

Equipment

- Stool, Machemer
- Vitrectomy machine with endoillumination light source and foot pedal controls; to be placed at surgeon's right side with foot pedal for right foot
- Surgical operating microscope (e.g. Zeiss) with foot pedal controls; to be placed at surgeon's left side with foot pedal for left foot
- Vitrectomy surgical pack, 20-gauge (containing high-speed 2500 probe vitrector [Alcon, Fort Worth, Texas], infusion lines, infusion cannula, Luer locks for air and fluid lines, etc.)
- Shielded bullet endoilluminating light pipe
- Binocular indirect ophthalmomicroscope (BIOM), AVI, or other indirect inverter lens system mounted to surgical scope, with foot pedal inverter control to surgeon's left side for left foot, next to microscope pedal
- Machemer irrigating or non-irrigating contact lens, flat plano concave contact lens, or other contact lens for magnified viewing of the macular region if needed for managing pathology posteriorly
- Patient cart for supine positioning, with wrist rest or Chan wrist rest at head of bed
- Surgical table and trays for surgical technologist on surgeon's right side
- Indirect ophthalmoscope, placed behind surgeon at head of bed
- Laser unit for intraocular laser and indirect laser, and appropriate microscope filters for endolaser
- Cryoprobe (straight) and cryotherapy machine (e.g. Frigitronic Cryo Machine)

Preparation of ocular surface

- Eyelash-trimming scissors with bacitracin ointment
- Povidone iodine 5% drops for conjunctival surface
- Povidone iodine 10% for periocular skin preparation
- Cotton-tipped applicators for preparation of eyelid and eyelash margins with povidone iodine
- Cover unoperated eye with wet eye pad or gauze and plastic shield

Drapes

- Large blue surgical drape with a hole for the operative eye (Cardinal Health, no. 8441); used to cover head and patient
- 3M 1060 surgical clear plastic drape without hole for the operative eyelid. Surgeon to cut hole in drape, to allow drape to be wrapped around lashes and eyelid margin
- Rolled surgical towel placed around head drapes to create a 'moat' for placing instruments, cotton-tipped applicator, etc.

Gloves

- Sterile gloves for nurse or surgeon performing ocular surface preparation prior to draping

Sterile surgical gloves for surgeon and assistant (author prefers Regent Biogel Neotech gloves)

Local anesthetic

1 : 1 mixture of lidocaine 2% with bupivacaine (Marcaine) 0.75%, approximately 10 cc (5 cc for local retrobulbar block and 5 cc for administration during the case or after the case for postoperative analgesia)

General anesthetic

Per anesthesiologist

Pack nose with 4×4 gauze in each nostril prior to draping to prevent gas or mucus from accumulating beneath drape or from seeping under drape to the operative ocular surface

Infusion solutions

Phakic eyes: Balanced Salt Solution Plus

Aphakic or pseudophakic eyes: balanced salt solution (BSS)

Diabetic eyes

Phakic: add 3 mL of D50 to Balanced Salt Solution Plus

Aphakic or pseudophakic: add 3 mL of D50 to BSS

For pars plana lensectomy: second infusion line with BSS

Lens line for handheld Machemer irrigating lens: BSS

Adrenaline (epinephrine) for infusion if requested for diabetic eye: 1 : 1000 0.5 mL in infusion bottle

Adrenaline for intraocular irrigation: 1 : 10 000 0.25 mL of adrenaline in 1 : 1000 mixed in 2.25 mL of BSS

Medications

Sterile Goniosol or methylcellulose

BSS in a squeeze bottle for topical application to the corneal surface

Topical tetracaine 0.5% if needed for topical anesthesia

Intravenous dexamethasone (Decadron): 8–10 mg intravenous (one) per surgeon preference for decreasing inflammation

Postsurgical subconjunctival injections

Dexamethasone 4 mg/mL: 0.5 mL

Cefazolin (Ancef) 100 mg/mL: 0.5 mL

Clindamycin 25 mg/mL: 0.5 mL (to be used in case of penicillin or cefazolin allergy)

Postsurgical topical medications at the conclusion of surgery

1 ggt of povidone iodine 5%

1 drop of atropine 1%

Bacitracin ointment

Dressings

Two sterile eye pads, paper tape, plastic shield

Bracelet for intraocular gas with warning against the use of nitrous oxide (for eyes with air or gas)

Suture

7-0 Vicryl no. 546 (for sclerotomy closure and conjunctival closure)

4-0 white silk no. S2782 (for scleral buckle mattress sutures)

2-0 silk ties no. A185H (for isolating rectus muscles during scleral buckle placement)

5-0 Mersilene no. 1764 (for sew-on lens ring for direct lenses)

Instruments

- Lid speculum (the author prefers a closed Lieberman speculum)
- Calipers
- Microvitreoretinal (MVR) blade no. 5560
- 20- and 28-diopter lenses
- Contact lenses such as plano concave or Machemer lens
- Wide-angle viewing lenses such as BIOM or AVI lenses
- 0.12 forceps
- Two needle drivers
- Westcott conjunctival scissors
- Cautery eraser tip, 18-gauge, for conjunctival and scleral surface
- Cautery, 23-gauge blunt or sharp tip for intraocular use
- Straight or angled forceps (e.g. Nugent forceps) without teeth for scleral buckle manipulation
- Flynn extendable silicone soft-tipped cannula (for fluid–air exchange)
- Scleral plugs (set of four including 20-gauge and 19-gauge)
- Chang forceps for epiretinal or internal limiting membrane (ILM) dissection, Sordouille or deJuan forceps for proliferative vitreoretinopathy (PVR) cases, Tano asymmetric forceps
- Membrane Micropick (PSI/Eye-Ko Assurance Products, St Charles, Missouri, no. 9029)
- 20-Gauge steel cannula with Luer lock for injecting fluid into the vitreous cavity, i.e. for indocyanine green, trypan blue, or triamcinolone acetonide
- Flexible iris retractors, for example Grieshaber iris retractors (if needed to dilate a miotic pupil)
- Phacofragmatome for pars plana lensectomy (fragmatome accessory pack, Alcon, no. 1021HP)
- Cotton-tipped applicators or Weck-Cel sponges
- Perfluoro-*n*-octane, Perfluoron, perfluorocarbon liquid (PFL) (Alcon) for use if needed for retinal detachment repair or giant retinal tear repair
- AntiFog Clear Field no. 300–006 (antifog solution for indirect viewing system, e.g. BIOM or AVI)

Supplies for gas exchange if needed

- 60-cc syringe for intraocular gas
- Sterile 0.22-μm filters, Millex-GS no. E4429–22 (Millipore, Carrigtwohill, Ireland)
- Sterile tubing for transferring gas from pressurized canister to syringe
- Sulfur hexafluoride (SF_6) or perfluoropropane (C_3F_8) gas for intraocular use (Alcon)

INDICATIONS

The indications for vitrectomy surgery are continuously expanding. Table 2.1 lists a number of indications for vitrectomy surgery today categorized by retina or vitreous pathology or by disease entity.

THE HISTORY OF VITREOUS SURGERY

Surgical intervention to remove the vitreous or vitreous opacities has served as a source of intrigue for many generations. The vitreous was the last intraocular frontier to receive common exploration because of the lack of knowledge about the physiologic roles of the vitreous and the fear of complications caused by inadvertent violation of the vitreous, for example during cataract surgery.[1] Posterior vitreous surgery through the pars plana was first reported by von Graefe in 1863 and described as vitreous transection of a vitreous

TABLE 2.1 Indications for vitrectomy surgery

Indication

Vitreous opacity or pathology

Vitreous hemorrhage	Proliferative retinopathies	Proliferative diabetic retinopathy Idiopathic (Eale diseases) Ischemic venous or arterial occlusive disease Sickle cell disease

Vitreous strands or
  debris
	Trauma
	Subarachnoid hemorrhage (Terson
	  syndrome)
	Associated with retinal tears, or
	  retinal detachment
	Inflammatory
	Related to posterior vitreous
	  detachment (if severe)
	Post-infectious
		Endophthalmitis
		Toxoplasmosis
		Toxocariasis
		Progressive outer retinal necrosis
		Acute retinal necrosis

Endophthalmitis		
Amyloidosis		
Severe asteroid hyalosis		

Cyclitic or pupillary
  membrane
	Idiopathic
	Inflammatory
	Post-infectious
	Persistant hyperplastic primary
	  vitreous	

Retinal detachment

Rhegmatogenous	Simple rhegmatogenous retinal
	  detachment
	Complex rhegmatogenous retinal
	  detachment
	Giant retinal tear
	Dialysis
	Proliferative vitreoretinopathy
	Post-infectious
		Progressive outer retinal necrosis
		Acute retinal necrosis
		Cytomegalovirus

Tractional retinal detachment	Proliferative diabetic retinopathy Vitreomacular traction Traumatic	

TABLE 2.1 Indications for vitrectomy surgery—cont'd

Indication
Epiretinal membranes

Idiopathic
Proliferative diabetic
    retinopathy
Traumatic
Proliferative
    vitreoretinopathy

Macular hole
Idiopathic
Traumatic
Myopic
Related to retinal
    detachment

Intraocular foreign body

Glaucoma
Phacolytic glaucoma
Malignant glaucoma or
    aqueous misdirection
Pupillary block
    glaucoma if due to
    luxation or
    dislocation of the lens
Ghost cell glaucoma
Neovascular glaucoma
    when associated
    with vitreous
    hemorrhage

Cataract

Luxated or dislocated lens	Pseudoexfoliation	
	Trauma	
	Persistant hyperplastic primary vitreous	
	Metabolic diseases	Marfan's syndrome

Retained lens fragments

Luxated or dislocated intraocular lens implant

membrane with a needle and removal of an intraocular foreign body (IOFB) with forceps.[2,3] Ford was the first to describe aspiration of opacified vitreous to improve vision in 1890.[4] Approximately 70 years later, in 1960, Michaelson reported cutting a dense vitreous membrane using a transscleral approach and a needle.[5] In 1964, Dodo reported cutting vitreous membranes in patients with dense vitreous hemorrhage.[6]

Anterior vitreous surgery was described quite late, and in 1950 Landegger reported cataract extraction with removal of opacified vitreous and vitreous replacement with cerebrospinal fluid or cadaver vitreous.[7] In 1958, Dodo reported vitreous replacement as a treatment for severe vitreous opacity.[8]

The treatment of retinal detachment using transscleral techniques was first described by Deutschmann in 1895, when he reported using a small transfixation knife to cut the vitreous and retina in order to reduce vitreous traction on the retina.[9]

Nearly complete removal of all the vitreous was described by Kasner in 1968, when he removed essentially all of the opacifed vitreous from an eye with amyloidosis via the open sky technique (Fig. 2.1).[10,11] The concept of removing almost all of the vitreous with relative safety and lack of devastating consequences to the eye paved the way for the modern development of vitreous surgery.

Machemer and coworkers developed the vitreous infusion suction cutter (VISC) to excise vitreous tissue and simultaneously replace it with BSS (Fig. 2.2).[12–14] The VISC required a 2-mm pars plana incision and the instrument tip was 1.7 mm in diameter and 30 mm in length. If the fiberoptic sleeve was placed over the instrument tip, a slightly larger pars plana incision was needed (Fig. 2.3). The instrument tip consisted of a smaller inner rotating tube and an outer tube with a port near the tip. The suction tube was the inner tube, and as vitreous was aspirated into the inner rotating tube, it was cut or sheared by the rotation of the inner tube past the edge of the hole in the outer tube. Suction was produced manually by pulling the plunger in a syringe connected to the VISC via plastic tubing. The infusion fluid passed through the outer tube and was connected via plastic tubing.

Douvas designed an infusion aspiration cutting instrument known as the rotoextractor (Fig. 2.4). It had exchangeable tips to allow end-cutting or side-cutting ports. The rotoex-

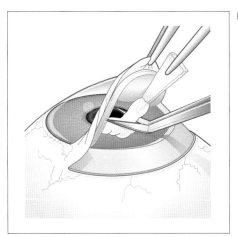

FIGURE 2.1 Open sky technique for vitrectomy, similar to that described by Kasner. (After Wilkinson and Rice 1997,[25] with permission.)

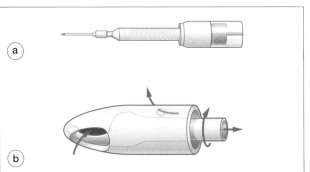

FIGURE 2.2 (**a**) Early version of the vitreous infusion suction cutter with handpiece containing the motor. (**b**) The tip of the instrument had a rotating shaft to act as a shearing blade. (After Wilkinson and Rice 1997,[25] with permission.)

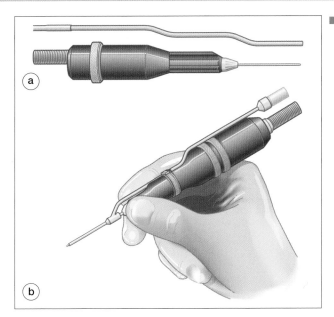

■ **FIGURE 2.3** (**a**) Illumination was provided by a fiberoptic bundle attached to the vitrectomy instrument. (**b**) Vitrectomy handpiece with attached fiberoptic sleeve. (After Wilkinson and Rice 1997,[25] with permission.)

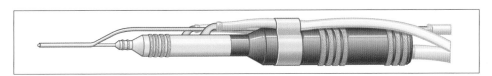

■ **FIGURE 2.4** The Douvas rotoextractor was initially designed for the removal of cataracts but was used widely for vitrectomy. (After Wilkinson and Rice 1997,[25] with permission.)

tractor had a 1.5-mm aspiration hole for removal of lens material and smaller 0.4-mm holes for removing vitreous.[15]

Peyman and coworkers designed the Vitrophage to aspirate vitreous into a tube and then excise it via an inner oscillating tube with a guillotine action. The infusion port was also at the end of the tip but located 180° apart from the aspiration port. A motor was used to drive both infusion and aspiration.[16]

Kreiger and Straatsma designed a vitreous excision instrument with a stereotactic micromanipulator (Fig. 2.5a,b).[17] The vitrectomy consisted of two concentric tubes. The inner tube was driven by a solenoid, and vitreous was aspirated into the side port when the inner tube was in the down position. Then the vitreous was cut when the inner tube was in the up position by shearing the vitreous between the inner tube and the outer tube hole (Fig. 2.5c).

O'Malley and Heintz developed the concept of three-port pars plana vitrectomy with 20-gauge instruments (Fig. 2.6).[18,19] It is this method of vitrectomy that has dominated the development of vitrectomy since that time and is currently used today. In addition to describing the vitrectomy instruments and techniques, O'Malley published the plugs and stiletto for entry incisions for the 20-gauge vitrectomy instrument system.[20]

O'Malley and Heintz also explored electrovitrectomy to allow electrodissection for severing vitreous strands and membranes.[21,22]

The large published series of Machemer served to set the stage for the management of vitreous and retinal pathology with pars plana vitrectomy.[23]

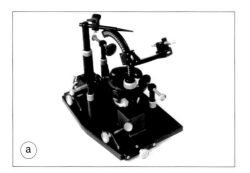

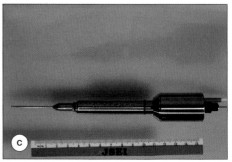

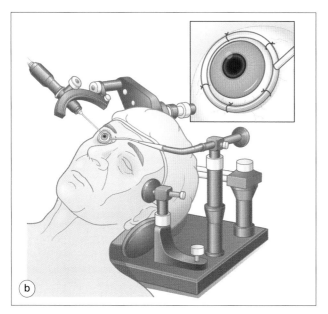

■ **FIGURE 2.5** (**a**) Stereotactic manipulator system designed by Kreiger and Straatsma. (**b**) Vitreous cutter designed by Kreiger and Straatsma. (**c**) The inner and outer tubes. (b, after Wilkinson and Rice 1997,[25] with permission.)

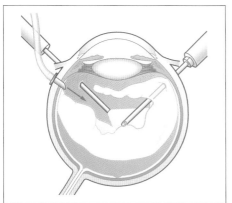

■ **FIGURE 2.6** Three-port pars plana vitrectomy pioneered by O'Malley with a separate infusion line, vitrectomy cutter, and light pipe. (After Wilkinson and Rice 1997,[25] with permission.)

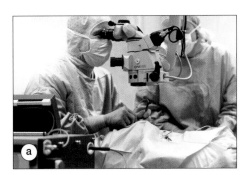
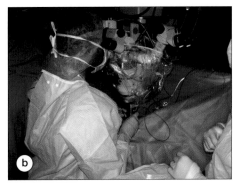

■ **FIGURE 2.7** Modern surgical microscopes. (**a**) Carl Zeiss surgical microscope, Opmi Visu 210. (**b**) Carl Zeiss surgical microscope with sterile plastic drape, binocular indirect ophthalmomicroscope (BIOM) lens assembly, BIOM inverter, and video camera attached opposite to the assistant scope. (a, courtesy of Carl Zeiss; b, courtesy of Abdhish R. Bhavsar, M.D.)

MODERN VITRECTOMY SURGERY

The development of the automated surgical microscope has allowed the continued development and growth of vitreous surgery.[24] With the ability to control the high-magnification image of the retina and vitreous cavity with a foot pedal for both focus and x–y movement, fine manipulation within the vitreous cavity became possible (Fig. 2.7).

Modern vitrectomy instruments utilized the positive design aspects of the earlier instruments and improved on them to permit development of lightweight disposable vitrectomy cutters with efficient aspiration and increasingly faster cut rates that are driven by pneumatic systems or electrical motors (Fig. 2.8). Heavier motor-driven cutters with extremely fast cut rates have also been developed.

Various contact and then non-contact lenses for viewing the retina and vitreous during vitrectomy surgery have been developed (Fig. 2.9a,b). The advent of wide-angle viewing with both contact (e.g. AVI and Volk) lenses and non-contact (BIOM and Volk systems) lenses has allowed more complete visualization of retinal and vitreous pathology of nearly the entire fundus at once (Fig. 2.9c–e).

A variety of forceps, scissors, picks, and aspiration cannulas have been developed (Fig. 2.10).

FLOW CONTROL AND VITREOUS CUTTER DYNAMICS

The rate of fluid flow through the vitrectomy port affects the vitreous flow and traction on the retina during vitrectomy surgery. Fluid flow through the vitrectomy port depends on the level of aspiration vacuum, the infusion pressure, the cutting rate, and the duty cycle of the cutter port. When the aspiration vacuum is increased or decreased, the fluid flow into the cutter can increase or decrease. If the infusion pressure is increased or decreased, the fluid flow into the cutter can increase or decrease. If the duty cycle is altered to keep the port opened or closed for different amounts of time, the flow can be altered. Fluidics and the technology of vitrectomy surgery are covered in Chapter 21, written by Steve Charles, M.D.

PREOPERATIVE PREPARATION

Appropriate informed consent is obtained by the surgeon for the surgical procedure that is anticipated. The author typically encourages family members of the patient, with the

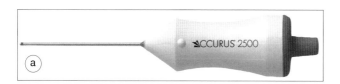

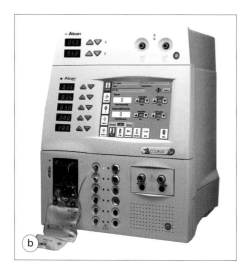

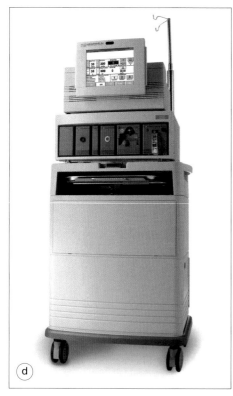

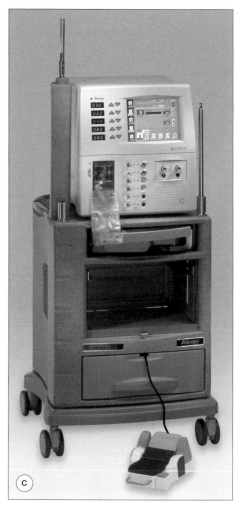

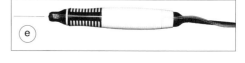

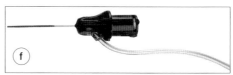

■ **FIGURE 2.8** (**a**) Alcon Accurus 20-gauge vitreous cutter, 2500 cuts per minute. (**b**) Alcon Accurus vitrectomy machine with standard and xenon light sources. (**c**) Alcon Accurus vitrectomy machine with stand. (**d**) Bausch & Lomb Millennium vitrectomy machine with stand. (**e**) Bausch and Lomb Lightning vitrectomy cutter. (**f**) Bausch & Lomb Lightning vitrectomy cutter tip. (a–c, courtesy of Alcon; d–f, courtesy of Bausch & Lomb.)

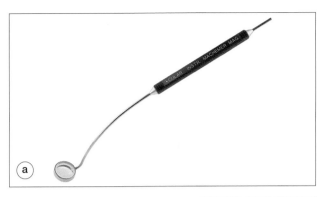

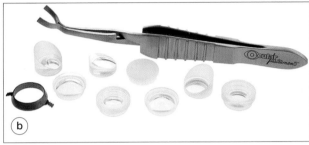

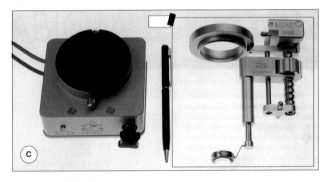

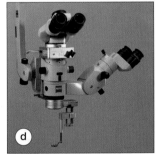

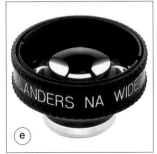

FIGURE 2.9 Standard contact, sew-on, and wide-angle viewing lenses and systems for vitrectomy. (**a**) Omvi Machemer Magnified Infusion Vitrectomy Lens for contact direct viewing of the fundus. (**b**) OLVS-3 Landers Vitrectomy Lens Ring System: standard sew-on lenses for contact direct viewing of the fundus with a variety of flat, magnified, and angled lenses. (**c**) binocular indirect ophthalmomicroscope (BIOM) wide-angle viewing system with inverter and lenses. (**d**) BIOM wide-angle viewing system attached to Zeiss surgical microscope. (**e**) OLIV-WFNA Landers Wide Field Vitrectomy Lens: wide-angle viewing contact lens. (a, b, and e, courtesy of Ocular Instruments; c and d, courtesy of Insight Instruments.)

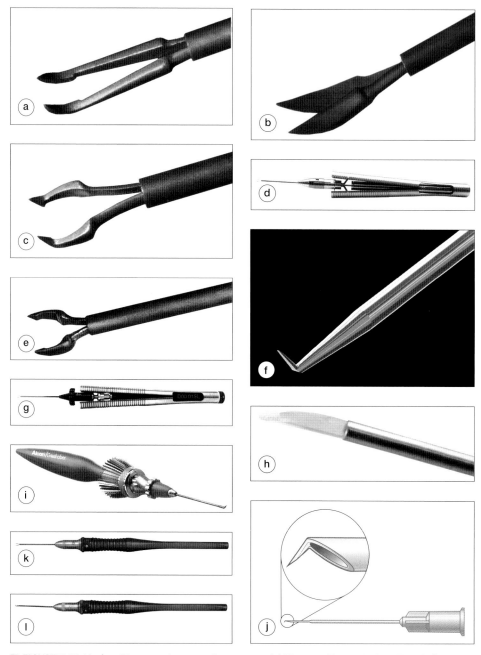

FIGURE 2.10 Modern 20-gauge vitrectomy instruments. (**a**) 23-gauge Kryptonite Low Mass Pick Forceps. (**b**) Diamond Black horizontal scissors. (**c**) Disposable Morris/Witherspoon full-view internal limiting membrane (ILM) forceps. (**d**) Forceps squeeze handle, reusable forceps tip. (**e**) Kryptonite microserrated Tano asymmetric microforceps. (**f**) Rice ILM elevator. (**g**) Syntrifugal large handle. (**h**) Tano diamond-dusted membrane scraper. (**i**) Revolution 20-gauge scissors. (**j**) Membrane Micropick, 20-gauge tapered to 30-gauge, disposable. (**k**) ET8202 TL end-gripping forceps, tapered. (**l**) ET8219 TL vertical scissors. (a–h, courtesy of Synergetics; i, courtesy of Alcon/Greishaber; j, courtesy of PSI/Eye-Ko; k and l, courtesy of Bausch & Lomb.)

approval of the patient, to participate in the care of the patient and in the informed consent discussion. This can help with the retention of information and allows the family members to discuss the surgery with the patient after they have left the medical office. Appropriate preoperative history is obtained and physical examination done by the patient's family physician or internist.

PROCEDURE

2.1

Anesthesia is achieved either by local retrobulbar block (the author typically uses a 50:50 mixture of 0.75% bupivacaine [Marcaine] and 2% lidocaine) with a Nadbath block or lid block or by general anesthesia. The author recommends avoiding the use of nitrous oxide if general anesthesia is administered, because of the possibility of placing an air or gas bubble into the eye at the end of the procedure. Nitrous oxide can diffuse into the air- or gas-filled eye and then dissipate postoperatively, which can lead to a gas underfill. In addition, the use of nitrous oxide in an eye with a preexisting gas bubble can make the gas bubble expand and can thereby raise the intraocular pressure (IOP).

The periocular surface is prepared with povidone iodine and then several drops of 5% povidone iodine are applied on to the conjunctival surface. The author prefers that the eyelashes are trimmed so that they do not rub across the surgical field or conjunctival surface during the surgery. The eyelashes are also scrubbed with povidone iodine 5% (Fig. 2.11). Tincture of benzoin is then applied to the periocular region to aid with adherence of the drapes around the eyelids and up to the bridge of the nose. This prevents air or fluid from under the drape or from the other eye from entering the surgical field.

The drapes are then applied to isolate the surgical field around the operative eye. The author prefers a large blue drape with a hole for the preoperative eye (Cardinal Health, no. 8441) and a 3M 1060 drape. The lid speculum is placed in such a manner that the eyelids and lashes are isolated from the surgical field and the 1060 drape is placed around and under the lashes (Fig. 2.12). This prevents the lashes from contacting the surgical instruments as they are passed into and out of the sclerotomy sites.

This chapter describes surgical techniques for 20-gauge vitrectomy surgery. For 23-gauge and 25-gauge vitrectomy surgery, please see, respectively, Chapter 3 (*23-Gauge vitrectomy*, by Howard F. Fine, M.D., Pawan Bhatnagar, M.D., and Richard F. Spaide, M.D.) and Chapter 4 (*25-Gauge vitrectomy*, by Anurag Gupta, M.D., and Steven Schwartz, M.D.).

The author begins by 'painting' the bulbar conjunctival surface with a cotton-tipped applicator soaked with 5% povidone iodine in case there are any bacteria expressed from the eyelids during the draping procedure. However, the author is not aware of any data to support this technique.

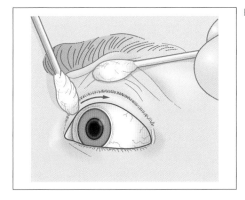

■ **FIGURE 2.11** Technique for scrubbing eyelash margins with povidone iodine during surgical preparation.

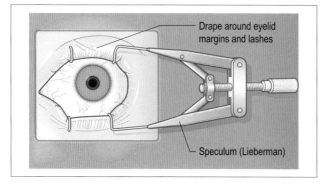

FIGURE 2.12 Draping technique with 3M 1060 drape placed such that the eyelid margins and lashes are isolated from the surgical field.

Drape around eyelid margins and lashes

Speculum (Lieberman)

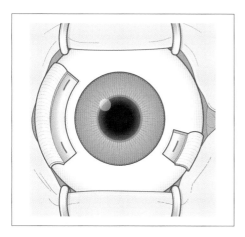

■ **FIGURE 2.13** Conjunctival peritomy temporally and superonasally for placement of sclerotomies.

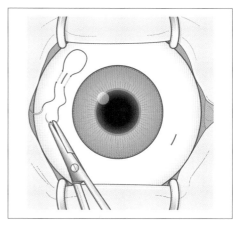

■ **FIGURE 2.14** Placement of 7-0 Vicryl mattress suture through partial-thickness sclera for infusion cannula.

The operating microscope is brought into position so that the ocular surface and operating field are visualized. Low magnification is used so that all the sclerotomy sites and cornea can be visualized in the same field of view. The author prefers to place the surgical microscope to the surgeon's left side with the foot pedal to the left side. If an automated inverter is used for a non-contact wide-angle viewing system, for example BIOM, then the foot pedal is placed just to the left of the operating microscope pedal. The vitrectomy foot pedal is placed to the surgeon's right foot.

A conjunctival peritomy is performed with Westcott scissors and 0.12 forceps at 1 mm posterior to the surgical limbus for approximately four clock hours temporally and approximately two clock hours superonasally. Relaxing incisions are made radially (Fig. 2.13). Wet-field cautery is performed to achieve hemostasis. In preparation for the infusion cannula sclerotomy site, a 7-0 Vicryl suture is placed with a needle driver in a mattress fashion inferotemporally (Fig. 2.14) at 3–4 mm posterior to the surgical limbus (3–3.5 mm for aphakic or pseudophakic eyes, 3.5–4 mm for phakic eyes) (Fig. 2.15). A sclerotomy is created by passing an MVR blade perpendicularly through the sclera between the 7-0 Vicryl sutures so that the blade travels approximately 5–6 mm through the sclera. Care is taken to pass the MVR blade toward the center of the vitreous cavity to avoid damaging the lens. A 4-mm pars plana infusion cannula is tested prior to insertion into the eye to ensure free

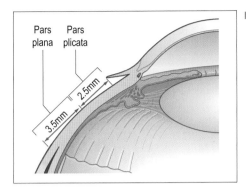

Pars plana   Pars plicata

3.5mm   2.5mm

■ **FIGURE 2.15** Placement of sclerotomies with respect to pars plana and pars plicata and with respect to phakic status: sclerotomies placed between 3.0 and 3.5 mm posterior to the surgical limbus for aphakic or pseudophakic eyes and 3.5–4.0 mm posterior to the surgical limbus in phakic eyes.

flow of BSS; it is then turned off and the infusion is stopped. The infusion cannula is inserted through the sclerotomy site so that the hub is flush with the scleral surface and then temporarily tied with the preplaced mattress suture. The position of the infusion cannula is confirmed by direct visualization of the infusion cannula and shaft by placing a light pipe externally and shining the light through the cornea while indenting the infusion cannula toward the center of the vitreous cavity. If the infusion cannula tip and shaft are free of retina or membranes, then the vitrectomy can proceed. If the infusion cannula tip and shaft are not clearly visualized or if there are membranes obscuring the infusion cannula, then either the cannula should be removed from the eye and the MVR blade should be passed again through the sclerotomy to ensure a patent sclerotomy site or, in the case of pseudophakic or aphakic eyes, an MVR blade can be passed through the superonasal sclerotomy site and under direct visualization the membranes can be carefully dissected away from the infusion cannula tip and shaft. Alternatively, a 6-mm pars plana infusion cannula can be used.

As the author prefers to have complete control of the IOP during surgery, he prefers to use an infusion cannula that can be sutured to the sclera, which minimizes the risk of displacement of the infusion cannula and subretinal or suprachoroidal injection of fluid, air, or gas, or sudden hypotony caused by exit of the infusion cannula from the eye. However, if you choose to use them, there are self-retaining infusion cannulas that do not require a suture.

Additional sclerotomy sites are created with the MVR blade superonasally and superotemporally at 3–4 mm posterior to the surgical limbus (3–3.5 mm for aphakic or pseudophakic eyes, 3.5–4 mm for phakic eyes).

Care is taken during the entire case to ensure control of the IOP. The sclerotomy sites are not left open for any length of time with either air infusion or fluid infusion, because the eye can become hypotonous, which increases the risk of choroidal hemorrhage. In addition, while the retina is detached, keeping a sclerotomy open can increase the risk of retinal incarceration. It is sound practice to place scleral plugs through the superior sclerotomy sites whenever the endoilluminating light pipe, vitrectomy, or other instruments are not occupying the sclerotomy sites.

The author prefers to use the BIOM wide-field viewing system (Fig. 2.9c,d), although the AVI and Volk contact indirect viewing systems are also available (Fig. 2.9e). The main advantage of a non-contact system is independence from an assistant, who would be necessary for a contact system. The BIOM indirect lens assembly is then brought into an appropriate position so that the lenses are aligned with the visual axis through the cornea. The BIOM lens is focused by rotating the 'corkscrew' knob on the arm attached to the lens.

2.2

The vitrectomy cutter is placed through one of the superior sclerotomy sites, and the light pipe is placed through the other superior sclerotomy site. The BIOM lens is then focused for optimal viewing by rotating the 'screw' on the arm attached to the lens. The vitrectomy cutter is placed so that the port is visible during the entire surgery. The light pipe is also placed in the vitreous cavity so that the tip is visible during the entire surgery. The core vitreous is removed by keeping the vitreous cutter in the central vitreous cavity. Rapid movement of the vitreous cutter during the surgery is avoided so that minimal traction on the vitreous occurs. If the posterior hyaloid is attached, then it is elevated off of the posterior retinal surface by aspirating anterior to the optic nerve with the vitreous cutter (Fig. 2.16). This is most effectively performed with a flat plano concave contact lens or a Machemer lens. The cutter is then used to elevate the posterior hyaloid in each quadrant and the hyaloid is separated from the retina out to the posterior vitreous base 360°, typically with the BIOM lens. The posterior hyaloid and the core vitreous are then removed thoroughly. During the vitrectomy, the light pipe is oriented such that the vitreous strands are illuminated at the vitreous cutter port. In addition, the retinal surface is illuminated so that proper orientation can be maintained within the vitreous cavity and so that the retina can be adequately visualized during the vitrectomy (Fig. 2.17). If the retina is not visualized during the surgery,

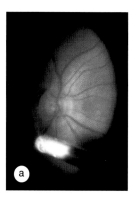

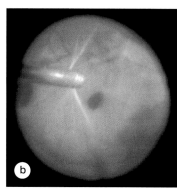

■ **FIGURE 2.16** (**a**) Elevation of posterior hyaloid in peripapillary region with the vitrectomy instrument. (**b**) Elevation of the posterior hyaloid anterior to the macular region. (Courtesy of Abdhish R. Bhavsar, M.D.)

a

b

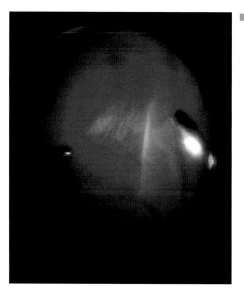

■ **FIGURE 2.17** Maintaining an adequate view of the retina during peripheral vitrectomy by using a shielded bullet endoilluminating light pipe oriented to illuminate both the cutter port and the retina, as in this example of a giant retinal tear. (Courtesy of Abdhish R. Bhavsar, M.D.)

then it is possible to contact the retina with the instruments and create retinal tears, retinal detachment, retinal hemorrhage, and even choroidal hemorrhage if sufficient force is used.

After the intraocular procedures necessary to repair the retina or vitreous pathology have been addressed, indirect ophthalmoscopy with 360° scleral depression is performed to ensure that there are no retinal tears or breaks. If there are any retinal tears, these are treated with cryoretinopexy at this time (Fig. 2.18). It is important to perform 360° scleral depression with indirect ophthalmoscopy, because retinal tears can be missed even when using the AVI or BIOM wide-angle viewing systems during the vitrectomy.

If there are any retinal tears, then fluid–air exchange is performed. If fluid–air exchange is necessary, then it is performed at this time, with a soft-tipped silicone cannula. The author prefers to use a Flynn extendable soft-tipped cannula with gentle aspiration anterior to the optic nerve. Approximately 5–7 min is allowed to elapse while the residual fluid reaccumulates in the posterior pole, and then it is removed once again with the soft-tipped cannula. This permits a more complete fluid–air or fluid–gas exchange. One of the superior sclerotomy sites is closed with 7-0 Vicryl suture by placing three passes through each sclerotomy site (Fig. 2.19), and then it is permanently tied with at least three square knots (the author usually places about five square knots). The other superior sclerotomy site is then temporarily closed with a 7-0 Vicryl suture in the same manner, but the knot is not tied. If gas exchange is desired, then the gas is prepared by the assistant in a 60-cc syringe. The appropriate concentration of gas desired is prepared by flushing the tube attached to the gas cylinder by opening the regulator briefly. Then a 60-cc syringe with a sterile 0.22-μm filter is attached to this tubing. The appropriate amount of gas is injected into the syringe as the regulator is opened on the gas cylinder. For example, if one desires a final concentration of 18% gas, then a volume of 10.8 cc of gas is injected into the syringe. With the same 20-μm filter in place, an additional volume of 49.2 cc of sterile air is withdrawn into the syringe for a total final volume of 60 cc. This yields a concentration of 18% gas. The distal end of the infusion tubing is clamped and the plug is removed from the remaining superior sclerotomy site. The syringe containing the gas is then connected to the infusion tubing via a Luer lock. The gas is injected slowly as the air is discharged passively through the open sclerotomy

2.3
2.4

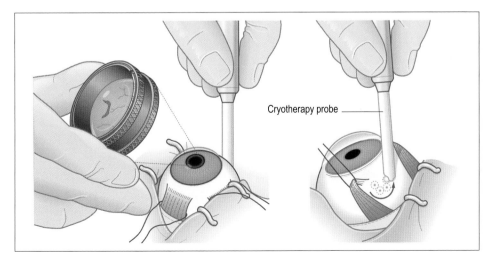

Cryotherapy probe

FIGURE 2.18 Indirect ophthalmoscopy with scleral depression and cryoretinopexy of a retinal tear. (After Wilkinson and Rice 1997,[25] with permission.)

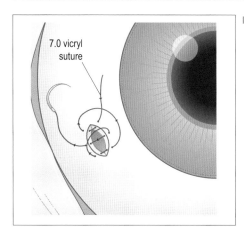

7.0 vicryl
suture

FIGURE 2.19 Suturing the sclerotomy sites with 7-0 Vicryl suture with three throws through partial-thickness sclera.

site with the loosened 7-0 Vicryl suture. After approximately 50 cc of gas has been injected, the assistant is asked to stop injecting gas. The remaining superior sclerotomy site is closed with the preplaced 7-0 Vicryl suture with at least three square knots.

While the infusion cannula is in place, the IOP can be adjusted appropriately either by injecting additional gas or by removing excess gas so that the IOP is approximately 15–20 mmHg. Measurement of the IOP can be performed by either palpation or by Tono-Pen (Medtronic, Minneapolis, Minneapolis). The infusion cannula is removed from the sclerotomy site by the assistant while the surgeon maintains traction on the preplaced mattress suture with two needle drivers and then ties the knot permanently with at least three square knots (the author usually places about five knots). By closing this sclerotomy site as the infusion cannula is removed, loss of gas from the vitreous cavity is prevented.

If fluid–air exchange is not needed, then the superior sclerotomy sites are closed with 7-0 Vicryl suture by placing three passes through each sclerotomy site and then they are permanently tied with at least three square knots (the author usually places about four or five square knots).

If the eye is to be left in the fluid-filled state, then the globe is palpated to ensure that a physiologic IOP, between 15 and 20 mmHg, is present. Alternatively, a Tono-Pen can be used to measure the IOP. While the infusion cannula is in place, the IOP can be adjusted appropriately by either increasing or decreasing the IOP setting on the vitrectomy machine (under global control or vented gas forced infusion).

If air, gas, or silicone oil tamponade is necessary for the treatment of the underlying pathology in pseudophakic or aphakic patients, the author typically performs an inferior peripheral punctate iridectomy with the vitrectomy instrument to prevent postoperative pupillary block caused by the gas or oil bubble.

If the eye is to be left in the air- or gas-filled state, and air has been placed into the vitreous cavity, then the preplaced 7-0 Vicryl mattress suture around the infusion cannula is loosened. The infusion cannula is then turned off and removed from the sclerotomy site by the assistant while the surgeon maintains traction on the preplaced mattress suture with two needle drivers and then ties the knot permanently with at least three square knots (the author usually places about five knots). If a gas bubble is to be placed, then the author typically uses 25–28% SF_6 gas for shorter term tamponade and 14–18% C_3F_8 gas for longer term tamponade. An SF_6 bubble will last about 2 weeks and a C_3F_8 bubble will last about 6–8 weeks. I prefer to perform gas–air exchange after closing one of the sclerotomy sites with 7-0 Vicryl suture, with three throws through the incision. The other superior sclerotomy site is then temporarily closed with 7-0 Vicryl suture, and the air infusion line is disconnected from the infusion tubing. Next, the 60-cc gas syringe prepared with the appropriate concentration of gas desired is connected to the distal end of the infusion tubing, but proximal to the infusion cannula tubing for injection of gas into the eye (Fig. 2.20). The suture for the remaining superior sclerotomy site that has been temporarily tied is then loosened so that as the gas is injected through the infusion line into the vitreous cavity, air can exit through that site. The author asks the assistant to inject 50 cc of gas slowly so that a complete gas–air exchange is performed. This leaves 10 cc of gas in the syringe to be used if necessary after the infusion cannula is removed from the eye. The IOP is then measured either by Tono-Pen or by palpation to determine that the IOP is physiologic or between 15 and 20 mmHg. The IOP can be adjusted by injecting additional gas or by removing gas using the syringe. The infusion cannula is then removed from the sclerotomy site by the assistant while the surgeon maintains traction on the preplaced mattress suture with two needle drivers. This prevents escape of the gas from the sclerotomy site. The 7-0 Vicryl suture is then tied permanently with at least three square knots (the author usually places about four or five knots).

If silicone oil is used for tamponade, then the author closes one of the superior sclerotomy sites permanently and passes a mattress suture through the remaining superior sclerotomy site with 7-0 Vicryl suture. A cut 18-gauge angiocath (Fig. 2.21) is then used to inject silicone oil through the remaining superior sclerotomy site while air is still flowing through the infusion cannula. This maintains the IOP while the silicone oil is placed into the eye. The oil infusion is stopped when the oil meniscus reaches the lens in phakic patients, the intraocular lens in pseudophakic patients, or the iris plane in aphakic patients. The IOP is palpated to ensure that it is approximately 15 mmHg, and this can be adjusted if necessary by injecting or removing some of the silicone oil. The angiocath is then removed from the eye by the assistant while the surgeon closes the preplaced mattress suture. The infusion line is clamped and is then removed from the eye while the preplaced mattress suture is permanently tied. Care is taken to irrigate the scleral surface with BSS or saline solution to prevent any silicone oil from remaining in the subconjunctival space.

The conjuctiva is closed with 7-0 Vicryl suture with buried knots. Subconjunctival injections of dexamethasone and an antibiotic such as cefazolin can be administered. These injections are administered using a 25-gauge rather than a 30-gauge needle to decrease the risk of scleral penetration and inadvertent intraocular injection. Local anesthetic also can be administered into the retrobulbar space for postoperative analgesia by entering the subconjuctival space, placing the cannula along the scleral surface, and extending the cannula until it reaches the posterior scleral surface. The author typically prefers to perform the injection with a 3-cc syringe and a 20-gauge blunt-angled cannula containing a 1:1 mixture of 0.75% bupivacaine (Marcaine) and 2% lidocaine.

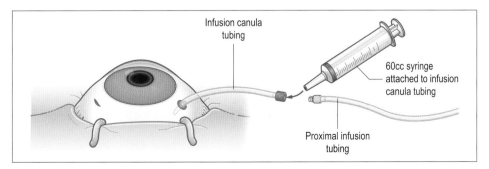

FIGURE 2.20 Attaching a 60-cc syringe containing the desired gas mixture to the infusion cannula via a Luer lock.

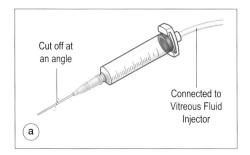

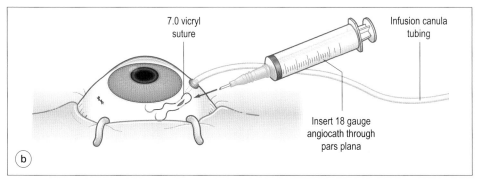

FIGURE 2.21 (**a**) Cutting an 18-gauge angiocath for placement through a sclerotomy site. (**b**) Placement of silicone oil through a pars plana sclerotomy site with preplaced 7-0 Vicryl suture.

The lid speculum and drapes are removed from the eye. A drop of 5% povidone iodine, 1% atropine, and antibiotic ointment (e.g. bacitracin) are placed on the surface of the eye. A sterile patch and shield are placed over the eyelids and taped into position.

The patient is then escorted to the recovery room. Once the patient is stable and situated in the recovery room, typically within about 5 min, postoperative positioning can be undertaken, if necessary. For example, the patient can be positioned in the face-down position or on one side or the other side, depending on the location of the retinal tears. For example, if the retinal tear is located in a nasal quadrant, then the patient is positioned such that the nasal portion of the operated eye is located upward or in the least dependent position. To clarify, if the retinal tear is located at the 2 o'clock position in the right eye, then the patient is positioned in the right side down position (Fig. 2.22a).

After an appropriate recovery period, typically 45–60 min, the patient can be discharged home. If the patient is to remain an inpatient, then he or she is typically transferred to the inpatient unit at this time. The author usually admits patients for overnight IOP monitoring or for positioning if they have a history of severe or advanced glaucoma, if they have a macular hole and can benefit from nurse education on face-down positioning after surgery, if their home is a great distance away, or if they have surgery late in the evening.

The basic skill of performing a vitrectomy is the essential skill for addressing all the myriad of pathologies that involve the vitreous and retina (Table 2.1).

Retinal detachment

The management of primary retinal detachment can be performed by scleral buckle techniques as described in Chapter 1 (*Scleral buckling surgery*, by Charles P. Wilkinson, M.D., and Abdhish R. Bhavsar, M.D.), by pneumatic retinopexy (Chapter 12, by W. Sanderson Grizzard, M.D., and Mark E. Hammer, M.D.), by vitrectomy surgery (as described in this

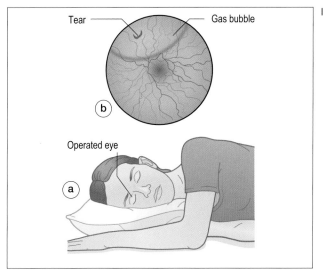

Tear — Gas bubble

(b)

Operated eye

(a)

FIGURE 2.22 (**a**) Right side down position if retinal tear is located in the nasal retina of the right eye. (**b**) Right eye from patient depicted in Figure 2.20 with right side down position with gas bubble tamponade of the nasal retina and retinal tear.

chapter), or by a combination of both vitrectomy and scleral buckle techniques.[25] Vitrectomy surgery is particularly helpful in cases of vitreous opacity such as vitreous hemorrhage. Although a number of retina surgeons prefer to repair retinal detachments with vitrectomy surgery alone, the author typically does not repair retinal detachments with vitrectomy alone. Even when the author performs vitrectomy surgery for retinal detachments, he typically at least places a band (i.e. 42 band) or a tire (i.e. 276 or 287 tire). The author believes that vitrectomy surgery alone without radical anterior vitreous base dissection is unlikely to relieve all potential vitreous traction. It is for this reason that he typically places a scleral band or scleral buckle at the same time during those cases in which he is also performing a vitrectomy for retinal detachment. Of course, for those cases that have primary scleral buckle surgery, vitrectomy is not necessary.

If a scleral buckle is going to be placed during the same surgery as the vitrectomy surgery, then the author typically places the scleral buckle first. A 360° conjunctival peritomy is performed at 1 mm posterior to the limbus and then Tenon's is separated in each quadrant by passing a curved Stevens scissors around the globe in each quadrant. Each of the four rectus muscles is isolated with a muscle hook, and then a long 4-0 silk suture tie is passed beneath the insertion of each muscle. A single knot is placed in each suture approximately 1–2 inches from the muscle insertion. Then the shorter end of the suture distal to the knot is cut at the knot. This leaves one loose end of each suture so that one can control the movement of the suture and the globe by differentially pulling on each suture, typically with two sutures (controlling two muscles) in a single hand.

Each of the scleral quadrants is inspected to note any pathology or scleral thinning.

The 4-0 silk sutures for the scleral buckle are placed in a mattress fashion within partial-thickness sclera with at least one suture in each quadrant. The anterior pass is placed at the spiral of Tillaux and the posterior pass is placed between 5 and 9 mm posterior to the first anterior pass. The location of the posterior pass depends on which tire or band is chosen. If a 41 or 42 band is chosen, then the posterior pass is 5–6 mm posterior to the anterior pass. If a 276 or 287 tire is chosen, then the posterior pass is 9 mm posterior to the anterior pass. Each suture is then temporarily and loosely tied with three loops. This allows for the suture to hold its knot when it is tightened and tied later in the case.

The scleral band or tire is then placed beneath each of the rectus muscles and silk mattress sutures. If a 276 or 287 tire is placed, then the 240 band is placed at the same time.

The buckle is left loosely in position and will be tightened later in the case. This prevents folding of the retina prior to reattaching the retina and also prevents the possible lack of visualization of the retina at the posterior crest of the buckle, which can occur if the buckle is tightened excessively.

After beginning the vitrectomy as described in the *Procedure* section above, it is of critical importance to ensure that the infusion cannula is free from the retina and not located in the subretinal space when performing vitrectomy surgery in patients with retinal detachment. After this is confirmed and after the endoilluminating light pipe and vitrector are placed through their respective sclerotomy sites, the infusion cannula can be opened. This prevents the vitreous and retina from becoming incarcerated in the sclerotomy sites at the beginning of the surgery.

Care is taken during the entire case to ensure control of the IOP. The sclerotomy sites are not left open for any length of time, either with air infusion or with fluid infusion, because the eye can become hypotonous, which increases the risk of choroidal hemorrhage. In addition, while the retina is detached, keeping a sclerotomy open can increase the risk of retinal incarceration. It is sound practice to place scleral plugs through the superior sclerotomy sites whenever the endoilluminating light pipe, vitrectomy, or other instruments are not occupying the sclerotomy sites.

The author prefers to use the BIOM wide-angle viewing system for all retinal detachment surgery. This allows a panoramic view during the entire case and allows vitreoretinal traction and tears to be addressed globally. Occasionally, a plano concave contact lens is used to address epiretinal membranes or hemorrhage that may require removal from the surface of the retina. The core vitreous is removed with the vitrector and shielded bullet endoilluminating light pipe. After the posterior hyaloid is removed with the vitreous cutter and the vitreous is completely removed from the retinal tears (Fig. 2.23), then the tears are marked with endodiathermy to achieve retinal whitening at the borders of the tears. This serves to enable visualization of the tears later in the case.

A retinotomy site for internal drainage of subretinal fluid is created with the endodiathermy tip or the vitrectomy instument to create a single small hole within an area of subretinal fluid, usually in the superior midperipheral retina to allow internal drainage of the subretinal fluid. If the detachment involves only the inferior retina, then the author typically performs the retinotomy site in either the nasal or temporal midperipheral retina, depending on which side the main causative retinal tears are located. For example, if the main tear is on the nasal side, then the author would perform the retinotomy on the nasal side. The author typically makes a round retinotomy hole with the vitrectomy instrument by gently aspirating the retina in the area of the desired retinotomy site, and then switches to the cutting mode while the retina is just within the tip of the vitrector and then makes one cut (Fig. 2.24a). The vitrector is withdrawn from the eye, and then the internal border

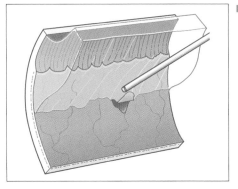

■ FIGURE 2.23 Removal of vitreous from the retinal tear to relieve traction.

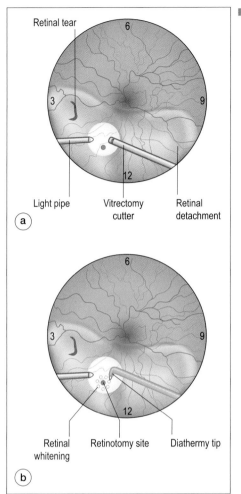

FIGURE 2.24 (**a**) Creating a retinotomy site for internal drainage of subretinal fluid in nasal midperipheral detached retina (surgeon's view). (**b**) Performing endodiathermy to mark the border of the retinotomy site in detached retina (surgeon's view).

of the retinotomy site is marked with the endodiathermy instrument to allow visualization of the hole during the remainder of the case (Fig. 2.24b).

Indirect ophthalmoscopy with 360° scleral depression is then performed to ensure that all the retinal tears or breaks have been identified and marked with endodiathermy. If there are additional retinal tears, then these can be marked with endodiathermy for endolaser after fluid–air exchange or they can be treated with cyroretinopexy at this time (Fig. 2.18). It is important to perform 360° scleral depression with indirect ophthalmoscopy, because retinal tears can be missed even when using the AVI or BIOM wide-angle viewing systems during the vitrectomy.

In pseudophakic or aphakic patients, the author typically performs an inferior peripheral punctate iridectomy with the vitrectomy instrument to prevent postoperative pupillary block caused by the gas or oil bubble.

Fluid–air exchange is then performed. The author prefers to use a Flynn extendable soft-tipped cannula. The subretinal fluid is aspirated during the fluid–air exchange. The globe is tilted toward the direction of the retinotomy site to allow the fluid in the subretinal space to drain toward the retinotomy site by gravity, and then it is aspirated (Fig. 2.25). When the retina is completely reattached, then

2.5

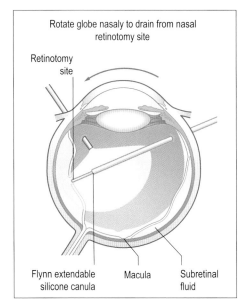

Rotate globe nasaly to drain from nasal retinotomy site

Retinotomy site

| Flynn extendable silicone canula | Macula | Subretinal fluid |

■ **FIGURE 2.25** Internal drainage of subretinal fluid using Flynn extendable silicone soft-tipped cannula while tilting the eye toward the nasal side to allow gravitational drainage of subretinal fluid to the nasal side.

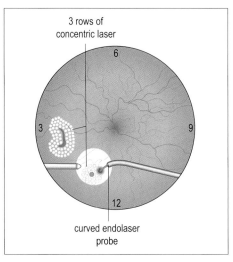

3 rows of concentric laser

curved endolaser probe

■ **FIGURE 2.26** Application of endolaser to surround retinal tear with three rows of concentric laser and retinotomy site with two rows of concentric laser with curved endolaser probe (surgeon's view).

the fluid remaining in the vitreous cavity is removed with the Flynn extendable soft-tipped cannula by gentle aspiration anterior to the optic disc.

2.5

Endolaser is then applied with a curved endolaser probe to treat around each of the retinal tears with three rows of concentric laser. The author typically surrounds the retinotomy site with one or two rows of concentric laser (Fig. 2.26). A curved endolaser probe allows one to treat more peripherally, particularly in phakic eyes. The author usually treats the peripheral retina with three or four rows of concentric laser, especially in pseudophakic eyes, as prophylaxis against future retinal tears or to prevent any missed small retinal tears from leading to recurrent retinal detachment. The endolaser treatment is performed to achieve moderate retinal whitening. Overzealous laser can lead to choroidal effusion, retinal holes, or even retinal or choroidal hemorrhage.

The residual fluid that has reaccumulated posteriorly is then removed with the Flynn extendable soft-tipped cannula by gentle aspiration at the retinotomy site and anterior to the optic disc.

If a buckle has been placed, then scleral buckle 4-0 silk mattress sutures are permanently tied and the knots trimmed. The knots are rotated posteriorly to potentially help reduce the risk of exposure. The band is tightened to achieve 360° indentation. The ends of the tire are trimmed so that they are apposed. The ends of the band are trimmed at the sleeve. The author typically places scleral buckles so that the ends of the tire, the ends of the band, and the sleeve are located in the superonasal quadrant. This location permits easy access during the surgery and potentially decreases the risk of exposure compared with placing the sleeve and buckle ends on the temporal side.

Once again, the residual fluid that has reaccumulated posteriorly is then removed with the Flynn extendable soft-tipped cannula by gentle aspiration at the retinotomy site and anterior to the optic disc. The retina is also examined to ensure that there is no active pathology to address and that the retina has remained attached.

Complete gas–air exchange is performed. The author typically uses 25–28% SF_6 gas for shorter term tamponade and 14–18% C_3F_8 gas for longer term tamponade. An SF_6 bubble will last about 2 weeks and a C_3F_8 bubble will last about 6–8 weeks. I prefer to perform gas–air exchange after closing one of the sclerotomy sites with 7-0 Vicryl suture, with three throws through the incision. The other superior sclerotomy site is then temporarily closed with 7-0 Vicryl suture, and the air infusion line is disconnected from the infusion tubing. Next, the 60-cc gas syringe prepared with the appropriate concentration of gas desired is connected to the distal end of the infusion tubing for injection of gas into the eye. The suture for the remaining superior sclerotomy site that has been temporarily tied is then loosened so that as the gas is injected through the infusion line into the vitreous cavity, air can exit through that site. I ask the assistant to inject 50 cc of gas slowly so that a complete gas–air exchange is performed. This leaves 10 cc of gas in the syringe to be used if necessary after the infusion cannula is removed from the eye. The IOP is then measured either by Tono-Pen or by palpation to determine that the IOP is physiologic or between 15 and 20 mmHg. The IOP can be adjusted by injecting additional gas or by removing gas using the syringe. The infusion cannula is then removed from the sclerotomy site by the assistant while the surgeon maintains traction on the preplaced mattress suture with two needle drivers. This prevents escape of the gas from the sclerotomy site. The 7-0 Vicryl suture is then tied permanently with at least three square knots (the author usually places about five knots).

The conjunctiva is closed with 7-0 Vicryl suture with buried knots. Subconjunctival injections of dexamethasone and an antibiotic such as cefazolin can be administered. These injections are administered using a 25-gauge rather than a 30-gauge needle to decrease the risk of scleral penetration and inadvertent intraocular injection. Local anesthetic also can be administered into the retrobulbar space for postoperative analgesia by entering the subconjunctival space, placing the cannula along the scleral surface, and extending the cannula until it reaches the posterior scleral surface. I typically prefer to perform the injection with a 3-cc syringe and a 20-gauge blunt-angled cannula containing a 1:1 mixture of 0.75% bupivacaine (Marcaine) and 2% lidocaine.

The lid speculum and drapes are removed from the eye. A drop of 5% povidone iodine, 1% atropine, and antibiotic ointment (e.g. bacitracin) are placed on the surface of the eye. A sterile patch and shield are placed over the eyelids and taped into position.

The patient is then escorted to the recovery room. Once the patient is stable and situated in the recovery room, typically within about 5 min, postoperative positioning can be undertaken, if necessary. For example, the patient can be positioned in the face-down position or on one side or the other side, depending on the location of the retinal tears. For example, if the retinal tear is located in a nasal quadrant, then the patient is positioned such that the nasal portion of the operated eye is located upward or in the least dependent position. To clarify, if the retinal tear is located at the 2 o'clock position in the right eye, then the patient is positioned in the right side down position (Fig. 2.22a).

After an appropriate recovery period, typically 45–60 min, the patient can be discharged home. If the patient is to remain an inpatient, then he or she is typically transferred to the inpatient unit at this time. The author usually admits patients for overnight IOP monitoring or for positioning if they have a history of severe or advanced glaucoma, if they have a macular hole and can benefit from nurse education on face-down positioning after surgery, if their home is a great distance away, or if they have surgery late in the evening.

Care is taken during the entire case to ensure control of the IOP. The sclerotomy sites are not left open for any length of time, either with air infusion or with fluid infusion, because the eye can become hypotonous, which increases the risk of choroidal hemorrhage. In addition, while the retina is detached, keeping a sclerotomy open can increase the risk of retinal incarceration. It is sound practice to place scleral plugs through the superior sclerotomy sites whenever the endoilluminating light pipe, vitrectomy, or other instruments are not occupying the sclerotomy sites.

Retinal detachment with giant retinal tear

The basic principles in the section above are followed regarding performing a scleral buckle and pars plana vitrectomy. I typically employ a 276 tire, 240 band, and 270 sleeve for the scleral buckle when performing surgery for giant retinal tears. After the scleral buckle has been placed and left loosely in position and the sutures are left loosely in position, the scleral buckle is left loosely around the globe to prevent retinal slippage or folding of the retina later in the case when the retina is reattached. Then the vitrectomy is performed. Care is taken to remove all of the vitreous traction from the posterior pole, the giant retinal tear, any other retinal tears, and the anterior vitreous. Occasionally, vitreous can be prolapsed posterior to the flap of the giant retinal tear and this vitreous should be removed.

2.6
2.7

Once the vitreous is removed by vitrectomy, the posterior border of the giant retinal tear is marked with endodiathermy for later visualization during the case, especially for visualization during fluid–air exchange (Fig. 2.27). The use of PFL for the repair of giant retinal tears has been pioneered by Stanley Chang, M.D.[26,27] PFL is used to reattach the retina and to unfold the giant retinal tear. A single bubble of PFL is formed by placing the cannula near the posterior segment of the vitreous cavity, over the disc or nasal to the disc, while injecting very slowly. By keeping the cannula within the existing bubble, a single bubble is allowed to form, which minimizes the formation of extraneous bubbles. As the PFL bubble is enlarged, the subretinal fluid is squeegeed out of the subretinal space, the giant retinal tear is unfolded, and the retina is reattached (Fig. 2.28). Three rows of endolaser are applied to the posterior border of the giant retinal tear. The author typically also places three rows of concentric laser to the remainder of the retinal periphery.

The scleral buckle sutures are then permanently tied, trimmed short, and rotated posteriorly (to potentially reduce the risk of exposure of the sutures). The buckle is tightened moderately, but care is taken to avoid placing a very 'high' buckle in order to reduce the risk of retinal slippage. Keeping the PFL in the vitreous cavity during this process of tying up the buckle can also reduce the risk of retinal slippage.

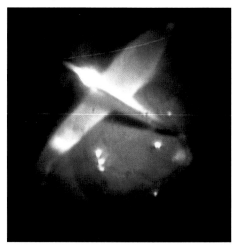

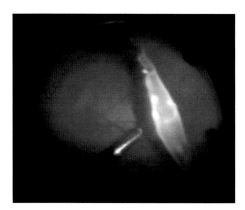

■ **FIGURE 2.27** Application of endodiathermy to the posterior border of a giant retinal tear with blunt endodiathermy probe (surgeon's view). (Courtesy of Abdhish R. Bhavsar, M.D.)

■ **FIGURE 2.28** Placement of perfluorocarbon liquid (PFL) bubble in the posterior pole slowly while forming a single bubble by keeping the tip of the cannula within the bubble. As the PFL bubble is enlarged, the giant retinal tear is unfolded, the subretinal fluid is squeegeed out of the subretinal space, and the retina is reattached. (Courtesy of Abdhish R. Bhavsar, M.D.)

In pseudophakic or aphakic patients, the author typically performs an inferior peripheral punctate iridectomy with the vitrectomy instrument to prevent post-operative pupillary block caused by the gas or oil bubble.

2.8

A fluid–air exchange is then performed. The fluid remaining in the vitreous cavity is removed first with the Flynn extendable soft-tipped cannula to help prevent retinal slippage. The PFL is then removed from the vitreous cavity, and the anterior border of the giant retinal tear is dried using the same cannula. Air is allowed to flow within the vitreous cavity for approximately 5 min to allow sublimation of any residual PFL.

Either gas–air or silicone oil–air exchange is performed to provide longer term tamponade. The author prefers gas tamponade with 16–18% C_3F_8 gas. The gas for intraocular injection is prepared by flushing the tube attached to the gas cylinder by opening the regulator briefly. Then a 60-cc syringe with a sterile 20-μm filter is attached to this tubing. The appropriate amount of gas is injected into the syringe as the regulator is opened on the gas cylinder. For example, if one desires a final concentration of 18% gas, then a volume of 10.8 cc of gas is injected into the syringe. With the same 20-μm filter in place, an additional volume of 49.2 cc of sterile air is withdrawn into the syringe for a total final volume of 60 cc. This yields a concentration of 18% gas. One of the superior sclerotomy sites is closed with 7-0 Vicryl suture, with three throws through the incision. The other superior sclerotomy site is then temporarily closed with 7-0 Vicryl suture, and the air infusion line is disconnected from the infusion tubing. Next, the 60-cc syringe containing the gas is connected to the distal end of the infusion tubing for injection of gas into the eye. The suture for the remaining superior sclerotomy site that has been temporarily tied is then loosened so that as the gas is injected through the infusion line into the vitreous cavity, air can exit through that site. I ask the assistant to inject 50 cc of gas slowly so that a complete gas–air exchange is performed. This leaves 10 cc of gas in the syringe to be used if necessary after the infusion cannula is removed from the eye. The IOP is then measured either by Tono-Pen or by palpation to determine that the IOP is physiologic or between 15 and 20 mmHg. The IOP can be adjusted by injecting additional gas or by removing gas using the syringe. The infusion cannula is then removed from the sclerotomy site by the assistant while the surgeon maintains traction on the preplaced mattress suture with two needle drivers. This prevents escape of the gas from the sclerotomy site. The 7-0 Vicryl suture is then tied permanently with at least three square knots (the author usually places about five knots).

If silicone oil is used for tamponade, then the author closes one of the superior sclerotomy sites permanently and passes a mattress suture through the remaining superior sclerotomy site with 7-0 Vicryl suture. A cut 18-gauge angiocath (Fig. 2.29) is then used to inject silicone oil through the remaining superior sclerotomy site while air is still flowing through the infusion cannula. This maintains the IOP while the silicone oil is placed into the eye. The oil infusion is stopped when the oil meniscus reaches the lens in phakic patients, the intraocular lens in pseudophakic patients, or the iris plane in aphakic patients. The IOP is palpated to ensure that the IOP is approximately 15 mmHg, and this can be adjusted if necessary by injecting or removing some of the silicone oil. The angiocath is then removed from the eye by the assistant while the surgeon closes the preplaced mattress suture. The infusion line is clamped and is then removed from the eye while the preplaced mattress suture is permanently tied. Care is taken to irrigate the scleral surface

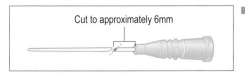

Cut to approximately 6mm

■ **FIGURE 2.29** Cut 18-gauge angiocath for placement of silicone oil into vitreous cavity.

with BSS or saline solution to prevent any silicone oil from remaining in the subconjunctival space.

The conjunctiva is closed with 7-0 Vicryl suture with buried knots. Subconjunctival injections of dexamethasone and an antibiotic such as cefazolin can be administered. These injections are administered using a 25-gauge rather than a 30-gauge needle to decrease the risk of scleral penetration and inadvertent intraocular injection. Local anesthetic also can be administered into the retrobulbar space for postoperative analgesia by entering the subconjunctival space, placing the cannula along the scleral surface, and extending the cannula until it reaches the posterior scleral surface. I typically prefer to perform the injection with a 3-cc syringe and a 20-gauge blunt-angled cannula containing a 1:1 mixture of 0.75 % bupivacaine (Marcaine) and 2% lidocaine.

The lid speculum and drapes are removed from the eye. A drop of 5% povidone iodine, 1% atropine, and antibiotic ointment (e.g. bacitracin) are placed on the surface of the eye. A sterile patch and shield are placed over the eyelids and taped into position.

The patient is then escorted to the recovery room. Once the patient is stable and situated in the recovery room, typically within about 5 min, postoperative positioning can be undertaken, if necessary. For example, the patient can be positioned in the face-down position or on one side or the other side, depending on the location of the retinal tears. For example, if the retinal tear is located in a nasal quadrant, then the patient is positioned such that the nasal portion of the operated eye is located upward or in the least dependent position. To clarify, if the retinal tear is located at the 2 o'clock position in the right eye, then the patient is positioned in the right side down position (Fig. 2.22a).

After an appropriate recovery period, typically 45–60 min, the patient can be discharged home. If the patient is to remain an inpatient, then he or she is typically transferred to the inpatient unit at this time. The author usually admits patients for overnight IOP monitoring or for positioning if they have a history of severe or advanced glaucoma, if they have a macular hole and can benefit from nurse education on face-down positioning after surgery, if their home is a great distance away, or if they have surgery late in the evening.

Pars plana lensectomy

It may be necessary to perform a pars plana lensectomy during the surgery as a planned procedure or as needed during surgery for opacity of the lens that precludes thorough vitrectomy surgery. The first step in performing a lensectomy is to place the infusion cannula and sclerotomies as described above. The MVR blade can then be used to enter the equator of the lens through the superonasal and superotemporal sclerotomy sites. A May infusion cannula or other angled infusion cannula can then be used to infuse BSS into the lens during the lensectomy through one of the superior sclerotomy sites. The phacofragmatome is then placed through the other superior sclerotomy site for performing the lensectomy. It is essential to have the May infusion cannula irrigating within the capsular bag during the lensectomy to prevent plugging of the phacofragmatome. The lens nucleus is removed with a to-and-fro movement to sculpt the inner nucleus, and then epinuclear material is removed in a similar manner (Fig. 2.30). The capsule is maintained as intact as possible to prevent fragments of the lens from dislocating posteriorly. Many times, however, the posterior capsule does not remain intact and some lens fragments are displaced posteriorly. The anterior capsule should be kept intact if future placement of an intraocular lens is considered. The posterior surface of the anterior capsule can be 'polished' using the vitrector with gentle aspiration to remove any residual lens epithelial cells. The remainder of the posterior capsule can be removed with the vitrector.

If there are any residual fragments remaining posteriorly, they can be removed using the BIOM or AVI wide-angle viewing systems and the phacofragmatome with the posterior infusion turned on rather than the May infusion cannula. When removing lens fragments from the posterior segment, the phacofragmatome is placed on aspiration without applying

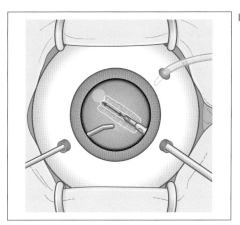

■ **FIGURE 2.30** Pars plana lensectomy with May infusion cannula and phacofragmatome using to and fro movement to remove the lens nucleus, epinucleus, and some cortical material.

ultrasound when gently aspirating the fragments from the posterior vitreous cavity. These fragments are then elevated in the anterior vitreous cavity, where the ultrasound power can be used to complete the phacofragmentation of the lens material without risk to the retina. The author prefers to set the phacofragmatome on variable vacuum on the foot pedal with a pulse rate of 10. This prevents the lens material from shooting away from the tip when using the ultrasound. It is essential to remove all of the lens fragments to prevent postoperative inflammation, phacolytic glaucoma, or cystoid macular edema.

Epiretinal membrane

Vitrectomy and the dissection of epiretinal tissue are described by George A. Williams, M.D., and Kimberly Drenser, MD, PhD, in Chapter 5 (*Epiretinal membrane surgery*). I prefer to use a flat plano contact lens with an episcleral lens ring for initial viewing, performing core vitrectomy and membrane dissection. Then I prefer to use the BIOM wide-angle viewing system for removal of the peripheral vitreous, endolaser (if necessary), and gas exchange (if necessary).

Macular hole

Vitrectomy surgery for repair of macular holes is described in Chapter 6 (*Macular hole surgery*) by Neil E. Kelly, M.D., and Abdhish R. Bhavsar, M.D. I prefer to use a flat plano contact lens with an episcleral lens ring for initial viewing, performing core vitrectomy, epiretinal membrane dissection, injection and removal of indocyanine green in the fluid-filled eye, and ILM dissection. Then I prefer to use the BIOM wide-angle viewing system for removal of the peripheral vitreous, endolaser (if necessary, to treat lattice degeneration or a retinal hole, for example), fluid–air exchange, and gas exchange.

Surgery for proliferative diabetic retinopathy

Vitrectomy surgery for diabetic retinopathy, particularly proliferative diabetic retinopathy, is the subject of Chapter 7 (*Proliferative diabetic retinopathy and vitreous hemorrhage*) by Edgar G. Thomas, M.D. I prefer to use delamination techniques with curved horizontal scissors to dissect epiretinal fibrovascular tissue. Fibrovascular attachments to the retina are divided with the scissors. I generally prefer to use the aspiration endodiathermy instrument to remove hemorrhage from the retinal surface with passive aspiration and to diathermize any areas of continued active hemorrhage. Achieving hemostasis early in the surgical case is particularly imperative in diabetic retinopathy, because hemorrage can be quite sudden and severe. Once there is a moderate amount of intraoperative hemorrhage on the retinal surface, it can be difficult to remove with fibrin and multiple areas of adhesion to the retina. I typically perform fluid–air exchange and internal drainage of subretinal fluid, if necessary, with a Flynn extendable soft-tipped aspiration cannula. I commonly use intraocular gas, 25–28% SF_6 or 14–18% C_3F_8, if there are any retinal tears or breaks.

Surgery for posterior segment trauma

Vitrectomy surgery for posterior segment trauma is the subject of Chapter 8 (*Surgical management of open-globe injuries*) by William F. Mieler, M.D., and Michael P. Rubin, M.D. For removal of an IOFB, I prefer to use the IOFB forceps, which requires a larger than 20-gauge sclerotomy site. A common mistake when removing IOFBs involves making the sclerotomy site for removal of the IOFB too small to comfortably remove the IOFB. Therefore once I know which sclerotomy site I will be using to remove the IOFB, I enlarge that site by almost twice the length of an MVR blade. Of course, if the IOFB is larger than this, then the sclerotomy site may require additional enlargement.

Surgery for proliferative vitreoretinopathy

Vitrectomy surgery for PVR is covered nicely by Allan E. Kreiger, M.D., in Chapter 9 (*Surgery for proliferative vitreoretinopathy*). Dr Kreiger was my vitrectomy surgery mentor and particularly so with respect to the principles of surgery for PVR. One critical point in performing surgery for PVR involves creating a sufficient retinotomy or retinectomy for relaxing the retina in cases of retinal foreshortening. I typically recommend performing a slightly larger retinotomy or retinectomy than one may think will be sufficient, because a common cause of failure of vitrectomy surgery for PVR is the creation of retinotomies or retinectomies that are too small in extent.

Surgery for submacular hemorrhage

The displacement of submacular hemorrhage by vitrectomy surgery is well covered by Keye L. Wong, M.D., in Chapter 10 (*Surgery for submacular hemorrhage*). I too prefer to use a 38-gauge cannula for creating a punctate retinotomy site for injecting tissue plasminogen activator into the submacular space. I typically perform this injection just superior to the superotemporal arcade. My usual pattern of postoperative positioning of patients undergoing this surgery is to have them positioned on their back for 1 hour post surgery to allow adequate time for the tissue plasminogen activator to act on the submacular hemorrhage. This is followed by upright positioning overnight until the following day. It is hoped that this will result in displacement of the hemorrhage inferiorly out of the macular region. Then face-down positioning is used for 5 days to help squeegee any remaining subretinal hemorrhage out of the macular region and to tamponade the retinotomy sites to ensure that the retina is reattached at these sites.

Drainage of choroidal hemorrhage, detachment, or effusion

Bruce Taylor, M.D., Richard Winslow, M.D., Maurice G. Syrquin, M.D., Gregory Kozielec, M.D., and Marcus Allen, M.D., describe their approach to the drainage of choroidal hemorrhage, detachment, or effusions in Chapter 14. If there is a choroidal hemorrhage, detachment, or effusion that also requires repair by vitrectomy surgery, as described, then I recommend performing the drainage of the choroidal hemorrhage or effusion prior to performing the vitrectomy. However, I do typically place an anterior chamber maintainer or infusion cannula into the anterior chamber through a limbal paracentesis prior to the choroidal drainage. This maintains positive pressure and maintains the IOP.

Surgical vitreous implants

The approach to surgical vitreous implants is covered in Chapter 15 (*Vitreoretinal surgery*) by Alex Bui, M.D., Sachin Mudvari, M.D., and Everett Ai, M.D. There are a number of pharmacotherapies that can be delivered by surgical vitreous implants, and the surgical technique is described in Chapter 15.

Vitreous biopsy for endophthalmitis or cytology

Vitrectomy and vitreous biopsy for endophthalmitis or cytology are nicely described by Robert Josephberg, M.D., in Chapter 16.

Vitrectomy surgery for retinopathy of prematurity

Vitrectomy surgery for retinopathy of prematurity is well covered by Michael T. Trese, M.D., in Chapter 19.

Surgery for intraocular tumors

Surgery for intraocular tumors is nicely described by Bertil Damato, M.D., and Carl Groenewald, M.D., in Chapter 20. While most intraocular tumors are typically treated with surgical approaches that do not require vitrectomy surgery, there a few circumstances when vitrectomy surgery can be utilized in the management of intraocular tumors. These approaches are described in Chapter 21 (*Vitrectomy technology and techniques*) by Steve Charles.

POSTOPERATIVE CARE

Most cases of vitrectomy surgery today are performed on an outpatient basis. When that is the case, the patient is typically instructed to keep the patch and shield in place over the operated eye until the next morning. Then the postoperative drops can be started. The author typically prescribes a cycloplegic, such as homatropine 5%, 1 drop q.h.s., to prevent postoperative ciliary spasm and pain, and a topical steroid, such as prednisolone acetate 1%, 1 drop q.i.d., to decrease postoperative inflammation. The author does not routinely prescribe antibiotic drops, because there is no evidence that they reduce the risk of endophthalmitis. In addition, the routine use of unnecessary antibiotics may increase the development of bacterial resistance throughout the environment. If it was necessary to remove the central corneal epithelium during the vitrectomy because of corneal epithelial edema, then the author recommends Pred Healon (Healon 0.001% plus prednisolone sodium phosphate 0.25%), 1 drop q.i.d., as well as a topical antibiotic, such as ofloxacin, a fluoroquinolone, 1 drop q.i.d., to avoid corneal infection.

The drops are typically continued for approximately 1 month. However, the cycloplegic drop can be discontinued within about 2 weeks after surgery. The topical steroid drop is typically tapered over a few weeks. For example, after 3 weeks of q.i.d. dosing, then the frequency can be reduced to 1 drop b.i.d. for 1 week, then 1 drop once a day for 1 week, and then the drop can be discontinued.

If the IOP is elevated over 30 mmHg postoperatively, then the author recommends initiating antiglaucoma medications. The only class of medication that is typically avoided is the prostaglandin analogs, because they may potentially increase inflammation and induce cystoid macular edema.

Postoperative positioning, as needed when intraocular gas tamponade is used, is described above.

It is typically not necessary to restrict activity to any significant degree. The author recommends that patients do not do any gardening or get dirt into their eyes for approximately 1 week after surgery. With heavy physical exertion, such as running, some patients may experience a throbbing sensation around the eye after surgery for a few weeks.

Postoperative medications (author's typical regimen) are as follows.

- Homatropine 5%: 1 gtt q.h.s.
- Prednisolone acetate: 1% 1 gtt q.i.d.
- In case the corneal epithelium was removed during surgery
  - Topical antibiotic such as ocufloxacin, moxifloxacin, or gatifloxacin: 1 gtt q.i.d.
  - Pred Healon (Healon 0.001% plus prednisolone sodium phosphate 0.25%): 1 gtt q.i.d.

Please see Box 2.1 for outpatient orders or discharge orders, Box 2.2 for inpatient post-operative orders, Box 2.3 for inpatient discharge orders, and Box 2.4 for postoperative instructions.

COMPLICATIONS

Intraoperative complications may include retinal tear or detachment (approximately up to 10%), iatrogenic posterior retinal tears (approximately 20% in patients with proliferative diabetic retinopathy), scleral perforation, choroidal effusion or choroidal hemorrhage, cataract from direct instrument contact with the lens (0.5%), and suprachoroidal or subretinal injection of fluid or gas.[28,29] Intraoperative retinal tears or detachment should be treated appropriately with cryoretinopexy or laser retinopexy.

Possible postoperative complications may include the following: retinal tear or detachment (approximately 1%), elevated IOP or secondary glaucoma, primary or secondary angle closure glaucoma, hypotony, cataract (eventually develops in almost all patients within a few years), endophthalmitis (less than 1%), choroidal effusion (5–43%), choroidal hemorrhage (less than 1%), vitreous hemorrhage (25–30% in patients with proliferative diabetic

---

Box 2.1 Outpatient or discharge orders (Circle appropriate orders)

Outpatient orders or discharge orders may include the following.
- Date: _____
- Time: _____
- Allergies: _____
  Discharge today
- Position
  - Face down for 1 week, then q.i.d. 15 min; sleep right/left side down q.h.s. for 1 week
  - Face down for 3 days, q.i.d. 1 h each time; sleep right/left side down q.h.s. for 1 week
  - Upright 2 days, then _____
  - Other: _____
  - No position necessary
- Eye protection
  - Shield to operated eye: _____ at all times, _____ q.h.s.
  - Glasses during day, shield q.h.s.
- Take off eye patch and start drops on morning after surgery
- Activity
  - No restrictions
  - No strenuous activity for 1 week
- Eye medications (operated eye)
  - Homatropine 5% 1 gtt q.h.s.
  - Cyclopentolate 1% 1 gtt q.h.s.
  - Prednisolone acetate 1% 1 gtt q.i.d.
  - Pred Healon 1 gtt q.i.d.
  - Timolol 0.5% 1 gtt b.i.d.
  - Cosopt 1 gtt b.i.d.
  - Brimonidine 0.2% 1 gtt b.i.d./t.i.d.
  - Acetazolamide 250 mg/500 mg sequel, 1 tablet p.o. daily, b.i.d., q.i.d.
  - Ocufloxacin/gatifloxacin/moxifloxacin 1 gtt q.i.d.
- Other medications: _____
- Follow-up appointment (please call my office to confirm: [telephone number])
  - office A _____ tomorrow/_____ other
  - office B
  - office C
- Postoperative instruction sheet: _____
- Signature: _____

Box 2.2 Inpatient postoperative orders

Inpatient or in-house postoperative orders may include the following.
- Date: _____
- Time: _____
- Allergies: _____
  Admit to inpatient unit
- Reason for admission
  - Face-down position
  - Intraocular pressure monitoring
  - Pain control
- Vital signs: _____ every shift
- Intravenous per anesthesia _____; other _____
- Intravenous fluids until adequate p.o. intake
- Diet: advance as tolerated to _____
- Activity
  —Ad lib ____
  —Bed rest ____
  —Bathroom privileges ____
  —Sit to eat ____
- Position
  - Face down for 1 week, then q.i.d. 15 min; sleep right/left side down q.h.s. for 1 week
  - Face down for 3 days, q.i.d. 1 h each time; sleep right/left side down q.h.s. for 1 week
  - Upright 2 days, then _____
  - Other: _____
  - No position necessary
- Eye protection
  - Shield to operated eye: ____ at all times, ____ q.h.s.
  - Glasses during day, shield q.h.s.
- Take off eye patch and start drops on morning after surgery
- Activity
  - No restrictions
  - No strenuous activity for 1 week
- Eye medications (operated eye), start tomorrow morning
  - Homatropine 5% 1 gtt q.h.s.
  - Cyclopentolate 1% 1 gtt q.h.s.
  - Prednisolone acetate 1% 1 gtt q.i.d.
  - Pred Healon 1 gtt q.i.d.
  - Timolol 0.5% 1 gtt b.i.d.
  - Cosopt 1 gtt b.i.d.
  - Brimonidine 0.2%/0.1% 1 gtt b.i.d./t.i.d.
  - Acetazolamide 250 mg/500 mg sequel, 1 tablet p.o. daily, b.i.d., q.i.d.
  - Ocufloxacin/gatifloxacin/moxifloxacin 1 gtt q.i.d.
- Other medications
  - Toradol 10 mg, 1 tablet p.o. q. 4–6 h p.r.n. for mild pain
  - Tylenol 650 mg p.o. q. 4 h p.r.n. for mild pain
  - Toradol 20 mg i.m./i.v. p.r.n. for pain once, then 10 mg i.m./i.v. q. 6 h p.r.n. for mild to moderate pain
  - Nubain 10 mg i.m. q. 4–6 h p.r.n. for moderate to severe pain
  - Dilaudid 1–2 mg i.m. q. 6 h p.r.n. for severe pain
  - Promethazine 12.5–50 mg i.m. q. 4–6 h p.r.n. for nausea (maximum 75 mg/24 h)
  - Diphenhydramine 25–50 mg p.o. q.h.s. p.r.n. for insomnia
- For patients with diabetes: one touch blood sugar per protocol; or _____
- Physician to cover medical concerns: _____
- Please check
  - visual acuity
  - intraocular pressure ____ q. 6 h
  - other: _____
  —(Notify physician of results)

Box 2.2 *Continued*

- Other: _____
- Follow-up appointment (please call my office to confirm: [telephone number])
  - office A _____ tomorrow/_____ other
  - office B
  - office C
- Postoperative instruction sheet: _____
- Signature: _____

Box 2.3 Inpatient discharge orders

What to expect after vitrectomy surgery
- Your eyelashes of the operative eye will be TRIMMED for the surgery. [This is the author's preference.]
- This may help to prevent infection and helps to decrease the accumulation of debris and discharge on the eyelids and lashes. The eyelashes will grow back in a few weeks.
- Your eye will be itchy, scratchy, or sore for a few weeks.
- Your eye will be bloody and red for at least a few weeks.
- Your eye will feel irritated or have a foreign body sensation for at least a few weeks.
- Your eye and surrounding area may be black and blue for a few weeks.
- Your eyelid may be swollen and may be hard to open for a few weeks.
- You can take whatever you normally take for pain (Advil, Tylenol, Motrin, etc.).
- Your vision may be limited after surgery and you may be able to see only hand movement for a few weeks after surgery, particularly if a gas bubble has been placed in your eye.
- If a gas bubble has been placed in your eye, then you may see a dark line moving across your vision, like a fluid level, and the bubble may break up into smaller bubbles. This is normal.

Box 2.4 Postoperative instructions

Postoperative instructions to patients may include the following.
- Call the office if there is any nausea or vomiting.
- Call the office if there is increased eye redness, pain, decreased vision, or excessive discharge.
- Call if you notice increased or new flashes or floaters or a new shadow or curtain across your vision.
- Physician's name and telephone number.

---

retinopathy), PVR (see Ch. 9), retinal folds, retinal slippage, cystoid macular edema, ptosis, anterior segment ischemia, rubeosis (most commonly in patients with severe proliferative diabetic retinopathy, 2–10%), or phthisis.[28,29] If a scleral buckle is placed, then there are potential risks of diplopia, infection, or exposure/extrusion or intrusion of the scleral buckle over time or intractable pain (rarely).[29] If silicone oil is used, then additional complications include keratopathy (15–80%), refractive change, glaucoma, hypotony (up to 20% in cases of PVR), cataract (75% after 2 years), recurrent epiretinal membranes, or perisilicone proliferation.

If a retinal tear or detachment occurs postoperatively, prompt treatment should be given. If the IOP is elevated, then appropriate antiglaucoma medications should be administered. If pupillary block is present, then a laser peripheral iridotomy is performed. If endophthalmitis is suspected, then prompt treatment is indicated with Gram stain, cultures, and intravitreal antibiotics (see Ch. 17). Choroidal effusion and hemorrhage can be managed by observation in mild cases. In severe cases, oral steroids can be administered. If the choroidal effusion or hemorrhage is very severe, with 'kissing' choroidals, then drainage of the serous choroidal effusion can be undertaken as soon as it is necessary. Drainage of choroidal hemorrhage should be undertaken after 10–14 days so that the choroidal hemorrhage or clot is liquefied (see Ch. 14). If anterior segment ischemia is suspected as a result of new rubeosis, anterior segment inflammation, corneal edema with Descemet's folds, or rapidly progressing cataract, then the underlying cause is corrected if possible. The main etiology that can be corrected is an overly high scleral buckle, which should be divided or removed promptly.

PROGNOSIS

Although the prognosis and visual acuity recovery generally depend on the underlying pathology and preexisting state of the retina, vitrectomy is a relatively safe procedure and the prognosis is generally good.

REFERENCES

1. Michels RG, Machemer R, Mueller-Jensen K. Vitreous surgery—past, present and future. Adv Ophthalmol 1974; 29:22–85.
2. von Graefe A. Therapeutische Miscellen. Graefes Arch Ophthalmol 1863; 9:42–152.
3. von Graefe A. Ueber operative Eingriffe in die tieferen Gebilde des Auges. B. Perforation von abgeloesten Netzhaeuten und Glaskoerpermembranen. Arch Ophthalmol 1863; 9:85–104.
4. Ford V. Proposed surgical treatment of opaque vitreous. Lancet 1890; i:462–463.
5. Michaelson IC. Transscleral division of mid-vitreous membrane under visual control. Br J Ophthalmol 1960; 44:634–635.
6. Dodo T, Toda S. Vitreous replacement as a treatment of severe vitreous opacity. Acta Soc Ophthalmol Jpn 1958; 62:129–143.
7. Landegger GP. Clinical experiences with vitreous replacement. Am J Ophthalmol 1950; 33:915–921.
8. Dodo T. Window-making procedure for post-hemorrhage vitreous membrane. Acta Soc Ophthalmol Jpn 1964; 68:811–826.
9. Deutschmann R. Uber ein neues Heilverfahren bei Netzhautablosung. Cbl Augenheilk 1895; 19:849–928.
10. Kasner D, Miller GR, Taylor WH, et al. Surgical treatment of amyloidosis of the vitreous. Trans Am Acad Ophthalmol Otolaryngol 1968; 72:410–418.
11. Kasner D. Vitrectomy: a new approach to the management of vitreous. Highlights Ophthalmol 1968; 11:304–329.
12. Machemer R, Buettner H, Norton EWD. Vitrectomy: a pars plana approach. Trans Am Acad Ophthalmol Otolaryngol 1971; 75:813–820.
13. Machemer R, Parel JM, Norton EWD. Vitrectomy: a pars plana approach. Technical improvements and further results. Trans Am Acad Ophthalmol Otolaryngol 1972; 76(2):462–466.
14. Machemer R, Parel JM, Norton EWD. A new concept for vitreous surgery. I. Instrumentation. Am J Ophthalmol Otolaryngol 1972; 10:172–177.
15. Douvas N. Roto-extractor for congenital and traumatic cataracts (20 cases). Cataract Surgery Congress, Miami, Florida, 1973.
16. Peyman GA, Dodich NA. Experimental vitrectomy: instrumentation and surgical technique. Arch Ophthalmol 1971; 86:548–551.
17. Kreiger AE, Straatsma BR. Stereotaxic vitrectomy. Mod Probl Ophthalmol 1974; 12:411–423.
18. O'Malley C, Heintz RM. Vitrectomy via the pars plana—a new instrument system. Trans Pac Coast Otoophthalmol Soc Annu Meet 1972; 53:121–137.
19. O'Malley C, Heintz RM. Vitrectomy with an alternative instrument system. Ann Ophthalmol 1975; 7(4):585–588.
20. O'Malley C, Trip RM. Plugs and stiletto: entry incisions for a 20 gauge instrument system. Ophthalmic Surg 1977; 8(1):76–81.
21. O'Malley C, Heintz RM. Electrovitrectomy. Am J Ophthalmol 1973; 76(3):336–342.
22. O'Malley C, Heintz RM. Electrovitrectomy. 2. Principles and results. Br J Ophthalmol 1975; 59(10):580–585.
23. Machemer R. A new concept for vitreous surgery. II. Surgical technique and complications. Am J Ophthalmol 1972; 74:1022–1033.

24. Parel JM, Machemer R, Aumayr W. A new concept for vitreous surgery. V. An automated operating microscope. Am J Ophthalmol 1974; 77(2):161–168.
25. Wilkinson CP, Rice RE. Michels retinal detachment. 2nd edn. St. Louis: Mosby; 1997.
26. Chang S, Lincoff H, Zimmerman NJ, et al. Giant retinal tears. Surgical techniques and results using perfluorocarbon liquids. Arch Ophthalmol 1989; 107(5):761–766.
27. Verstraeten T, Williams GA, Chang S, et al. Lens-sparing vitrectomy with perfluorocarbon liquid for the primary treatment of giant retinal tears. Ophthalmology 1995; 102(1):17–20.
28. Michels RG, Wilkinson CP, Rice TA. Vitreous surgery. In: Retinal detachment. St. Louis: Mosby; 1990:863–888.
29. Michels RG, Wilkinson CP, Rice TA. Complications of retinal detachment. In: Retinal detachment. St. Louis: Mosby; 1990:959–1057.

3 23-Gauge vitrectomy

Howard F. Fine, Pawan Bhatnagar, and Richard F. Spaide

23-Gauge vitrectomy systems were created to combine the advantages of both 20- and 25-gauge systems. The primary benefit of 25-gauge vitrectomy is the self-sealing, sutureless sclerotomy. This promotes faster wound healing, improves patient comfort, decreases inflammation, diminishes conjunctival scarring, reduces postoperative astigmatic change, and may lessen surgical opening and closing times.[1–10] However, compared with traditional 20-gauge systems, 25-gauge vitrectomy may be associated with higher rates of hypotony and choroidal detachment[10–14] due to wound leakage. Secondly, 25-gauge vitrectomy may be associated with increased incidences of intra- and postoperative retinal tears and detachments, secondary to a lack of adequate peripheral vitrectomy from overly flexible instruments and excessive vitreoretinal traction at sclerotomy sites.[12,15,16] The advantages of traditional 20-gauge instruments over smaller 25-gauge versions are that a larger bore translates into greater instrument functionality with stiffer shafts, faster and more efficient cutters, brighter light pipes, extrusion cannulas which provide greater suction, scissors with a more pronounced curve, and multipurpose instruments with greater functionality.

23-Gauge systems combine the best of both 20- and 25-gauge worlds with sutureless, self-sealing sclerotomies and robust, high-functionality instruments.

INDICATIONS AND CONTRAINDICATIONS

The indications for 23-gauge vitrectomy surgery are similar to those for 20-gauge surgery and include: non-clearing vitreous hemorrhage or opacity; epiretinal membrane; macular hole; retained lens fragments; retinal detachment; tractional retinal detachment; diagnostic vitrectomy; intraocular foreign body; retained oil or heavy liquid; vitreomacular traction; and miscellaneous procedures (subretinal surgery, etc.) (Box 3.1).

Contraindications for 23-gauge vitrectomy also overlap contraindications for 20-gauge surgery including: failure to obtain appropriate informed consent; bleeding diathesis or anticoagulation; corneal or other opacity precluding adequate visualization; scleromalacia or other conditions that may prevent adequate wound healing; suspected neoplasm which could seed the orbit, such as retinoblastoma; and other medical contraindications to anesthesia or surgical procedures (Box 3.2).

Additionally, not all 20-gauge vitrectomy surgical tools are currently available in a 23-gauge version, such as the fragmatome and some silicone oil injection/extrusion devices. In these cases, the surgeon may opt to use 20-gauge instrumentation or use a hybrid system with a mixture of 20- and 23-gauge sclerotomies and instruments (Box 3.2).

SURGICAL TECHNIQUE

Preoperative preparation

Written, informed consent concerning the benefits of undergoing the surgical procedure, potential risks, and alternatives must be obtained. There should be a detailed discussion with the patient concerning postoperative expectations including potential visual outcome, postoperative instructions including medications, positioning, limitations on activity and air travel (dependent on air or gas tamponade), and follow-up visits.

Box 3.1 Indications for 23-gauge vitrectomy surgery

- Vitreous hemorrhage
- Epiretinal membrane
- Macular hole
- Retained lens fragment
- Retinal detachment
- Tractional retinal detachment
- Diagnostic vitrectomy
- Intraocular foreign body
- Retained oil or heavy liquid
- Non-clearing vitreous hemorrhage
- Symptomatic posterior vitreous detachment
- Vitreomacular traction
- Miscellaneous procedures—submacular surgery, etc.

Box 3.2 Contraindications for 23-gauge vitrectomy surgery

Contraindications to vitrectomy surgery

- Failure to obtain appropriate informed consent
- Bleeding diathesis or anticoagulation
- Corneal or other opacity precluding adequate visualization
- Scleromalacia or other condition which may prevent adequate wound healing
- Suspected neoplasm which could seed the orbit, such as retinoblastoma
- Other medical contraindication to anesthesia or surgical procedure

Contraindications specific to 23-gauge vitrectomy

- Silicone oil cases
- Dropped nucleus cases
- Extensive proliferative vitreoretinopathy
- Severe diabetic tractional retinal detachment
  (Note that a single sclerotomy can be 20-gauge to overcome these limitations.)

Patients should be nil per os (nothing by month) for at least 8 hours, or as directed by the anesthesia team. Appropriate medical clearance is essential. Discussion with the anesthetist to avoid nitrous oxide anesthesia if intravitreal gas tamponade is planned is important.

Procedure
Opening

3.1
3.2
3.3
3.4
3.5

Patients should receive sedation and then a retro- or peribulbar block, such as with a 5 mL injection of a 50:50 mixture of 4% lidocaine and 0.75% bupivacaine. Supplemental anesthesia is administered as necessary. Patients' skin and lashes should be prepped with 5% povidone iodine (Betadine) solution and the ocular surface with povidone iodine solution, followed by draping and placement of a lid speculum.

Vitrectomy opening with 23-gauge instrumentation differs by manufacturer. Currently, the two major manufacturers of 23-gauge instrumentation are Alcon (Fort Worth, Texas) and Dutch Ophthalmic Research Center (DORC; Zuidland, The Netherlands).

For the Alcon system (Fig. 3.1), displace the conjunctiva in the posterior–anterior location or circumferentially with a cotton swab or conjunctival forceps. Insert the trocar/cannula 4.0 mm posterior to the limbus in phakic patients or 3.5 mm in pseudophakes. Beveling this could help reduce the risk of postoperative hypotony. Remove the trocar

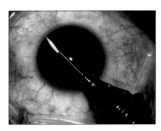

FIGURE 3.1 Alcon 23-gauge instrumentation: a 23-gauge trocar with beveled tip. (Courtesy of Alcon, Inc.)

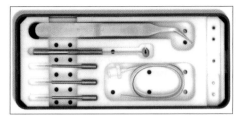

FIGURE 3.2 DORC 23-gauge instrumentation: blue infusion cannula, three blunt inserters (top right), flat plate (middle right), cannula forceps (bottom), two closure plugs (bottom left), infusion cannula (middle left), and two instrument cannulas (top left). (Courtesy of DORC.)

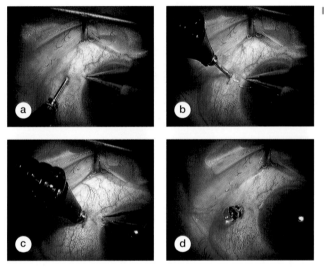

FIGURE 3.3 Alcon 23-gauge opening. (**a**) Displace the inferotemporal conjunctiva and insert the trocar/cannula in a beveled fashion 3.5 mm posterior to the limbus. (**b**) Once the beveled tip is engaged, redirect the trocar/cannula perpendicular to the sclera and aimed at the mid-vitreous cavity. (**c**) Insert the trocar/cannula to the hub. (**d**) Remove the trocar, and then connect the infusion tubing. (Courtesy of Alcon, Inc.)

while stabilizing the cannula with a forceps. The primed infusion tubing can then be inserted and emits an audible click when appropriately connected. Confirming that the trocar is in the vitreous rather than the suprachoroidal space can be achieved with an oblique view through the pupil with light pipe illumination. The infusion tubing can be secured with tape to the drapes and the infusion begun. The superotemporal and superonasal cannulas can be inserted in a similar fashion. Plugs may be used to maintain intraocular pressure and prevent vitreous or retinal incarceration in the cannula (Fig. 3.2).

For the DORC system (Fig. 3.3), displace the inferotemporal conjunctiva approximately 1–3 mm with the pressure plate. This plate has a central opening 3.5 mm from the edge through which the 23-gauge 45° stiletto blade is inserted at an angle of approximately 25°, 3.5 mm posterior to the limbus. The blunt microtrocar/cannula is then inserted, maintaining apposition of the conjunctival and scleral openings with the pressure plate. In similar fashion, the superotemporal and superonasal cannulas can be inserted, and plugs may be used to maintain intraocular pressure as needed (Fig. 3.4).

Intraoperative techniques

A discussion of the myriad of techniques available intraoperatively is beyond the scope of this text. Most 23-gauge instruments behave like their 20-gauge counterparts and can be

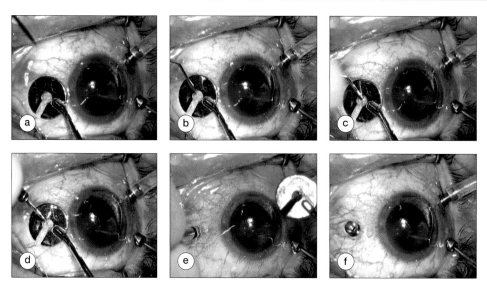

■ **FIGURE 3.4** DORC 23-gauge opening. (**a**) Displace the conjunctiva with the toothed pressure plate (Dutch Ophthalmic USA, Kingston, NH). (**b**) Caliper measurements are not needed as the central opening of the circular pressure plate is 3.5 mm from the edge. (**c**) Insert the 45° 23-gauge stiletto blade (BD Medical-Ophthalmic Systems, Franklin Lakes, NJ) at a 20–30° angle through the conjunctiva and sclera at the pars plana, creating a tunneled sclerotomy. (**d**) Next, without releasing the pressure plate, insert the metal trocar through the wound using a blunt inserter. (**e**) The inserter can be removed by stabilizing the trocar at its flanged lip with the notched edge of the pressure plate. (**f**) Configuration once the trocars have been inserted. Removal of the trocars is performed by grasping the flanged lip with the trocar forceps, followed by brief pressure over the sclerotomy site with a cotton swab. (Courtesy of DORC.)

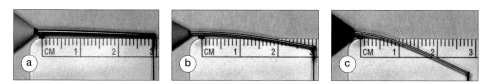

■ **FIGURE 3.5** The flexibility of cutters is demonstrated by suspending a syringe filled with 20 mL of water from the (**a**) 20-gauge, (**b**) 23-gauge, and (**c**) 25-gauge cutters held horizontally.

used in a similar fashion with less concern for instrument flexibility than in 25-gauge cases (Figs 3.5–3.8).

Closing

Closing with both the Alcon and DORC 23-gauge systems is similar. Plugs are placed in the cannula. The cannula should be removed with gentle traction using a forceps, and the displaced conjunctiva repositioned to its normal location with a cotton swab or smooth forceps immediately after cannula removal. The infusion may be clamped or turned down temporarily during cannula removal to reduce fluid or air egress through a sclerotomy. Numerous techniques are available for air–gas exchange. One such method is injection of gas with a 30-gauge needle just prior to removal of the last remaining cannula. Care should be taken to check for sclerotomy leakage at a physiologic pressure. Signs of leakage include significant conjunctival bleb formation, inability to maintain a physiologic pressure, and observation of fluid or gas egress through sclerotomies. Leaking sclerotomies should be

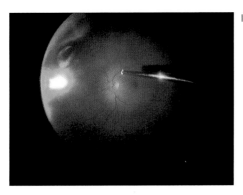

■ **FIGURE 3.6** An example of the wide-field light pipes available with 23-gauge instrumentation.

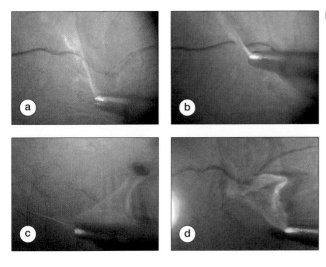

■ **FIGURE 3.7** Sequential intraoperative photographs (**a–d**) showing peeling of the internal limiting membrane using 23-gauge end-gripping forceps. The internal limiting membrane was elevated without the use of stains and peeled through the macula.

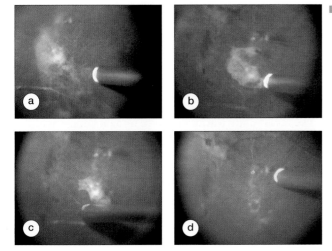

■ **FIGURE 3.8** Sequential intraoperative photographs (**a–d**) showing dissection of diabetic membranes without the use of intraocular scissors. The membranes were elevated with the use of suction and then delaminated with the vitrector for en bloc resection.

closed by suturing the sclera directly, which may require a small conjunctiva incision. Usual postoperative care such as atropine drops, antibiotic/steroid ointment, and a patch and shield are customary.

SCLEROTOMY LEAKAGE

Tunneled sclerotomies for vitrectomy surgery were described in 1996, but still required opening of the conjunctiva,[12] and were frequently associated with bleeding from sclerotomy sites and wound leakage requiring sutures.[2] Many modifications have been made to improve the technique.[1,3–8] Traditional 20-gauge sclerotomies have a 1.15-mm width, requiring sutures. Sutureless 25-gauge vitrectomy utilizes a non-tunneled roughly 0.5-mm sclerotomy, and tunneled 23-gauge vitrectomy employs a 0.72-mm sclerotomy.[17] If the scleral thickness 3.5 mm posterior to the limbus is 0.6 mm, then a 25° tunneled wound would be roughly 1.4 mm long (thickness/sine [angle]).

There is evidence in the literature that non-tunneled 25-gauge sclerotomies frequently do not self-seal. One series reported a 14% incidence of hypotony requiring additional gas or saline tamponade within 2–6 hours postoperatively.[11] Gupta indicated that 22% (9 of 41) of fluid-filled eyes which underwent 25-gauge vitrectomy required sclerotomy suture placement or suffered postoperative hypotony.[12] In a review of 140 consecutive 25-gauge cases, Lakhanpal et al. published that 7.1% of eyes (10 of 140) required a suture for adequate closure and 3.8% (5 of 140) demonstrated postoperative choroidal detachment.[10] Even these figures underestimate the true incidence of hypotony in vitrectomized eyes after 25-gauge surgery as the authors note that 18.6% of patients (26 of 140) in the series did not undergo vitrectomy: 11 patients with intralesional injection for choroidal neovascularization, 8 patients with arteriovenous manipulation for branch vein occlusion, and 7 patients with epiretinal membrane. Hypotony, even if transient, is not a benign condition and may increase the postoperative risks for serious complications including retinal or vitreal incarceration, suprachoroidal hemorrhage, and endophthalmitis.[13,14] However, some surgeons now use a gas fill to plug 25-gauge sclerotomies,[18] which can increase the risk of cataract and secondary retinal tears and adds operative time, or perform only a limited peripheral vitrectomy.

RETINAL TEAR AND DETACHMENT

Excessive instrument flexibility hampers thorough removal of the peripheral vitreous. Ibarra et al. noted that a 'more prominent residual vitreous skirt could cause significant anterior vitreoretinal traction and subsequent retinal tears or detachments beyond the immediate postoperative period with an increased incidence of 25-gauge cases'.[15] Ibarra's series included a subsequent detachment rate of 2.2% (1 case in 45). Gupta and colleagues[12] reported an incidence of intraoperative retinal tears of 2.9% (2 of 70) but no postoperative detachments. Fujii et al. also described a 2% (1 of 35) postoperative detachment rate.[16] The apparent increased rate of retinal detachments following 25-gauge surgery could also be related to decreased illumination from smaller bore light pipes causing missed breaks intraoperatively,[12] but newer illumination systems may obviate this issue. In this series of 77 patients, no intraoperative sclerotomy site tears were noted and no patient without a prior retinal detachment developed a subsequent detachment.

INSTRUMENTS AND DEVICES

Preoperative preparation

- Dilation drops (i.e. phenylephrine hydrochloride 2.5%, tropicamide 1%)
- Proparacaine hydrochloride 0.5%
- Alcohol swabs

- Retro- or peribulbar block (i.e. 5 cc of a 50 : 50 mixture of 4% lidocaine with 0.75% bupivacaine in a syringe with a retrobulbar needle)
- Povidone iodine (Betadine) solution

Intraoperative instrumentation

- Operating microscope
- Sterile drapes
- Lid speculum
- Caliper
- Needle holders
- Forceps (i.e. internal limiting membrane forceps, end-gripping, tying forceps, etc.)
- Scissors (i.e. vertical, horizontal, curved)
- Brush
- Endodiathermy
- Endolaser
- Extrusion cannulas (i.e. flute-tipped, soft-tipped, etc.)
- Pic
- Heavy liquid (i.e. Perfluoron [Alcon])
- Intraocular tamponade (i.e. silicone oil, inert gases such as sulfur hexafluoride [SF_6] and perfluoropropane [C_3F_8])
- Vannas and Westcott scissors
- Weck-Cel sponges
- Balanced salt solution
- 23-gauge entry system (Dutch Ophthalmic Research Center)
  - Infusion cannula
  - Infusion line
  - Stiletto microvitreoretinal blade
  - Transconjunctival pressure plate
  - Closure plugs
- 23-gauge entry system (Alcon)
  - Trocar/cannulas
  - Infusion line
  - Closure plugs
- Viewing system (such as binocular indirect ophthalmomicroscope [BIOM], AVI hand-held lenses)

Postoperative medications and equipment

- Steroid drops (i.e. prednisolone acetate 1%)
- Antibiotic drops (i.e. moxifloxacin HCl 0.5% [Alcon], gatifloxacin 0.3% [Allergan])
- Dilating drops (i.e. cyclogyl 1%, atropine sulfate 1%)
- Eye shield
- Sunglasses
- Postoperative positioning gear (i.e. head rests, positioning chairs, etc.)

CONCLUSION

23-Gauge systems provide for efficient vitrectomy with robust, stiff, functional instruments in a sutureless manner, reducing inflammation and scarring, and possibly improving wound healing and patient comfort. The indications for 23-gauge surgery nearly match the list for traditional 20-gauge surgery, with possible exceptions including phacofragmentation and silicone oil extraction/infusion. The learning curve is not steep and surgeons familiar with 25-gauge systems will quickly master opening and closing techniques. Beveled sclerotomies may reduce well-reported risks of postoperative hypotony seen in 25-gauge systems, but care should be taken to ensure there is no wound leak at the conclusion of each case. The stiff 23-gauge instruments and robust cutters are likely to reduce the occurrence of retinal tears and detachment seen with more flexible 25-gauge instruments. The transconjunctival 23-gauge vitrectomy system combines the best of 20- and 25-gauge worlds: functional, robust instrumentation and sutureless, self-sealing sclerotomies.

REFERENCES

1. Chen JC. Sutureless pars plana vitrectomy through self-sealing sclerotomies. Arch Ophthalmol 1996; 114(10):1273–1275.
2. Milibak T, Suveges I. Complications of sutureless pars plana vitrectomy through self-sealing sclerotomies. Arch Ophthalmol 1998; 116(1):119.
3. Kwok AK, Tham CC, Lam DS, et al. Modified sutureless sclerotomies in pars plana vitrectomy. Am J Ophthalmol 1999; 127(6):731–733.
4. Schmidt J, Nietgen GW, Brieden S. Self-sealing, sutureless sclerotomy in pars plana vitrectomy. Klin Monatsbl Augenheilkd 1999; 215(4):247–251.
5. Jackson T. Modified sutureless sclerotomies in pars plana vitrectomy. Am J Ophthalmol 2000; 129(1):116–117.
6. Assi AC, Scott RA, Charteris DG. Reversed self-sealing pars plana sclerotomies. Retina 2000; 20(6):689–692.
7. Rahman R, Rosen PH, Riddell C, et al. Self-sealing sclerotomies for sutureless pars plana vitrectomy. Ophthalmic Surg Lasers 2000; 31(6):462–466.
8. Theelen T, Verbeek AM, Tilanus MA, et al. A novel technique for self-sealing, wedge-shaped pars plana sclerotomies and its features in ultrasound biomicroscopy and clinical outcome. Am J Ophthalmol 2003; 136(6):1085–1092.
9. Yanyali A, Celik E, Horozoglu F, et al. Corneal topographic changes after transconjunctival (25-gauge) sutureless vitrectomy. Am J Ophthalmol 2005; 140(5):939–941.
10. Lakhanpal RR, Humayun MS, de Juan E Jr, et al. Outcomes of 140 consecutive cases of 25-gauge transconjunctival surgery for posterior segment disease. Ophthalmology 2005; 112(5):817–824.
11. Gupta A, Gonzales CR, Lee SY, et al. Transient post-operative hypotony following transconjunctival 25 gauge vitrectomy. ARVO 2003; abstract 2026.
12. Gupta OP, Weichel ED, Fineman MS, et al. Postoperative complications associated with 25-gauge pars plana vitrectomy. Retina Society abstract 2005.
13. Meyer CH, Rodrigues EB, Schmidt JC, et al. Sutureless vitrectomy surgery. Ophthalmology 2003; 110(12):2427–2428.
14. Lam DS, Yuen CY, Tam BS, et al. Sutureless vitrectomy surgery. Ophthalmology 2003; 110(12):2428–2429.
15. Ibarra MS, Hermel M, Prenner JL, et al. Longer-term outcomes of transconjunctival sutureless 25-gauge vitrectomy. Am J Ophthalmol 2005; 139(5):831–836.
16. Fujii GY, De Juan E Jr, Humayun MS, et al. Initial experience using the transconjunctival sutureless vitrectomy system for vitreoretinal surgery. Ophthalmology 2002; 109(10):1814–1820.
17. Eckardt C. Transconjunctival sutureless 23-gauge vitrectomy. Retina 2005; 25(2):208–211.
18. Charles S. Debating the pros and cons of 23-g vs. 25-g. vitrectomy. Retinal Physician 2006; 3(1):24–25.

THE LIBRARY
THE ... ...MENT CENTRE
THE ... ...AL
HALIFAX HX3 ...

4 25-Gauge vitrectomy

Anurag Gupta and Steven D. Schwartz

Traditional pars plana vitrectomy involves the creation of 20- or 19-gauge incisions in the pars plana after surgical dissection of the conjunctiva. The scleral incisions and the overlying conjunctiva are sutured closed on completion of the surgical procedure. In 2002, a vitrectomy system was introduced that allows for the creation of 25-gauge sclerotomies that do not require surgical closure of sclerotomies or conjunctiva on completion of the procedure.[1] The system is based on the use of microcannulas introduced through the conjunctiva and sclera using an insertion trocar. On completion of the surgery, the microcannulas are simply removed from the eye as the pars plana incisions are intended to be self-sealing. This surgical system obviates the need for opening and closing the conjunctiva and closing the sclerotomies with sutures.

SURGICAL SYSTEMS

The first 25-gauge transconjunctival sutureless vitrectomy system was developed in 2002 by Bausch & Lomb Surgical (St Louis, Missouri), and was given the acronym TSV-25. The TSV-25 is based on the much heralded Millennium platform that was initially developed for use with standard 20- or 19-gauge vitrectomy. The modifications for the TSV-25 start with the use of the entry alignment system (EAS), which includes three microcannulas, a sharp insertion trocar, a specialized infusion cannula, cannula plugs, and a plug forceps (Fig. 4.1). The vitreous cutter uses the Millennium electric handpiece with a 25-gauge cutter tip.

Shortly after the commercial introduction of the TSV-25, a microcannula package was developed by Dutch Ophthalmic Research Center International b.v. (DORC; Zuidland, The Netherlands) for use with the Accurus vitrectomy system by Alcon Surgical (Fort Worth, Texas). In addition to including the microcannulas and insertion trocars, the DORC package also included a 25-gauge pneumatic cutter for use with the Accurus system.

Alcon Surgical quickly developed their own proprietary 25-gauge vitrectomy system for the Accurus. The vitrectomy handpiece is a 25-gauge pneumatic vitreous cutter that is ergonomically indistinguishable from other 20-gauge ocutomes offered by Alcon Surgical. This system allows for easy, atraumatic insertion of the cannulas due to very sharp insertion trocars (Fig. 4.2). The cannulas have also been modified to allow for easier removal on completion of the vitrectomy.

INSTRUMENTATION

As the popularity of the 25-gauge vitrectomy systems increases, a larger armamentarium of surgical instruments is being developed. Almost all of the companies that manufacture microsurgical instruments for standard 20-gauge vitrectomies have added a line of 25-gauge instruments to their catalogs. A complete selection of forceps, scissors, picks, light pipes, and laser probes is currently available. Disposable instruments have found a niche due to the delicate nature of the tools. As technology improves, combination illuminated instruments and automated scissors may soon become available.

Table 4.1 itemizes a standard 25-gauge vitrectomy instrumentation list.

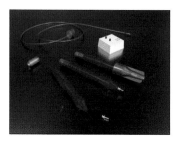

FIGURE 4.1 Entry alignment system (Bausch & Lomb Surgical).

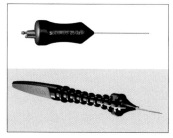

FIGURE 4.2 25-Gauge vitreous cutter handpiece (top) and trocar with microcannula (bottom) (Alcon Surgical).

TABLE 4.1 Instrumentation list for 25-gauge vitrectomy

Instrument		
Operating microscope with inverter		
Viewing system	Wide angle	Binocular indirect ophthalmomicroscope (BIOM) Handheld lens (i.e. AVI lens)
	High magnification	Drop-on macular lens Lander irrigating lens
Vitrectomy system with 25-gauge capability	Bausch & Lomb Millennium Alcon Accurus	
Illumination system with light pipe	Standard illumination Xenon light source	Photon from Synergetics (1 and 2) Xenon from Alcon
Handheld instrumentation	25-gauge forceps (Greishaber, Alcon, DORC, Synergetics) 25-gauge soft tip aspiration (Greishaber, Alcon, DORC, Synergetics) 25-gauge endolaser (Alcon, Iridex)	
Miscellaneous standard vitrectomy instruments	Lid speculum 0.12 mm Castroviejo forceps Calipers	
Medications	Preoperative dilation drops	2.5% Phenylephrine 1% Tropicamide
	Intraoperative subconjunctival medications	Third generation cephalosporin Dexamethasone (4 mg/cc)
	Postoperative	Prednisolone acetate 1% Atropine 1% Fluoroquinolone

INDICATIONS

25-Gauge vitrectomy systems can be used for a wide variety of vitreoretinal disorders. The biggest advantages are seen in patients with surgical conditions such as isolated non-clearing vitreous hemorrhages, and those that primarily involve the macula such as macular holes, puckers, vitreomacular traction syndrome, simple tractional retinal detachments, and sheathotomies. As the surgeon becomes more experienced with this system, surgical indications may expand to include more complex and peripheral pathology such as repair of rhegmatogenous retinal detachments, treatment of retinopathy of prematurity and other pediatric disorders, removal of cortical lens fragments, and intraocular lens repositioning. The system is particularly useful in patients who have either had previous ocular surgery, or have underlying conditions that would cause conjunctival dissection to be of increased complexity. This is especially true when the patient has had previous filtering surgery for glaucoma as 25-gauge vitrectomy minimizes conjunctival trauma.

The limitations of surgical indications are shrinking as the available instrumentation for 25-gauge vitrectomy expands. Although there are no absolute contraindications for the 25-gauge vitrectomy system, careful consideration must be given before its use in patients with complex retinal detachments with proliferative vitreoretinopathy, retained nuclear lens fragments, and pathology that may require the use of silicone oil. Many of these restrictions may be overcome with the conversion of one or more ports to standard 20-gauge sclerotomies.

PREOPERATIVE PREPARATION

In anticipation of vitreoretinal surgery, patients are dilated preoperatively. A standard combination of 2.5% phenylephrine and 1% tropicamide may be used to provide adequate dilation for the 25-gauge vitrectomy. At our institution, one drop of each medication is instilled in the lower conjunctival fornix every 5 min for 15 min.

Once the patient has been brought to the operating room, anesthesia is administered based on surgeon preference. The patient is then prepped and draped in sterile ophthalmic fashion, with particular attention paid to the instillation of 5% or 10% povidone iodine into the conjunctival fornices. A lid speculum is inserted and the patient is prepared to undergo 25-gauge vitrectomy.

SURGICAL TECHNIQUE

4.1

The mechanics of the 25-gauge vitrectomy system are quite different from 20-gauge vitrectomy. While there is a significant decrease in the amount of intraoperative time spent on the non-cognitive portions of the surgery (i.e. surgical opening and closing), the actually intraocular approach to vitreoretinal disorders is much more complex. Vitreoretinal surgeons must modify their surgical approach when first using the 25-gauge vitrectomy system. There is a steep learning curve as it typically takes a surgeon about 10 cases to become comfortable with 25-gauge vitrectomy.

Techniques for cannula insertion have evolved over the past few years as our experience with the systems has increased. The initial insertion of the microcannulas was directly through the conjunctiva and sclera. As reported at the American Academy of Ophthalmology in 2002, there was a 20% rate of postoperative hypotony.[2] This led to a modification of the insertion technique to its current methodology. Prior to insertion of the microcannula on the trocar, the conjunctiva is laterally displaced using a fine-toothed forceps or a cotton-tipped applicator (Fig. 4.3). On creation of the wound, the conjunctival incision no longer directly overlies the sclerotomy. This resulted in a significant decrease in the rate of hypotony as conjunctiva and Tenon's capsule cover the sclerotomy when the trocars are removed at the end of the case.[3]

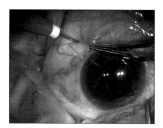

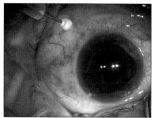

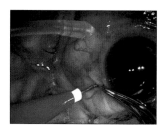

■ **FIGURE 4.3** Maximal displacement of conjunctiva before trocar and microcannula are inserted through the pars plana is essential.

■ **FIGURE 4.4** The 25-gauge infusion cannula is inserted within the first microcannula placed.

■ **FIGURE 4.5** The second microcannula is inserted with conjunctival displacement.

After the first trocar is inserted an appropriate distance from the limbus, typically in the inferotemporal quadrant, the infusion cannula is placed within the microcannula (Fig. 4.4). Proper placement is ensured under direct visualization through the pupil. A second microcannula is placed in either of the superior quadrants (Fig. 4.5). If the patient has had a previous vitrectomy, a microcannula plug is required to maintain intraocular pressure while the third trocar is inserted. In a non-vitrectomized eye, this is often an optional step. Once all the microcannulas are in position, the appropriate surgical instruments are introduced.

The greatest variation from standard 20-gauge pars plana vitrectomy occurs during the intraocular portion of the surgery. There is a great deal of flexibility to all of the instruments used during 25-gauge vitrectomy due to the small size (diameter) of the instrument shafts. This flexibility does not permit the surgeon to move and rotate the globe as freely during surgery as with the larger 20-gauge instrumentation. The microcannulas must be used as fulcrums around which intraocular contents are manipulated. Access to the peripheral vitreous gel is much more difficult, and may require scleral depression for more complete removal. One of the distinct advantages of a cannula system is the ability to move the infusion cannula to any port, allowing the surgeon to engage peripheral gel from multiple angles, a technique used more often with the 25-gauge systems.

The actual movement of instruments through the microcannulas is very different for surgeons who are not used to performing vitrectomies with a cannula system. The usual proprioceptive clues from resistance of movement through open sclerotomies are absent, requiring a hypervigilance to the actual intraocular positioning of instruments at all times to avoid inadvertent contact with the retina.

Vitreous gel is removed more slowly with the smaller-gauge vitreous cutters. In order to partially compensate for the decreased speed of vitrectomy, both the infusion pressure and aspiration are often raised while performing the core vitrectomy. With the TSV-25 from Bausch & Lomb Surgical, the authors generally prefer the following settings: vacuum 550, cut rate 1500, and bottle height 90 cm. For the Accurus system from Alcon Surgical, the authors prefer a vacuum from 550 to 600, cut rate 1500, and forced infusion pressure of 40 mmHg. These settings are general starting guidelines and are often changed based on the patient's ocular condition.

When performing dissection at the vitreoretinal interface, movements that have become familiar with standard 20-gauge vitrectomy are no longer possible with the flexible 25-gauge instruments. Forceps and scissors must be advanced to the area of interest and then rotated around the microcannula fulcrum to avoid unintended stress and possible bending or breaking of the instruments. While certain vitreous cutters, such as the Lightning cutter used with the TSV-25, work even when the shaft is bent to almost 90°, great care must be taken to not overflex the instruments since they may break. A full complement of aspiration cannulas and laser probes has been developed for the 25-gauge systems and may be used depending on surgeon preference.

After completing the vitrectomy and accomplishing the goals of surgery, surgical closure is quite rapid. The authors recommend first ensuring free flow of fluid or air through both of the superior sclerotomies. One microcannula is removed with forceps (Fig. 4.6). The infusion is then turned off and the other microcannula is removed in rapid succession to minimize the amount of fluid or air that escapes into the subconjunctival space. Finally, the remaining microcannula is removed together with the infusion cannula in a single maneuver (Fig. 4.7). We wait for 2–3 min to ensure that the globe maintains an adequate intraocular pressure. If the eye is hypotonous at this time, the volume is augmented with fluid or gas accordingly using a 30-gauge needle to inject through a separate pars plana site.

POSTOPERATIVE CARE

At the conclusion of the surgery, the eye is lightly pressure patched with an antibiotic/steroid combination ointment, gauze eye pads, and a hard shield. The patient is discharged home from the recovery area once stabilized depending on the route of anesthesia administration with strict instructions not to manipulate the patch. On postoperative day one the patch is removed and the eye is examined with special attention paid to intraocular pressure and signs of intraocular infection. Subsequent follow-up is based on the preoperative diagnosis and surgeon preference.

COMPLICATIONS

Any of the complications that can occur with 20-gauge vitrectomy surgery can occur with 25-gauge vitrectomy surgery. Please refer to Chapter 2, *Vitrectomy surgery*, by Abdhish R. Bhavsar, M.D. Of particular note, with 25-gauge surgery there appears to be an increased rate of hypotony as described above. In addition, some authors are concerned about a potentially higher rate of endophthalmitis with 25-gauge surgery, although this is controversial.

OUTCOMES

Intraoperatively, use of the 25-gauge vitrectomy system may allow for much faster surgical times as the need for involved conjunctival dissection and sclerotomy creation is eliminated.[4] The decrease in surgical time is most appreciated when the eye has had a previous pars plana vitrectomy as performing a core vitrectomy with the 25-gauge systems occurs at a slower rate when compared to 20-gauge standard vitrectomy. It has been postulated

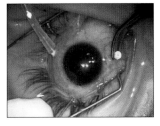

FIGURE 4.6 The microcannula is removed with a non-toothed forceps.

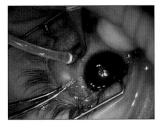

FIGURE 4.7 The last microcannula and infusion cannula are removed together.

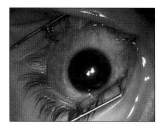

FIGURE 4.8 Immediate postoperative appearance of the eye. Note the lack of ocular inflammation, chemosis, or hemorrhage.

that the decreased flow and volume of infusion fluid may lead to decreased rates of postoperative cataract formation.[5]

Perhaps the greatest advantage of the 25-gauge vitrectomy systems is seen in the immediate postoperative period. Often times—due to the almost complete absence of periorbital swelling, conjunctival chemosis, and hyperemia, or intraocular inflammation—it is difficult to distinguish which eye had surgery, even on postoperative day one (Fig. 4.8). Even more important, patient satisfaction with this surgical system is very high because of the lack of pain or foreign body sensation associated with suture placement. Vision recovery with the 25-gauge system has been reported to be quicker than that with the 20-gauge system in patients with comparable conditions.[6] The transient postoperative astigmatism sometimes noted due to 20-gauge sclerotomy closure with tight sutures in the immediate postoperative period is negligible with the 25-gauge systems, maintaining the patient's preoperative refractive error.[7] Because of the decrease in surgically induced trauma, patients often do not require extensive postoperative medications and there is a much quicker resumption of normal activities.

REFERENCES

1. Fujii GY, De Juan E Jr, Humayun MS, et al. A new 25-gauge instrument system for transconjunctival sutureless vitrectomy surgery, Ophthalmology 2002; 109:1807–1812; discussion 1813.
2. Schwartz SD. Advances in vitreoretinal surgery. Orlando, FL: American Academy of Ophthalmology; 2002.
3. Gupta A, Gonzales C, Lee S, et al. Transient post-operative hypotony following transconjunctival 25-gauge vitrectomy, Association for Research in Vision and Ophthalmology (ARVO) Annual Meeting, Fort Lauderdale, FL; 2003.
4. Lakhanpal RR, Humayun MS, de Juan E Jr, et al. Outcomes of 140 consecutive cases of 25-gauge transconjunctival surgery for posterior segment disease. Ophthalmology 2005; 112:817–824.
5. Gupta A, Chen C, Savar L, et al. 25-Gauge transconjunctival vitrectomy: cataract progression, Investig Ophthalmol Vis Sci (ARVO Abstracts) 2005; 46:54–58.
6. Rizzo S, Genovesi-Ebert F, Murri S, et al. 25-Gauge, sutureless vitrectomy and standard 20-gauge pars plana vitrectomy in idiopathic epiretinal membrane surgery: a comparative pilot study. Graefes Arch Clin Exp Ophthalmol 2006; 244:472–479.
7. Yanyali A, Celik E, Horozoglu F, Nohutcu AF. Corneal topographic changes after transconjunctival (25-gauge) sutureless vitrectomy. Am J Ophthalmol 2005; 140:939–941.

5

Epiretinal membrane surgery

George A. Williams and Kimberly Drenser

INSTRUMENTS

20-Gauge vitrectomy

A standard three-port vitrectomy is the most common setup for performing a vitrectomy with membrane peeling. A 3-mm infusion port, light pipe, vitrector, microvitreoretinal (MVR) blade, soft-tipped extrusion cannula, and intraocular forceps are needed for the surgery. We most commonly use the Eckhardt forceps, although a variety of fine-tipped forceps are available. Indocyanine green (ICG) is helpful, although not required, in staining and visualizing the internal limiting membrane (ILM), if that is also removed. Additionally, a diamond-dusted forceps may be helpful with more dense membranes which may shred with a fine-tipped forceps.

Alternatively, a two-port surgery can be used for removing an epiretinal membrane (ERM). In this case, the infusion cannula is not placed and an irrigating light pipe is used to maintain the intraocular pressure. The additional instruments are unchanged.

Sclerotomies are closed with 7-0 Vicryl suture. The conjunctiva is approximated and secured with 6-0 plain gut suture.

25-Gauge vitrectomy

A three-port setup is used with the 25-gauge system. Both Bausch & Lomb and Alcon have 25-gauge systems available, and both use a trocar system for the ports. The required instrumentation includes an infusion cannula, light pipe, vitrector, MVR blade (or 25-gauge 1½ inch needle on a tuberculin syringe), and intraocular forceps (an expanding list of forceps is becoming available for 25-gauge surgery). An extrusion cannula (a soft-tipped option is being developed, but the available hard-tipped cannula is sufficient) may be needed if a fluid–air exchange is performed. The ILM can be stained with ICG, trypan blue, or triamcinolone acetonide (Kenalog), introduced into the eye via a 25-gauge blunt cannula on a syringe. Sutures are generally not required for wound closure.

SURGICAL TECHNIQUE

The goal of this surgery is to completely remove all epiretinal tissues which are exerting tractional forces on the underlying retina at the posterior pole. Two key planes must be accurately identified to ensure successful surgery. The true posterior hyaloid must be identified and freed from its peripapillary attachments and the posterior pole. Next, the ERM must be identified and removed away from the surface of the retina without damaging the underlying nerve fiber layer. An overly aggressive membrane stripping will result in permanent damage to the neurosensory tissues. Conversely, a partial removal of the epiretinal tissue has a higher rate of ERM recurrence and may not alleviate the patient's symptoms.

Preoperative optical coherence tomography (OCT) will often guide the surgical approach. OCT will frequently identify areas where the ERM has a space between itself and the underlying retina due to wrinkling of the retina under traction (Figs 5.1 and 5.2). These areas are ideal for making a flap in the ERM as there is some degree of safety that the ERM may be incised without damaging the retina. Evidence of vitreomacular traction

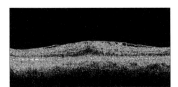

FIGURE 5.1 OCT demonstrating an epiretinal membrane without significant macular edema. Note the distortion exerted on the full-thickness retina.

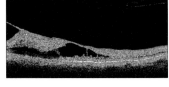

FIGURE 5.2 OCT demonstrating an epiretinal membrane with significant macular edema. Considerable distortion of the retina is present.

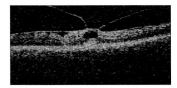

FIGURE 5.3 OCT demonstrating vitreomacular traction syndrome and underlying epiretinal membrane. A subfoveal cyst is present.

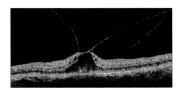

FIGURE 5.4 OCT demonstrating vitreomacular traction syndrome with significant macular edema. An obvious epiretinal membrane is not present.

(VMT), best seen with OCT (Figs 5.3 and 5.4), alerts the surgeon to vitreous schisis which is most likely present and emphasizes that care must be taken to ensure the true hyaloid face has been disinserted in its entirety. These cases also tend to have abnormally tight vitreomacular adhesions overlying the fovea. Direct inspection of the fovea is necessary as the posterior hyaloid is surgically disassociated from the macula.

This surgery can be performed with a 20-gauge two-port setup, a 20-gauge three-port setup, or a 23-gauge or 25-gauge three-port setup. The traditional approach for this surgery uses a 20-gauge three-port vitrectomy. After a conjunctival peritomy is performed, an infusion port is secured in the inferotemporal sclera. Sclerotomies are placed with an MVR blade (19- or 20-gauge) at the 10 and 2 o'clock positions, 3.5 mm posterior to the limbus (3 mm if the patient is aphakic or pseudophakic). A core vitrectomy is performed with an intraocular light pipe and the vitrector. Current vitrectomy machines allow for multiple settings. We prefer a surgeon-controlled setting that allows for control of both the vacuum and cutting rate with the foot pedal, allowing for maximal control during the surgery. A wide-field viewing system allows for a complete vitrectomy with simultaneous panretinal viewing, but is not mandatory. A posterior pole contact lens is used for detailed work at the posterior pole, including disinserting the posterior hyaloid from the optic nerve head and membrane dissection.

5.1

After a core vitrectomy is completed, the posterior hyaloid is dissociated from its posterior attachments with moderate suction. This can be achieved with the vitrector (cutting rate turned off) or a soft-tipped extrusion cannula. The port is engaged in the peripapillary hyaloid edge and anterior–posterior traction is used to free the hyaloid from its attachments. This is done circumferentially around the optic nerve head until the hyaloid is free 360° and a Weiss ring is apparent. It is important to avoid pulling the vitreous in horizontal planes as this creates excessive tension on the contralateral hyaloid attachments and may result in peripheral retinal tears. For very adherent posterior hyaloid attachments, the soft-tipped cannula allows a safer method for a more aggressive extrusion. Brushing the soft-tipped cannula in a back-and-forth motion radial to the optic nerve head is also useful in determining if a schitic layer of hyaloid is still present by causing the 'fish strike' sign. If there remains doubt as to the complete dissociation of the hyaloid from the posterior pole, various stains may be helpful.

Both ICG and triamcinolone will adhere to elevated edges of hyaloid and aid in identifying any remaining vitreous.

Once the posterior hyaloid is elevated, the vitrectomy is completed, removing the vitreous both centrally and peripherally. There is debate as to the extent of vitrectomy required for successful surgery. A limited vitrectomy does not appear to hinder ERM removal itself but may result in increased postoperative complications, such as retinal tear, retinal detachment, vitreous incarceration, and proliferative vitreoretinopathy. Non-vitrectomy surgery appears to have a higher rate of ERM recurrence as well.[1] We favor a more complete vitrectomy, with removal of the vitreous out toward the vitreous base insertion. We use a high-speed cutting rate and moderate vacuum, both adjustable with the surgeon's foot pedal.

The ERM generally is easily identified without the aid of stains, although the use of ILM and ERM staining ensures complete membrane removal. Once a satisfactory region for starting the membrane peel has been identified, a flap must be made. We generally perform a sharp dissection of the ILM with the MVR blade. A flap may also be made directly with a fine intraocular forceps. The ILM is grasped and the forceps is moved tangential to the retina until a tear is created. Care must be taken not to grasp and tear the underlying retina. Once the flap is started, a fine intraocular forceps is used to slowly remove the membrane. The forceps is always moved along the surface of the retina, avoiding movements in an anterior–posterior fashion, as this may result in tearing the underlying retina. Frequent relaxation and regrasping of the flap at its most distal edge will allow for the least traumatic removal.

Membrane staining (with ICG, trypan blue or triamcinolone) often reveals membrane complexity that is not appreciated otherwise and facilitates membrane removal.[2–7] ICG in particular will stain vitreous and the internal limiting membrane. It does not stain the ERM itself and will create a pattern of 'reverse staining', where the ERM is highlighted against a green background (ILM and/or residual vitreous). Toxicity to the retinal pigment epithelium (RPE) has been shown *in vitro* where high concentrations of ICG are used. Surgical concentrations are quite low (especially if a $1:19$-cc dilution is used) and the ICG staining is performed under fluid. Toxicity has not been demonstrated *in vivo*. Trypan blue is less useful as it stains all membranes and does not help to identify the various membrane planes. Use of triamcinolone for staining has also been reported.[6,7] The cohesive properties of triamcinolone make this less helpful in distinguishing the various layers in a complex membrane. Triamcinolone will also adhere to bare retina and may create confusion regarding the appropriate surgical plane.[8]

Removing the ILM in addition to the ERM confirms that a complete membrane stripping was attained. Starting the membrane removal at the ILM allows for simultaneous removal of the ILM and the overlying ERM. Epiretinal membranes are often multilayered and attempts to remove the ERM only may result in partial dissection of the membrane and a higher risk of recurrence.[9] Also, there is evidence that removal of the ILM at the time of ERM stripping results in less ERM recurrence.[10–12]

The bare retina will whiten with ILM removal, secondary to local axonal swelling. It is not uncommon to create small pinpoint hemorrhages along the surface of the nerve fiber layer as well. This is particularly true when underlying retinal edema is present and the nerve fiber layer becomes partially interdigitated with the overlying ERM. This will resolve during the postoperative period and does not create long-term retinal damage.

Occasionally, a macular cyst will become unroofed with removal of the ERM. This may result in a partial- or full-thickness macular hole. A full-thickness macular hole will require a fluid–air exchange and a subsequent gas–air exchange (sulfur hexafluoride [SF_6] or perfluoropropane [C_3F_8]).

Prior to closing the sclerotomies, indirect ophthalmoscopy with scleral depression should be performed to ensure that no retinal tears have developed during the course of surgery. Retinal tears most frequently occur posterior to the sclerotomies secondary to traction on the vitreous base with the introduction of instruments, but may occur anywhere in the retina. Any retinal tears should be treated at that time with cryotherapy or laser. The sclerotomies are closed with 7-0 Vicryl suture. The conjunctiva is approximated and secured with 6-0 plain gut suture.

OUTCOME

This is a very successful surgery with high anatomic success rates, high visual acuity success rates, and high patient satisfaction. Less than 5% of patients having surgery will feel that the procedure was not worthwhile.[12] Additionally, over 70% of patients have improved postoperative visual acuity, with visions of 20/50 or better.[4,12–14] Idiopathic membranes have a more favorable prognosis, achieving the best postoperative vison.[15] Although the rate of ERM recurrence appears to be lower with ILM peeling, there does not appear to be a difference in postoperative visual outcomes.[10,11]

Macular edema is also improved after removal of the ERM, although preoperative cystoid macular edema may herald less visual improvement.[11] The resolution of macular edema after ERM removal may be secondary to eliminating the tractional components acting on the retina.[14] Alternatively, improved microcirculation of the macula after membrane stripping may improve the retinal microenvironment and neuronal health.[16,17] It is most likely that both mechanisms play a role in the postoperative success of this surgery.

VIDEO

A complex membrane demonstrating vitreomacular traction, hyaloid schisis, epiretinal membrane, and macular edema. ICG staining shows densely adherent schitic hyaloid at the posterior pole. Subsequent ICG staining demonstrates reverse staining, with the ILM staining green and the overlying ERM remaining opaque. Both the ILM and ERM are removed simultaneously.

REFERENCES

1. Sawa M, Ohji M, Kusaka S, et al. Nonvitrectomizing vitreous surgery for epiretinal membrane long-term follow-up. Ophthalmology 2005; 112(8):1402–1408.

2. Kwok AK, Lai TY, Li WW, Woo DC, Chan NR. Indocyanine green-assisted internal limiting membrane removal in epiretinal membrane surgery: a clinical and histologic study. Am J Ophthalmol 2004; 138(2):194–199.

3. Kwok AK, Lai TY, Li WW, Yew DT, Wong VW. Trypan blue- and indocyanine green-assisted epiretinal membrane surgery: clinical and histopathological studies. Eye 2004; 18(9):882–888.

4. Sorcinelli R. Surgical management of epiretinal membrane with indocyanine-green-assisted peeling. Ophthalmologica 2003; 217(2):107–110.

5. Li K, Wong D, Hiscott P, Stanga P, Groenewald C, McGalliard J. Trypan blue staining of internal limiting membrane and epiretinal membrane during vitrectomy: visual results and histopathological findings. Br J Ophthalmol 2003; 87(2):216–219.

6. Tognetto D, Zenoni S, Sanguinetti G, Haritoglou C, Ravalico G. Staining of the internal limiting membrane with intravitreal triamcinolone acetonide. Retina 2005; 25(4):462–467.

7. Kimura H, Kuroda S, Nagata M. Triamcinolone acetonide-assisted peeling of the internal limiting membrane. Am J Ophthalmol 2004; 137(1):172–173.

8. Satofuka S, Inoue M, Shinoda K, Ishida S, Imamura Y, Ando Y. Adherence of intravitreally injected triamcinolone acetonide to the denuded retinal surface after internal limiting membrane peeling. Retina 2005; 25(5):672–673.

9. Sivalingam A, Eagle RC Jr, Duker JS, et al. Visual prognosis correlated with the presence of internal-limiting membrane in histopathologic specimens obtained from epiretinal membrane surgery. Ophthalmology 1990; 97(11):1549–1552.

10. Kwok AK, Lai TY, Yuen KS. Epiretinal membrane surgery with or without internal limiting membrane peeling. Clin Experiment Ophthalmol 2005; 33(4):379–385.

11. Geerts L, Pertile G, van de Sompel W, Moreels T, Claes C. Vitrectomy for epiretinal membranes: visual outcome and prognostic criteria. Bull Soc Belge Ophtalmol 2004; 293:7–15.

12. Scott IU, Smiddy WE, Feuer W, Merikansky A. Vitreoretinal surgery outcomes: results of a patient satisfaction/functional status survey. Ophthalmology 1998; 105(5):795–803.

13. Massin P, Paques M, Masri H, et al. Visual outcome of surgery for epiretinal membranes with macular pseudoholes. Ophthalmology 1999; 106(3):580–585.

14. Pournaras CJ, Kapetanios AD, Donati G. Vitrectomy for traction macular edema. Doc Ophthalmol 1999; 97(3–4):439–447.

15. Margherio RR, Cox MS Jr, Trese MT, Murphy PL, Johnson J, Minor LA. Removal of epimacular membranes. Ophthalmology 1985; 92(8):1075–1083.

16. Kadonosono K, Itoh N, Nomura E, Ohno S. Capillary blood flow velocity in patients with idiopathic epiretinal membranes. Retina 1999; 19(6):536–539.

17. Shinoda K, Kimura I, Eshita T, et al. Microcirculation in the macular area of eyes with an idiopathic epiretinal membrane. Graefes Arch Clin Exp Ophthalmol 2001; 239(12):941–945.

6 Macular hole surgery

Neil E. Kelly and Abdhish R. Bhavsar

INSTRUMENTATION

Equipment
- Stool, Machemer
- Posterior segment vitrectomy machine with endoillumination light source and foot pedal controls; to be placed at surgeon's right side with foot pedal for right foot
- Surgical operating microscope, i.e. Zeiss, with foot pedal controls; to be placed at surgeon's left side with foot pedal for left foot
- Vitrectomy surgical pack, 20-gauge (containing high-speed 2500 probe vitrector [Alcon, Fort Worth, Texas], infusion lines, infusion cannula, Luer locks for air and fluid lines, etc.)
- Shielded bullet endoilluminating light pipe
- Binocular indirect ophthalmomicroscope (BIOM), AVI or other indirect inverter lens system mounted to surgical scope, with foot pedal inverter control to surgeon's left side for left foot, next to microscope pedal
- Machemer irrigating or non-irrigating contact lens, flat plano concave contact lens, or other contact lens for magnified viewing of the macular region while creating a posterior vitreous detachment and while performing membrane dissection
- Patient cart for supine positioning, with wrist rest or Chan wrist rest at head of bed
- Surgical table and trays for surgical technologist on surgeon's right side
- Indirect ophthalmoscope, placed behind surgeon at head of bed
- Laser unit for intraocular laser and indirect laser, and appropriate microscope filters for endolaser
- Cryoprobe (straight) and cryotherapy machine (e.g. Frigitronic Cryo Machine)

Preparation of ocular surface
- Eyelash-trimming scissors with bacitracin ointment
- Povidone iodine 5% drops for conjunctival surface
- Povidone iodine 10% for periocular skin preparation
- Cotton-tipped applicators for preparation of eyelid and eyelash margins with povidone iodine
- Cover unoperated eye with wet eye pad or gauze and plastic shield

Drapes
- Large blue surgical drape with a hole for the operative eye (Cardinal Health, no. 8441); used to cover head and patient
- 3M 1060 surgical clear plastic drape with adhesive at the surgical region of the drape. A slit is cut in the drape for placing the lid speculum to open the eyelids. The drape is wrapped around the eyelashes and eyelid margin to prevent the margin of the lid from contact with the surgical surface
- Rolled surgical towel place around head drapes to create a 'moat' for placing instruments, cotton-tipped applicator, etc.

Gloves
- Sterile gloves for nurse or surgeon performing ocular surface preparation prior to draping
- Sterile surgical gloves for surgeon and assistant (second author prefers Regent Biogel Neotech gloves)

Local anesthetic
- 1:1 mixture of lidocaine 2% with bupivacaine (Marcaine) 0.75%, approximately 10 cc (5 cc for local retrobulbar block and 5 cc for administration during the case or after the case for postoperative analgesia)

General anesthetic
- Per anesthesiologist
- Pack nose with 4 × 4 gauze in each nostril prior to draping to prevent gas or mucus from accumulating beneath drape or from seeping under drape to the operative ocular surface

Infusion solutions
- Phakic eyes: Balanced Salt Solution Plus
- Aphakic or pseudophakic eyes: balanced salt solution (BSS)
- Diabetic eyes
  - Phakic: add 3 mL of D50 to Balanced Salt Solution Plus
  - Aphakic or pseudophakic: add 3 mL of D50 to BSS
- For pars plana lensectomy: second infusion line with BSS
- Lens line for handheld Machemer irrigating lens: BSS
- Adrenaline (epinephrine) for infusion if requested for diabetic eye with fibrovascular proliferation: 1:1000 0.5 mL in infusion bottle
- Adrenaline for intraocular irrigation if requested for diabetic eye with fibrovascular proliferation: 1:10 000: 0.25 mL adrenaline in 1:1000 mixed in 2.25 mL of BSS

Medications
- Sterile Goniosol or methylcellulose
- BSS in a squeeze bottle for topical application to the corneal surface
- Topical tetracaine 0.5% if needed for topical anesthesia
- Postsurgical subconjunctival injections
  - Dexamethasone 4 mg/mL: 0.5 mL
  - Cefazolin (Ancef) 100 mg/mL: 0.5 mL
  - Clindamycin 25 mg/mL: 0.5 mL (to be used in case of penicillin or cefazolin allergy)
- Postsurgical topical medications at the conclusion of surgery
  - 1 ggt of povidone iodine 5%
  - 1 ggt atropine 1%
  - Bacitracin ointment

Dressings
- Two sterile eye pads, paper tape, plastic shield
- Bracelet for intraocular gas with warning against the use of nitrous oxide

Suture
- 7-0 Vicryl no. 546 (for sclerotomy closure and conjunctival closure)
- 4-0 white silk no. S2782 (for scleral buckle mattress sutures, in cases of macular hole with retinal detachment)

- 2-0 silk ties A185H (for isolating rectus muscles during scleral buckle placement)
- 5-0 Mersilene no. 1764 (for sew-on lens ring for direct lenses)

Instruments
- Lid speculum (the second author prefers a closed Lieberman speculum)
- Calipers
- Microvitreoretinal (MVR) blade no. 5560
- 20- and 28-diopter lenses
- Contact lenses, such as plano concave or Machemer lens
- Wide-angle viewing lenses, such as BIOM or AVI lenses
- 0.12 forceps
- Two needle drivers
- Westcott conjunctival scissors
- Cautery eraser tip, 18-gauge, for conjunctival and scleral surface
- Cautery, 23-gauge blunt or sharp tip for intraocular use
- Flynn extendable silicone soft-tipped cannula (for air–fluid exchange)
- Scleral plugs (set of four including 20-gauge and 19-gauge)
- Chang forceps for epiretinal or internal limiting membrane (ILM) dissection, Sordouille or deJuan forceps, Tano asymmetric forceps
- Membrane Micropick (20-gauge tapered to 30-gauge, PSI/Eye-Ko Assurance Products, St Charles, Missouri, no. 9029)
- 20-Gauge steel cannula with Luer lock for injecting fluid into the vitreous cavity, i.e. for indocyanine green, trypan blue, or triamcinolone acetonide
- Flexible iris retractors, for example Grieshaber iris retractors (if needed to dilate a miotic pupil)
- Phacofragmatome for pars plana lensectomy (fragmatome accessory pack, Alcon, no. 1021HP)
- Cotton-tipped applicators or Weck-Cel sponges
- Perfluoro-*n*-octane, Perfluoron, perfluorocarbon liquid (PFL) (Alcon) for use if needed for retinal detachment repair or giant retinal tear repair
- AntiFog Clear Field no. 300-006 (antifog solution for indirect viewing system, e.g. BIOM or AVI)

Supplies for gas exchange
- 60-cc syringe for intraocular gas
- Sterile 0.22-μm filters, Millex-GS no. E4429-22 (Millipore, Carrigtwohill, Ireland)
- Sterile tubing for transferring gas from pressurized canister to syringe
- Sulfur hexafluoride (SF_6) or perfluoropropane (C_3F_8) gas for intraocular use (Alcon)

HISTORY

Macular holes had long been considered a relatively common and untreatable condition.[1] Trauma[2] and cystoid degeneration[3] were formerly considered the principal causes. Most researchers now agree that vitreoretinal traction is the probable cause of idiopathic macular holes, whether it be anterior–posterior vitreoretinal traction or tangential contraction of the pre-foveal cortical vitreous as described by Johnson and Gass.[4] In a post mortem study of eight eyes with idiopathic macular holes, Frangieh et al.[5] found surrounding retinal detachment, mild cystoid edema in the inner and outer plexiform layers, partial photoreceptor degeneration, thin fibroglial epiretinal membranes, small areas of retinal pigment epithelium (RPE) irregularity, and an occasional small operculum that was probably retinal tissue.

Macular holes were considered an inoperable condition because of the apparent missing tissue and photoreceptor degeneration. Schocket et al.[6] reported visual improvement following laser photocoagulation of macular holes. Blankenship and Ibanez-Langlois[7] reported successful treatment of retinal detachments secondary to macular holes without maculopexy. Most retinal surgeons had had the experience of repairing a retinal detachment with peripheral tears and a macular hole. Treating the peripheral tear and draining through the macular hole frequently resulted in very good vision, to which most observers would comment, 'it must have been an eccentric macular hole', because everyone knew that it was impossible to obtain good vision with a true macular hole.

THE GENESIS OF MACULAR HOLE SURGERY

Back in 1985 there was much new work being done with vitrectomy and the macula. The results of macular pucker surgery were starting to be published. Pneumatic retinopexy was in its infancy and we were starting to fix all kinds of retinal detachments with gas and cryotherapy. There was no treatment for idiopathic macular holes. It looked as though someone had taken a cookie cutter to the macula and removed a piece. The unfortunate patients with this condition were sent home, and told that nothing could be done.

Surrounding the hole there generally is a rim of elevated retina, with underlying fluid. I (NEK) thought that if we could flatten the elevated rim, with vitrectomy and gas, then vision might improve. I ran this idea by a more senior retina surgeon, and he told me to go ahead and give it a go. Therefore, in September 1985, I performed vitrectomy and did a fluid–gas exchange on a patient with a 20/200 idiopathic macular hole. The operation was unsuccessful, because I did not remove the posterior cortical vitreous, which was unknown by me and most surgeons in those days. Four years later this patient returned with a bullous retinal detachment that was caused by a retinal tear that developed when his vitreous detached. He still had his macular hole, but when we removed the remaining vitreous and repaired the detachment, his hole closed and his visual acuity returned to 20/60.

Undeterred by the initial failure, 2 years later I operated again on a patient with a macular hole and 20/200 visual acuity. This was successful and the hole closed with the visual acuity returning to 20/25. The third patient had her cataract removed because of decreased vision that was caused by her very large macular hole. About this time we were learning to remove the posterior cortical vitreous, and after her macular surgery, the vision returned to 20/40 and her macula looked absolutely perfect. At this point my partner Dr Robert Wendel and I knew that we were doing more than simply flattening the rim of fluid surrounding the hole.

We did more cases, and learned a lot. When doing fluid–gas exchange, if we noted a transparent, jelly-like substance around the optic nerve, we knew that the posterior cortical vitreous had not been removed, so we would refill the eye with balanced salt solution, and once again try to engage the vitreous with a silicone-tipped aspirator. When this bent, a finding that we called the 'fish strike' sign, we knew that we had engaged the vitreous, and with additional suction could separate it from the retina, and then remove it.

We also learned that, as reported by Frangieh and colleagues,[5] a majority of macular holes had an associated epiretinal membrane. In our first report on macular hole surgery (MHS)[8] we described these membranes as, 'thin, hard to see, and best recognized as multifaceted irregular light reflexes rather than the typical opaque tissue seen with idiopathic epiretinal membranes'. We described techniques to remove these membranes, which in retrospect are the internal limiting membranes that have provoked so much controversy over the last 15 years. After removing the membranes, we always filled the eye with 20% SF_6 gas, and had the patients remain head down for 1 week. We devised several devices to help the patients maintain this position.

Thus, we described MHS as a five-step procedure: vitrectomy, removal of posterior cortical vitreous, removal of any associated epiretinal membranes, fluid–gas exchange, and 1-week prone positioning.

After doing a few cases, I reported early results on five cases at a local retina meeting. A very famous, internationally known retina specialist later sent me a note stating that he didn't want to embarrass me, and therefore didn't say anything, but he felt that three of my cases really weren't macular holes.

In 1989 we presented at the Academy in New Orleans the results of the first 20 cases operated on for macular hole. Our results weren't as good as today, and our reception was even worse. The reviewer, in referring to some failures, said, 'and then Humpty Dumpy fell off the wall'. As I returned to my seat, a colleague said, 'Too bad it didn't work.' But it was a start.

RECENT CLASSIFICATION AND ETIOLOGY

In 1988, Gass[4] introduced the concept of tangential vitreous traction, and proposed a new classification for macular holes. He proposed that a layer of attached cortical vitreous was present, and could exert tangential traction on the fovea, resulting in the formation of macular holes. Gass' new classification described four stages of hole formation: Stage I, foveal detachment; Stage II, early hole formation; Stage III, fully developed macular hole with vitreofoveal separation; and Stage IV, macular hole with posterior vitreous detachment.

Stage I

Stage I holes may be thought of as premacular hole lesions. These have the appearance of a yellow dot (Stage Ia) or a yellow halo (Stage Ib). Gass stressed that other lesions can simulate the Stage I condition, and has cautioned that drusen, central serous retinopathy, adult vitelliform macular dystrophy and other conditions may simulate the Stage I lesion.

Patients with a Stage I hole experience mild blurring and distortion of vision. These lesions may spontaneously resolve or progress to Stage II. Spontaneous resolution of Stage I is probably due to spontaneous vitreous separation. On these occasions, the vision can improve and the metamorphopsia can decrease. The risk of progression to a Stage II or Stage III hole, once a Stage I hole has developed, is reported to be about 50%, although some dispute this finding.

Stage II

Stage II macular holes are characterized by a small retinal defect that can be either central or eccentric. In these cases the vision has generally deteriorated from the Stage I levels, and is usually in the 20/50 to 20/70 range. The time it takes for a hole to progress from Stage I to Stage II, or even Stage III, varies. Gass describes one patient whose hole took more than 3 years to develop. I have seen many patients who claim their vision was absolutely normal until it suddenly deteriorated and they presented with a Stage III hole. Fluorescein angiography of the Stage II hole demonstrates a small area of hyperfluorescence in the early stages of the angiogram.

Stage III

Stage III holes are characterized by a large central defect, in the range of 500 microns, with a surrounding rim of elevated retina. Most of these lesions have a small operculum suspended in the center of the defect; this may be hard to see. These cases do not have a vitreous detachment, except perhaps at the fovea where the operculum is slightly elevated off of the retinal surface. Sometimes it is difficult to determine whether or not the posterior hyaloid is attached, and a syneretic vitreous cavity frequently gives the appearance of a posterior vitreous detachment. Surgery can confirm the presence of an attached posterior hyaloid in these instances. Optical coherence tomography (OCT) demonstrates partial or complete absence of retinal tissue, and provides useful information about the relationship of the posterior hyaloid to the development of the hole. Fluorescein angiography in these cases reveals a larger area of hyperfluorescence during the early phases of the study.

Stage IV

Stage IV macular holes are characterized by a macular hole with posterior vitreous separation. Again, it is sometimes difficult to ascertain whether the hyaloid is detached or not. The presence of a Weiss ring and a small operculum on the posterior surface of the anteriorly displaced mobile posterior hyaloid is evidence of a vitreous detachment. In a large number of eyes undergoing MHS, a posterior vitreous detachment was present in approximately 8% of the cases.[8]

INDICATIONS FOR SURGERY

Because the operation is not successful in all cases, and because the postoperative positioning requirements are arduous, MHS is not recommended for every patient with a macular hole. The length of time that the hole has been present has an effect on visual results, and therefore a 90-year-old patient who has had a hole for 20 years would not be a good candidate. Conversely, a 60-year-old patient with recently developed bilateral holes would be an excellent candidate. Age, status of the fellow eye, vision, the length of time that the hole has been present, visual requirements, and ability to comply with postoperative positioning are factors that must be considered. However, one of my patients who had bilateral holes documented for a decade was gratified when his vision returned to 20/50 OU postoperatively. Stage I holes should not be operated on. Surgery for Stage II and Stage III holes gives good results. Longstanding large Stage IV holes will have a less than optimal visual result.

PREOPERATIVE PREPARATION

Appropriate informed consent is obtained by the surgeon for the surgical procedure that is anticipated. The author typically encourages family members of the patient, with the approval of the patient, to participate in the care of the patient and in the informed consent discussion. This can help with the retention of information and allows the family members to discuss the surgery with the patient after they have left the medical office. This is particularly important for educating the patient and family members about the significance of face-down positioning after surgery for optimizing the chances of closure of the macular hole. Appropriate preoperative history and physical examination are obtained by the patient's family physician or internist.

SURGERY FOR IMPENDING MACULAR HOLE

In Gass' landmark article in 1988, he proposed the undertaking of a feasibility study of vitreous surgery on eyes at high risk of developing macular holes. A month before the publication of their article, Smiddy and Michels published the results of their study of vitrectomy for impending macular holes.[9] They performed vitrectomy on 15 eyes with a high risk for developing macular hole. High-risk characteristics include: (1) macular cyst and vision of 20/50 or less; (2) cystic retina or RPE changes; and (3) slight visual loss, metamorphopsia and low detachment of the retina. Of the 15 eyes studied, 12 stabilized. Five had better vision, four had the same, and three were worse. Three of the eyes went on to develop full-thickness holes with significant visual loss.

In 1990, Jost and Hutton[10] published the results of a study of vitreous surgery on a group of 15 eyes believed to be at risk for macular hole formation. Ten out of 11 Stage I eyes improved, and two out of four Stage II eyes improved. Three of the eyes went on to develop a larger macular hole formation.

De Bustros and colleagues[11] studied vitrectomy for prevention of macular holes in symptomatic fellow eyes with Stage I macular holes. These patients were randomized to vitrectomy versus observation. They were unable to prove that vitrectomy for prevention of macular holes was worthwhile. Personally, I don't do surgery on impending holes. I believe that the possibilities of spontaneous resolution or the creation of a full-thickness hole are very real, and I prefer to wait and perform MHS only if a hole develops.

SURGERY FOR FULL-THICKNESS MACULAR HOLES

6.1

Surgery for full-thickness macular holes has been performed for several years. This type of MHS involves: (1) a standard pars plana vitrectomy; (2) removal of adherent cortical vitreous; (3) removal of any associated epiretinal and internal limiting membranes (there is controversy over the need for this procedure); (4) fluid–gas exchange; and (5) extended postoperative occiput-up (i.e. face-down) positioning to allow for gas tamponade. Following the standard vitrectomy, there is frequently a large syneretic vitreous cavity. After removal of all apparent vitreous, it is necessary to engage the posterior hyaloid. This adheres to the retina, and is best engaged by suction over the retina. This was done initially with a silicone-tipped aspirating needle; a suction force of 150–250 mmHg is usually required. Suction is applied directly over the retinal surface.

When the cortical vitreous is engaged, the needle flexes (Fig. 6.1). This has been called the 'fish strike' sign.[8] After the hyaloid is engaged, suction is continued and sometimes increased. Ultimately, the hyaloid will be stripped off the retinal surface up to the mid-vitreous cavity. The level of difficulty varies from patient to patient. Because of occasional adherence to the optic nerve head, a forceps may be needed to grasp the hyaloid and strip it off the disc surface. If the hyaloid is firmly adherent, its removal can cause small hemorrhages on the retinal surface. These do not have any adverse effects, and are comparable to the small retinal hemorrhages seen on the disc surface after spontaneous vitreous separation. After one is comfortable removing the posterior cortical vitreous, the vitreous cutter, using suction only, positioned over the optic nerve, and turned toward it, can be used to engage it (Fig. 6.2).

After the hyaloid is peeled back to the mid-vitreous cavity, it is excised and the vitreous skirt trimmed anteriorly, care being taken to avoid lens damage or other retinal

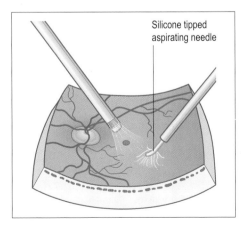

Silicone tipped aspirating needle

FIGURE 6.1 Fish strike sign: a soft-tipped, silicone aspirating needle bends when the posterior hyaloid is engaged with suction. (Original drawing courtesy of Neil E. Kelly, MD.)

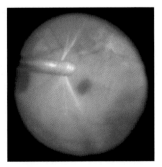

FIGURE 6.2 Engaging and elevation of the posterior hyaloid with the vitrectomy instrument. (Courtesy of Abdhish R. Bhavsar, M.D.)

complications. The stripping of the anterior hyaloid has sometimes caused peripheral retinal tears that become evident by a sudden onset of a small amount of vitreous bleeding. It is essential to check for this possibility with indirect ophthalmoscopy in every case. On occasion, it is difficult to know whether the hyaloid was detached preoperatively and removed at the time of anterior vitrectomy, or whether it was just difficult to engage it with the soft-tipped silicone needle. In these cases, a useful technique to ascertain the presence or absence of residual cortical vitreous is to proceed with a fluid–air exchange. If there is residual posterior hyaloid present, a transparent gelatinous substance is noted on the disc margin as the last few drops of BSS are aspirated from the surface of the retina. In these cases, a fluid–air exchange is performed and other attempts to remove the cortical vitreous are necessary.

After removal of the posterior hyaloid, the ILM and any associated epiretinal membranes are sometimes removed. The use of this controversial procedure was originally proposed by Kelly and Wendel.[8] Ray Margherio and colleagues[12] studied several hundred patients, half of which had the ILM removed and half that didn't. The results were fairly similar. Throughout the 1990s many reports were made extolling the virtues of removing or not removing the ILM. All in all, there seems to be a slightly higher rate of initial hole closure with removal, but on occasion it is not easy to do.

Various techniques have been used to remove the ILM. The least complicated way may be to make a linear scratch in the ILM with a barbed MVR blade or a Membrane Micropick (Fig. 6.3). A Michels membrane pick then can be slipped under the cut edge, and with horizontal, lamellar dissection, the ILM can be lifted, and later removed with an appropriate forceps (Fig. 6.4). This is not always easy to do; indocyanine green (ICG) dye has thus

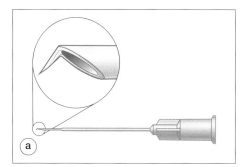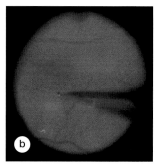

■ **FIGURE 6.3** (**a**) Membrane Micropick. (**b**) Initial incision in the internal limiting membrane with a Membrane Micropick after ICG staining. (a, original drawing courtesy of PSI/EYE KO Inc.; b, courtesy of Abdhish R. Bhavsar, M.D.)

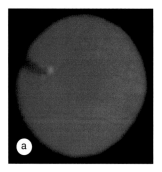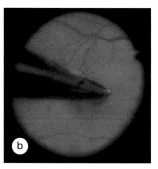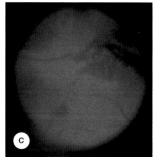

■ **FIGURE 6.4** (**a**) Intraoperative view prior to ILM staining with ICG. Continuing the dissection of ILM with the Chang forceps (**b**) across the macular hole and (**c**) around the macular hole. (Courtesy of Abdhish R. Bhavsar, M.D.)

been recommended. Various methods have been described, but what seems to work best is to layer a dilute, small quantity onto the retina after a fluid–gas exchange for a very short time. The dye is then removed, and a fluid–gas exchange is carried out. This allows a nice view of the ILM, and it is much easier to remove (Fig. 6.5). The only reason not to try this technique is that ICG has been thought to be slightly toxic to the retina. The visual results were reported to be not quite as good, but a recent paper[13] described excellent anatomic and visual results on 114 eyes undergoing ICG-assisted ILM peeling in MHS. The second author of this chapter prefers to perform ICG placement in the fluid-filled eye without prior fluid–air exchange to minimize the risk of dye pooling within the base of the macular hole, thus decreasing the potential risk of toxicity to the RPE in the foveal region. He advocates using four applications of ICG, with one application in each quadrant applied at two disc areas from the macular hole, by gently squirting the ICG from a tuberculin syringe with a 20-gauge cannula toward the retinal surface at a distance of about 5 mm. The ICG is then immediately removed from the vitreous cavity with the vitrectomy instrument. Trypan blue staining of the ILM seems to result in high closure rates and better visual results than ICG.[13] Other techniques have been described to remove the ILM. One of these involves injecting Healon between the ILM and the retina, as described by Morris and Witherspoon.[14] The ballooned-up ILM is thus easier to grab and remove. Normally, a disc-sized or larger area around the macular hole is freed of ILM if possible.

This sounds like a lot of work, but I am convinced that the success rate is higher, and I recommend it for Stage III and IV holes. A recent report of almost 600 eyes showed a higher success rate with removal of the ILM.[15] A recent Stage II hole can probably be closed without removal of the ILM.

After careful examination of the peripheral retina with indirect ophthalmoscopy and scleral depression, a total fluid–air exchange is performed. This takes several minutes, because BSS continues to cascade down the walls of the retina and appears over the disc and in the macular hole itself. The optic disc and the hole are repeatedly aspirated until fluid no longer accumulates. It is perhaps best to plug the sclerotomies and wait for a few minutes to allow residual fluid to accumulate. Afterwards, remove the BSS that has reaccumulated using a very fine, tapered tip extrusion needle (33-gauge). As the last few drops of fluid are removed from the hole, the edges of the hole often tend to shrink and approximate, and the retina flattens. After the last drop is removed, the head is then quickly turned sideways so as to elevate the macula from any recurring 'BSS lake'. An alternative method which the second author prefers involves using a Flynn extendable soft-tipped cannula to perform the fluid–air exchange, with aspiration anterior to the optic disc rather than within the macular hole, to help avoid any inadvertent disruption of the RPE within the fovea. As the sclerotomies are closed in the usual fashion (albeit with the head turned to the side), a gas–gas exchange with a non-expansile concentration of SF_6 (20%) is generally used (the second author prefers to use 28% SF_6).

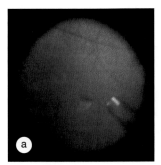
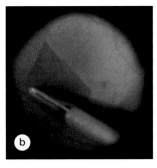

■ FIGURE 6.5 (**a**) Starting ILM dissection with Chang forceps after ICG staining. (**b**) Continuing ILM dissection with Chang forceps after ICG staining. (Courtesy of Abdhish R Bhavsar, M.D.)

a

b

Early in the development of MHS, various surgeons tried to increase their success rate by employing what were called adjuvants. Glaser et al.[16] reported the results of using transforming growth factor beta (TGF-β). A small amount of this material was applied to the base of the hole at the end of the fluid–gas exchange; C_3F_8 was also used for a longer tamponade. Later studies showed that this was not beneficial, and adjuvants are no longer used.

POSTOPERATIVE CARE

Postoperative strict occiput-up (face-down) positioning was initially prescribed for at least 1 week. Later, the time was reduced to 3–5 days. This seems to be very important, and is one of the most difficult aspects of the procedure for the patient and family members. Preoperative counseling is mandatory to ensure that the patient cooperates. Those that cannot are not good surgical candidates. This positioning entails such things as drinking through straws, using ointment that can be applied in the prone position, and examining the patient from the floor on the first postoperative visit, so that the head is not elevated. In postoperative examinations, one frequently observes a 'good positioning spot' (GPS) if compliance has been satisfactory (Fig. 6.6). This is an accumulation of red blood cells or other debris on the endothelium and indicates that the patient has been attentive to this positioning. The GPS cannot be seen with the slit lamp for the first few days after surgery because the patient's head should not be raised even in the surgeon's examination room. Usually the patient is kept in this position for 5–7 days.

As the bubble absorbs, and the former hole area can be seen, the success of the procedure can be assessed. If the edges of the hole are almost imperceptible, or not perceptible, the hole is closed and considered an anatomic success. If the edges of the hole are elevated, then the operation has failed and additional prone positioning probably would not be helpful. Paul Tornambe[17] has described MHS employing head-up positioning. He combines MHS with cataract extraction and a longer-acting gas. Occiput-up positioning is not necessary, and his results are good.

In my experience, if the hole persists postoperatively, a reoperation is necessary. Perhaps the ILM was not removed adequately, or perhaps the patient was not compliant with positioning. Robert Johnson[18] has, however, had success repeating the fluid–gas exchange with more positioning.

Postoperative medications can include a topical steroid, i.e. prednisolone acetate 1% 1 gtt q.i.d., and a cycloplegic, i.e. homatropine 5% 1 gtt q.h.s. An antibiotic is optional, however, as there is no level 1 evidence from a randomized clinical trial to show a

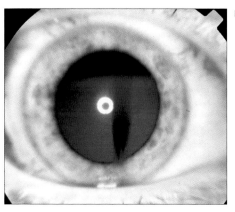

■ **FIGURE 6.6** Good position spot (GPS) blood and debris accumulates on endothelium if patient has been compliant with face-down positioning requirements. (Courtesy of Neil E. Kelly, M.D.)

reduction in endophthalmitis with postoperative antibiotic drops. The topical steroid can be continued for approximately 4 weeks and then tapered over 1–2 weeks.

RESULTS

Over the last 15 years there have been thousands of papers published on macular hole surgery results. Most are non-randomized, but indicate hole closure with visual improvement in 80–100% of patients.[19–21] Visual acuity of 20/40 or better occurs in 25–40% of cases. A small but significant number of patients achieve 20/20 vision.

The duration of symptoms affects the results of macular hole repair surgery. The greatest chance for anatomic success (Fig. 6.7) and for improvement in visual acuity (Fig. 6.8) occurs when symptoms have been present for less than 6 months. If the initial surgery fails, repeat surgery is successful in 80–100% of cases.[22]

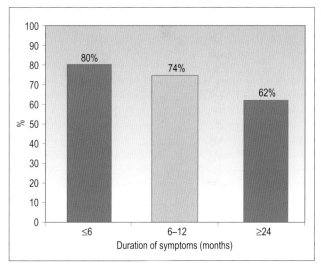

FIGURE 6.7 Anatomic success versus duration of symptoms. Proportion of eyes that were anatomically successful, stratified by duration of symptoms (m = months), demonstrating the inverse relationship between anatomic success and duration of symptoms in 170 consecutive cases. (Adapted from Wendel et al. 1993.[21])

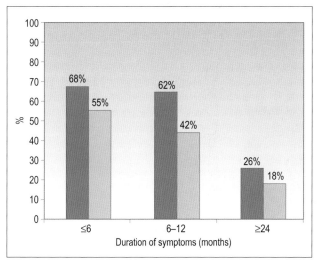

FIGURE 6.8 Visual acuity versus duration of symptoms. Percentage of eyes that improved by two (dark blue) and four (light blue) lines of visual acuity after surgery, stratified by duration of symptoms (m = months), demonstrating the inverse relationship between visual acuity improvement and duration of symptoms in 170 consecutive cases. (Adapted from Wendel et al. 1993.[21])

COMPLICATIONS OF SURGERY

Cataracts, pigmentary mottling, retinal tears and detachment, visual field defects, as well as vascular occlusion have all been experienced with MHS.

Cataracts will ultimately occur in 100% of patients undergoing MHS. These are of the nuclear sclerotic variety, sometimes develop slowly, and can affect vision more than one would think for their opaqueness. Therefore, if the hole is closed, the vision is frequently better following cataract surgery than was anticipated preoperatively. Posterior subcapsular cataracts that are gas related have not occurred, probably because of good positioning, which keeps the gas away from the lens.

Pigment mottling of the retina occurs occasionally, and can be mild or severe (Fig. 6.9). Poliner and Tornambe[23] report a high incidence of this complication, but others have not seen it as frequently. The higher incidence may be due to excessive tissue manipulation, such as in epiretinal membrane removal, or to light toxicity. Charles[24] believes that it is related to suction pressure at fluid–gas exchange.

Retinal tears and detachments have not been a major problem. For many years, it seemed that removing the posterior hyaloid was prophylactic for retinal detachment. I performed approximately 100 cases of MHS before the first detachment occurred. Currently, the incidence seems to be running around 1%, but reports as high as 17% have been made.[25] Because all the vitreous is gone, these can frequently be repaired with pneumatic retinopexy. A little more common, perhaps in the 2% range, is the development of retinal tears as the posterior hyaloid is removed. Laser or cryocoagulation along with fluid–gas exchange repairs these tears.

Visual field defects have been reported after macular hole surgery. Hutton et al.[26] documented 13 patients with visual field defects after MHS. The number of patients undergoing MHS was unknown. The defects were temporal. Gass et al.[27] prospectively studied 105 patients undergoing MHS, and found only one small asymptomatic defect develop.

Vascular occlusion, a devastating complication, has been reported.[8] This may be related to an expanding gas bubble, although expansile concentrations are not used. Great care must be taken when doing a total fluid–gas exchange in these generally older, frequently phakic, patients. It is wise to check the disc circulation with indirect ophthalmoscopy before putting on the dressing.

PATHOLOGY OF SUCCESSFUL MACULAR HOLE SURGERY

Funata et al.[28] reported the first clinicopathologic results on a patient who had undergone successful bilateral MHS. They showed that both holes were anatomically repaired, one with, and one without, glial proliferation. Defects in the ILM were present in both foveas related to the epiretinal membrane, or posterior hyaloid removal. The photoreceptors adjacent to the healed macular holes appeared normal. Both eyes eventually returned to 20/40 vision.

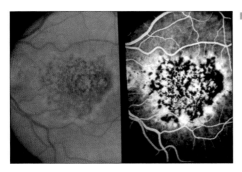

■ **FIGURE 6.9** Macular pigment mottling after macular hole repair surgery. (Courtesy of Neil E. Kelly, M.D.)

SUMMARY

Macular holes are now a treatable condition. In the 16 years since the concept of macula hole surgery was introduced at the American Academy of Ophthalmology meeting in New Orleans, and the presenter (the primary author of this chapter) was laughed off the stage, the technique has progressed to the point that I have heard busy surgeons stand up in meetings and say: 'I have not had a failure in 3 years.' Everything can be improved on, and MHS can be refined as I am sure many of those reading this chapter will do.

REFERENCES

1. Gass JD. Stereoscopic atlas of macular disease, 3rd edn. St Louis: Mosby, 1987; p 692.
2. Ogilivie FM. On one of the results of contusion injuries of the eye (holes at the macula). Trans Ophthal Soc UK 1900; 20:202.
3. Vogt A. Die Opthalmgkopie im Rottrein Ucht. Munchen Med Wschr 1925; 72:1101.
4. Johnson RW, Gass JDM. Idiopathic macular hole. Ophthalmology 1988; 95:917–924.
5. Frangieh GT, Green WR, Engle HM. A histopathologic study of macular cysts and holes. Retina 1981; 4:311–336.
6. Schocket SS, Lakhanpal V, Xiaoping M, et al. Laser treatment of macular hole and detachment. Ophthalmology 1988; 95:574–581.
7. Blankenship GW, Ibanez-Langlois S. Treatment of macular hole and detachment. Ophthalmology 1987; 94:333–336.
8. Kelly ME, Wendel RT. Vitreous surgery for idiopathic macular holes. Arch Ophthalmol 1991; 109:654–659.
9. Smiddy WE, Michels RG. Vitrectomy for impending macular hole. Am J Ophthalmol 1988; 105:371–376.
10. Jost BF, Hutton WL, Fuller DG, et al. Vitrectomy in eyes at risk for macular hole formation. Ophthalmology 1990; 97:843–848.
11. De Bustros S. Vitrectomy for prevention of macular holes. Results of a randomized multicenter clinical trial. Vitrectomy for Prevention of Macular Hole Study Group. Ophthalmology 1994; 101:1055–1059; discussion 1060.
12. Margherio RR, Margherio AR, Williams GA, et al. Effect of perifoveal tissue dissection in the management of acute idiopathic full-thickness macular holes. Arch Ophthalmol 2000; 118:495–498.
13. Lee KL, Dean S, Guest S. A comparison of outcomes after indocyanine green and trypan blue assisted internal limiting membrane peeling during macular hole surgery. Br J Ophthalmol 2005; 89(4):420–424.
14. Morris R, Witherspoon D. Video presentation at Vitreous Society meeting (ASRS), Alaska, 1998.
15. Kumagi K, Furukawa M, Ogino N, et al. Vitreous surgery with and without internal limiting membrane peeling for macular hole repair. Retina 2004; 24(5):721–727.
16. Glaser BM, Sjaarda RN, Kupperman BD, et al. Transforming growth factor beta in the treatment of full thickness macular holes. Ophthalmology 1991; 98:145–146.
17. Tornambe PE, Poliner LS, Grote K. Macular hole surgery without face down positioning. A pilot study. Retina 1998; 18(1):84–86.
18. Johnson RN, McDonald HR, Schatz H, Ai E. Outpatient postoperative fluid–gas exchange after early failed vitrectomy surgery for macular hole. Ophthalmology 1997; 104:2004–2013.
19. Park DW, Sipperley JO, Sneed SR, et al. Macular hole surgery with internal limiting peeling and intravitreal air. Ophthalmology 1999; 106:1392–1397.
20. Leonard LE, Smiddy WE, Flynn HW, Feuer W. Long-term visual outcomes in patients with successful macular hole surgery. Ophthalmology 1997; 104:1648–1652.
21. Wendel RT, Patel AC, Kelly NE, Salzano TC, Wells JW, Novick GD. Vitreous surgery for macular holes. Ophthalmology 1993; 100(11):1671–1676.
22. Smiddy WE, Sjaarda RN, Glaser BM, et al. Reoperation after failed macular hole surgery. Retina 1996; 16:13–18.
23. Poliner LS, Tornambe PE. Retinal pigment epitheliopathy after macular hole surgery. Ophthalmology 1992; 99:1671–1677.
24. Charles S. Academy course presentation. Advanced Vitrectomy Techniques, Dallas, 1992.
25. Park SS, Marcus DM, Duker JS, et al. Posterior segment complications after vitrectomy for macular hole. Ophthalmology 1995; 102:775–781.

26. Hutton WL, Fuller DG, Snyder WB, et al. Visual field defects after macular hole surgery. A new finding. Ophthalmology 1996; 103:215–228.

27. Gass CA, Haritoglou C, Messmer EM, Schaumberger M, Kampik A. Peripheral visual field defects after macular hole surgery; a complication with decreasing incidence. Br J Ophthalmol 2001; 85:549–551.

28. Funata M, Wendel RT, de la Cruz Z, et al. Clinicopathologic study of bilateral macular holes treated with pars plana vitrectomy and gas tamponade. Retina 1992; 12:289–298.

7 Proliferative diabetic retinopathy and vitreous hemorrhage

Edgar G. Thomas

DIABETIC VITRECTOMY SURGERY

Indications

Pars plana vitrectomy was developed in the early 1970s by Robert Machemer as a method for removing formed vitreous via an approach through the structureless part on the anterior portion of the globe using a closed system. Rationales for treatment with vitrectomy are varied due to the differences in pathoanatomy of this severe proliferative vascular disease. Indications for surgical intervention for proliferative diabetic retinopathy (PDR) are listed in Box 7.1. Management of the disease now involves the potential off-label use of pre-, intra-, and postoperative antiproliferative pharmacologic therapies which alter the disease process (Box 7.2). Recent understanding of the role of intraocular production of vascular endothelial growth factor (VEGF) and its causal relationship to the development of pre-retinal neovascularization has enhanced our understanding of the stimulus for neovascular growth.[1–3] Evidence now exists that after successful vitrectomy surgery for PDR, the levels of VEGF are significantly reduced, indicating a beneficial effect on causality.[4] Persistent high levels of VEGF postoperatively have also been correlated with the risk of anterior segment neovascularization and neovascular glaucoma.[5]

Management of diabetic complications in the early course of the disease, prior to those mentioned in Box 7.1, has been with improved hyperglycemic control, management of renal compromise and, when the criteria for treatment reached those based on the Diabetic Retinopathy Study (DRS) and the Early Treatment Diabetic Retinopathy Study (ETDRS), laser photocoagulation—either panretinal for proliferative disease or focal for macular edema. Surgery began as a large gauge, single multifunctional instrument (3.1 mm) inserted through the pars plana. Current surgery is now in evolution from 20-gauge (0.9 mm) to 25-gauge (0.55 mm), and possibly a new paradigm shift will take place as an intermediate size vitrector–cannula system at 23-gauge (0.7 mm) is now becoming available for clinical use. The latter system may eliminate the problems seen with the larger and smaller system vitrectors and allow sutureless microvitrectomy surgery with enhanced instrument rigidity.

Pharmacologic agents are now available with increasing scientific data to indicate their efficacy in enhancing the treatment of diabetic retinopathy. Purified ovine hyaluronidase (Vitrase) has been shown to be safe and effective in reducing vitreous hemorrhage density. A secondary benefit in vitreous liquefaction may enhance vitreous removal during vitrectomy. This drug has no effect on membrane adherence to the retina. Bevacizumab (Avastin), the monoclonal antibody to vascular endothelial growth factor (VEGF-A), may play a significant role in reducing preoperative neovascularization of the retina and iris, and facilitate membrane removal by reducing vascularity within the membranes. This effect facilitates membrane removal and intraoperative bleeding. Both of these drugs are not Food and Drug Administration (FDA) approved for these indications, but the body of evidence available indicates that they will play a significant role in the management of diabetic retinopathy.

BOX 7.1

- Chronic, non-clearing, vitreous hemorrhage
- Traction retinal detachment involving the macula
- Combined traction–rhegmatogenous retinal detachment
- Taut posterior hyaloid producing macular edema
- Macular pucker producing macular edema
- Secondary macular hole formation
- Neovascularization of the iris, neovascular glaucoma requiring intraocular laser treatment

BOX 7.2

- Purified ovine hyaluronidase (Vitrase) (Ista Pharmaceuticals)
- Bevacizumab (Avastin), monoclonal antibody to vascular endothelial growth factor (Genentech)
- Ranibizumab (Lucentis), antibody Fab fragment to vascular endothelial growth factor (Genentech)
- Triamcinolone acetonide (Kenalog)

PREOPERATIVE MEDICAL THERAPY

Vitrase

Data for safety and efficacy issues indicate that the off-label use of Vitrase, a purified ovine hyaluronidase, is safe and efficacious for the clearance of vitreous hemorrhage in patients with diabetes. A single intravitreous dose of Vitrase, 55 I.U., at the onset of a dense vitreous hemorrhage with vision <20/200, may clear the vitreous hemorrhage sufficiently to allow panretinal photocoagulation and delaying or, in some cases, avoiding the need for vitreous surgery.[6,7] A predictive model of hemorrhage clearance at 1 month, based on a change in vitreous hemorrhage density score, can help to predict which patients will clear the hemorrhage and which of those will require vitrectomy.[8,9]

Avastin

Avastin (bevacizumab), a monoclonal antibody to VEGF-A developed for metastatic colon cancer, has a major effect on suppressing vasculogenesis. Early reports of its off-label use are very encouraging, using it to reduce or eliminate iris neovascularization, facilitate surface membrane removal, and reduce postoperative bleeding and postoperative anterior segment neovascularization.[10]

PREOPERATIVE PREPARATION

Avoid patients with active ocular surface disease, specifically those with or being treated for conjunctivitis. Meticulous lid preparation and draping with the use of povidone iodine (Betadine) 5%[11,12] under sterile technique guidelines are prerequisites for reducing the risk of endophthalmitis. Ocular occluders may be used to place a separate discrete covering over the lid margins and lashes to prevent contamination of the instruments with bacteria as they cross over the lid margin, moving in and out of the eye.

INSTRUMENTATION

- Vitrectomy system: Accurus (Alcon) or Millennium (Bausch & Lomb)
- Microvitreoretinal (MVR) blade: 20-gauge system (Bausch & Lomb, Alcon)

- Trocar/cannula
    - 23-gauge systems (DORC, Bausch & Lomb, Alcon)
    - 25-gauge systems (DORC, Bausch & Lomb, Alcon)
- Vitrectors (same as above)
- 20-Gauge scissors, forceps, extrusion cannulas, light pipe, endolaser probes (multiple vendors)
- Light source for small gauge instrumentation
- Xenon (Synergetics, Alcon, Bausch & Lomb)
- 23-Gauge scissors, extrusion cannulas, light pipe, endolaser probes
- 25-Gauge scissors, extrusion cannulas, light pipe, endolaser probes
- Tornambe Torpedo 20-gauge
- Tornambe Torpedo 25-gauge mini-light
- Endolaser (multiple vendors: Iridex, Alcon, Lumenis, etc.)

Intraoperative
- Perfluorocarbon liquids for reattaching the retina, possible aid to dissection
- Viscoelastics for assisting membrane separation
- Triamcinolone acetonide (Kenalog) for vitreous or membrane visualization

Postoperative tamponade agents
- Gases
    - Sulfur hexafluoride (SF_6) (Alcon)
    - Perfluoropropane (C_3F_8) (Alcon)
- Liquid silicone oil
    - 1000 Centistoke (Alcon, Adato)
    - 5000 Centistoke (Adato)

Postoperative medications
- Subconjunctival injections
    - Vancomycin (multiple manufacturers) 20 mg/mL, 0.5 mL
    - Dexamethasone (Decadron, Merck) 4 mg/mL, 0.5–1 mL
- Intravenous injections
    - Acetazolamide, 250–500 mg, for control of or anticipated elevated intraocular pressure in patients with preexisting anterior segment neovascularization or intraocular gas
- Intravitreous injections
    - Triamcinolone acetonide (Kenalog), off-label, for inflammation, anti-angiogenesis
    - Bevacizumab (Avastin), off-label, 1.25 mg/0.05 mL, 0.05–0.1 mL
- Topical steroid
    - Prednisolone acetate 1.0%, 1 drop q.i.d.
    - Fluoroquinolone, third or fourth generation, 1 drop q.i.d., or
- Combination (generic)
    - Dexamethasone, polymyxin, bacitracin drops or ointment q.i.d.

SURGICAL TECHNIQUE

The choice of vitrectomy instrumentation will determine the next steps in the procedure. Conjunctival incision, suturing of the infusion cannula and making of large sclerotomies with an MVR blade are the requisites for 20-gauge surgery (see Chapter 2, *Vitrectomy surgery*, by Abdhish R. Bhavsar, M.D.). With the evolution of 25-gauge surgery in the past 3 years, transconjunctival insertion of the trocar/cannulas in the standard locations, at 3.5 mm for the phakic patient and at 3.0 mm for the pseudophakic or aphakic eye (see

Chapter 4, *25-Gauge vitrectomy*, by Anurag Gupta, M.D. and Steven D. Schwartz, M.D.), is now normal practice.

The paradigm maybe changing again to 23-gauge, an intermediate gauge between 20 and 25, and may yet be a further improvement in vitrectomy technology (see Chapter 3, *23-Gauge vitrectomy*, by Howard F. Fine, M.D., Pawan Bhatnagar, M.D., and Richard F. Spaide, M.D.). Analysis of vitreoretinal pathoanatomy is shown in Figure 7.1. Configuration of a macular traction detachment, a definite indication for surgical intervention, is shown in Figure 7.2. The management of a combined traction–rhegmatogenous retinal

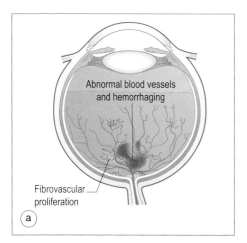

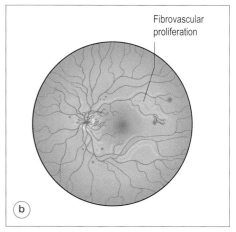

■ **FIGURE 7.1** Cross-sectional anatomy of the posterior segment showing the fibrovascular proliferation at the disc and at additional sites along the major vascular arcades with partial separation of the posterior cortical gel and vitreoschisis.

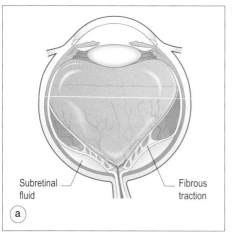

■ **FIGURE 7.2** Tractional retinal detachment with the posterior cortical gel elevating the retina in the region of the central macula and peripapillary region.

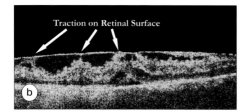

detachment depends on internal identification of the retinal break which is usually associated with an area of taught fibrovascular proliferation as shown in Figure 7.3. Another indication for surgical intervention is significant vitreopapillary traction causing obstruction of axoplasmic flow. This configuration is seen in Figure 7.4.

Insertion of the 20-gauge instruments requires an MVR blade to penetrate the sclera in the typical 10, 2, and 4 o'clock positions for the left eye, and 8, 10, and 2 o'clock positions for the right eye, with the infusion cannula sutured into the inferior temporal sclerotomy. The 23-gauge instruments require tangential insertion of the trocar/cannulas in the same positions and the 25-gauge instruments require the trocar/cannulas to be placed after the displacement of the conjunctiva with a cotton-tipped applicator or smooth forceps.

Wide-field viewing with the binocular indirect ophthalmomicroscope (BIOM), AVI or Volk systems is indispensable in being able to view the entire retinal surface in the areas of the membrane formation. With the older small field systems, one was not aware of distant traction and tears being induced that were not visible in the operative field, only to be found later in the procedure, at which point they were unavoidable. Contact systems add an additional factor, that of needing a competent assistant to hold the lens during the procedure, whereas the non-contact system (BIOM) does not require an assistant.

The vitrector instruments are placed through open sclerotomies for 20-gauge, and through the cannulas for the 23- and 25-gauge systems. Cannula insertion of instruments limits the number, type, and configuration of instruments that can be used and, in general, limited numbers of instruments still exist for the latter two. The angulation of any scissors, forceps and other instruments prevents passage through straight metal (23-gauge) or polymer (25-gauge) cannulas. Dependency of vitrector design to remove membranes—specifically fibrovascular tissue from the retinal surface—relates to cutter aperture proximity to the end of the cutter and is enhanced in both of these cutters. This allows the vitrector, in essence, to become scissors and interface within the planes of the tissue, avoiding direct trauma to the retina.

With 20-gauge scissors and forceps the standard segmentation with vertical scissors (Fig. 7.5) and delamination techniques with horizontal scissors (Fig. 7.6) can be performed without difficulty. Using the other smaller gauge systems requires membrane stripping

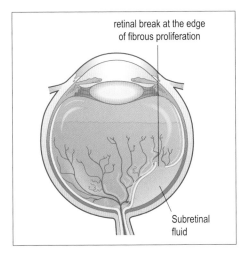

FIGURE 7.3 Rhegmatogenous retinal detachment due to a break at the edge of the fibrous proliferation showing a dome-shaped configuration.

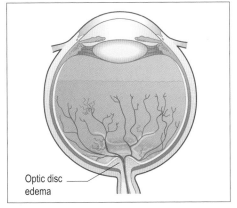

FIGURE 7.4 Epipapillary traction obstructing axoplasmic flow by pulling directly on the optic nerve.

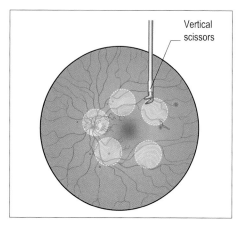

FIGURE 7.5 Separation of fibrovascular 'islands' after use of vertical scissors to segment the preretinal proliferation.

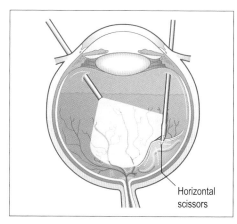

FIGURE 7.6 Delamination of the preretinal fibrovascular proliferation with horizontal scissors.

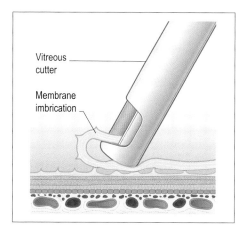

FIGURE 7.7 Indentation delamination with vitreous cutter tip removing the fibrovascular proliferation 'en toto'.

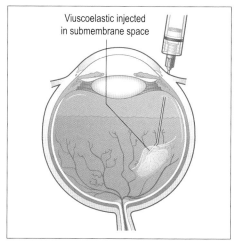

FIGURE 7.8 Injection of viscoelastic into the subhyaloid space is used to separate the retina and the posterior cortical gel from each other to facilitate membrane removal.

with either forceps to begin the process or indentation over the membranes to initiate membrane removal (indentation delamination) (Fig. 7.7). Disposable vitrectors and disposable and reusable forceps are available for these maneuvers (DORC, Alcon, Bausch & Lomb). Separation of the surface membranes with the use of a viscoelastic may also facilitate all of these techniques for managing fibrovascular membranes (Fig. 7.8).

Fragmentation, because of instrument size limitations, can only be done with 20-gauge and requires enlargement of one sclerotomy to accomplish when the smaller gauge instruments are used. Bimanual techniques may confer added advantages with the use of additional light sources to illuminate and eliminate the need for a single function light probe. Illuminated instruments, mostly 20-gauge, are available and supplemental light sources such as the Tornambe Torpedo or the Synergetics lighted infusion cannula help to illuminate the eye so that two instruments may be used simultaneously. This will facilitate the removal of membranes when access to the interface between the retina and the membranes is necessary for safe removal.

COMPLICATIONS

Complications consist of creating an intraoperative rhegmatogenous retinal detachment repaired by standard drainage, air–gas tamponade, and focal endophotocoagulation. Rarely is scleral buckling needed unless the breaks are peripheral and associated with vitreous base trauma with cannula or instrument insertion or removal. Intraoperative bleeding from surface or membrane sites is managed by increasing the intraocular pressure via machine directly or elevating the infusion bottle (less predictable). Achieving hemostasis by an immediate fluid–air exchange is beneficial, but if return to balanced salt solution (BSS) is anticipated, opacification of the posterior lens capsule is much more common acutely thereafter.

Postoperative complications relate to recurrent vitreous hemorrhage requiring vitreous cavity washout, repeat vitrectomy to identify and treat residual or recurrent membrane formation (rare), and anterior segment neovascularization requiring additional laser photocoagulation. Vitreous fluid–air exchange (AFX) is an office procedure with local retrobulbar anesthesia or subconjunctival anesthesia and a sequential sterile air (Millipore filtered)–fluid exchange via the pars plana using a 25-gauge needle with the standard povidone iodine preparation described above, followed by additional laser panretinal photocoagulation if indicated.

Treatment of anterior segment neovascularization and vitreous hemorrhage may also be approachable with intravitreous injection of bevacizumab (Avastin). This may allow vitreous hemorrhage to clear so that additional laser can be applied to reduce recurrence. There is no advantage in injecting Vitrase in a previously vitrectomized eye. Postoperative macular edema, epiretinal membrane formation, and macular holes should be managed as they are in non-diabetic patients.

VISUAL OUTCOME

In a study 10 years ago, eyes were evaluated that improved 73%, had usable vision (16%), and progressed to light perception (LP) or no light perception (NLP) vision (11%). Risk factors for eyes with LP and NLP vision included preoperative iris neovascularization (INV), postoperative INV, postoperative macular ischemia, and postoperative vitreous hemorrhage.[13] Vitrectomy for complications of severe proliferative diabetic retinopathy is especially valuable in improving the patient's overall visual function.[14] Patients with vitreous hemorrhage but without the sequelae of traction retinal detachment, severe macular edema, rhegmatogenous retinal detachment, and pre- or postoperative anterior segment neovascularization seem to have the best prognosis.

Brown et al's study[15] showed that reoperation for the sequelae of proliferative diabetic retinopathy may be as high as 8–9%. The primary causes for reoperation included rhegmatogenous retinal detachment, recurrent vitreous hemorrhage, and neovascular glaucoma. Severe preretinal and subretinal fibrous proliferation, as demonstrated histopathologically, accounted in large part for the poor result.

REFERENCES

1. Sydorova M, Lee MS. Vascular endothelial growth factor levels in vitreous and serum of patients with either proliferative diabetic retinopathy or proliferative vitreoretinopathy. Ophthalmic Res 2005; 37:188–190.
2. Burgos R, Simo R, Audi L, et al. Vitreous levels of vascular endothelial growth factor

are not influenced by its serum concentrations in diabetic retinopathy. Diabetologia 1997; 40:1107–1109.

3. Ishida S, Shinoda K, Kawashima S, Oguchi Y, Okada Y, Ikeda E. Coexpression of VEGF receptors VEGF-R2 and neuropilin-1 in proliferative diabetic retinopathy. Invest Ophthalmol Vis Sci 2000; 41:1649–1656.

4. Funatsu H, Yamashita H, Noma H, et al. Outcome of vitreous surgery and the balance between vascular endothelial growth factor and endostatin. Invest Ophthalmol Vis Sci 2003; 44:1042–1047.

5. Itakura H, Kishi S, Kotajima N, Murakami M. Persistent secretion of vascular endothelial growth factor into the vitreous cavity in proliferative diabetic retinopathy after vitrectomy. Ophthalmology 2004; 111:1880–1884.

6. Kuppermann BD, Thomas EL, de Smet MD, Grillone LR. Pooled efficacy results from two multinational randomized controlled clinical trials of a single intravitreous injection of highly purified ovine hyaluronidase (Vitrase) for the management of vitreous hemorrhage. Am J Ophthalmol 2005; 140:573–584.

7. Kuppermann BD, Thomas EL, de Smet MD, Grillone LR. Safety results of two phase III trials of an intravitreous injection of highly purified ovine hyaluronidase (Vitrase) for the management of vitreous hemorrhage. Am J Ophthalmol 2005; 140:585–597.

8. Thomas E, Grillone LR, McNamara TR, Gow JA, Pearson R, Hochberg AM. Preliminary evaluation of an early surrogate marker for successful laser treatment in ovine hyaluronidase-treated subjects with diabetes and severe vitreous hemorrhage. The US Food and Drug Administration (FDA), 2006 FDA Science Forum; 2006.

9. Bhavsar A, Grillone L, McNamara T, Gow J, Hochberg A, Pearson R. Predicting Response of Vitreous Hemorrhage and Outcome of Photocoagulation after Intravitreous Injection of Highly Purified Ovine Hyaluronidase in Patients with Diabetes. Invest Ophthalmol Vis Sci 2008; 25

10. Avery RL. Regression of retinal and iris neovascularization after intravitreal bevacizumab (Avastin) treatment. Retina 2006; 26:352–354.

11. Ferguson AW, Scott JA, McGavigan J, et al. Comparison of 5% povidone–iodine solution against 1% povidone–iodine solution in preoperative cataract surgery antisepsis: a prospective randomised double blind study. Br J Ophthalmol 2003; 87:163–167.

12. Ta CN. Minimizing the risk of endophthalmitis following intravitreous injections. Retina 2004; 24:699–705.

13. Mason JO 3rd, Colagross CT, Haleman T, et al. Visual outcome and risk factors for light perception and no light perception vision after vitrectomy for diabetic retinopathy. Am J Ophthalmol 2005; 140:231–235.

14. Smiddy WE, Feuer W, Irvine WD, Flynn HW Jr, Blankenship GW. Vitrectomy for complications of proliferative diabetic retinopathy. Functional outcomes. Ophthalmology 1995; 102:1688–1695.

15. Brown GC, Tasman WS, Benson WE, McNamara JA, Eagle RC Jr. Reoperation following diabetic vitrectomy. Arch Ophthalmol 1992; 110:506–510.

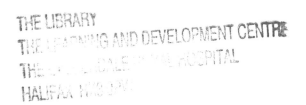
THE LIBRARY
THE LEARNING AND DEVELOPMENT CENTRE
THE ... HOSPITAL
HALIFAX ...

8 Surgical management of open-globe injuries

William F. Mieler and Michael P. Rubin

INSTRUMENTS AND DEVICES

- Topical anesthesia, dilating drops, fluorescein strips, antibiotics
- Protective eye shield
- Access to tetanus prophylaxis
- All standard office equipment for a complete ocular examination
- Slit lamp
- Gonioscopy lens
- Indirect ophthalmoscope
- Scleral depressor
- Photography (color photographs, fluorescein angiography)
- Access to radiology (x-rays, CT scan, MRI)
- Fully equipped operating room with vitrectomy system (20-, 23-, 25-gauge)
- Microinstruments, including illuminators, forceps, scissors, foreign body forceps
- Phacofragmentor (to remove the lens if necessary)
- Internal and external magnets
- Scleral buckling materials and associated sutures
- Perfluorocarbon liquids
- Indirect photocoagulation unit
- Silicone oil with viscous fluid injector
- Intraocular gases: sulfur hexafluoride (SF_6) and perfluoropropane (C_3F_8)

INDICATIONS AND CONTRAINDICATIONS

Ocular trauma is a major cause of visual impairment in the United States,[1] and levies a tremendous burden in both direct and indirect costs. There are approximately 2.4 million ocular injuries annually, with males approximately nine times more often affected than females and most victims are under the age of 40 years. The devastating effects of closed-globe trauma are more commonly encountered than those of open-globe injury (penetrating, perforating, and retained intraocular foreign body [IOFB]), but open-globe injuries represent a major cause of ocular morbidity.[2] Table 8.1 outlines ocular trauma terminology, while Table 8.2 provides an ocular injury classification scheme.[2] Because ocular trauma can manifest in virtually unlimited forms, along with numerous differing needs for assessment and treatment, uniform terminology and classification will help to arrange for a successful approach to surgical repair of these oftentimes challenging problems.

There really are relatively few contraindications to surgical repair of open-globe injuries. Generally, the problem is quite evident, and needs to be surgically addressed. At times the extent of the ocular damage is much worse than what was initially appreciated. It is imperative to provide a thorough evaluation of the patient, yet still exercise care to be certain that one does not cause a worsening of the problem during the course of the evaluation. Additionally, one needs to avoid imaging studies such as MRI when dealing with metallic IOFBs. These issues will be discussed in greater detail in the forthcoming sections.

TABLE 8.1 Ocular trauma terminology

Term	Definition
Eyewall	Sclera and cornea
Closed globe	The eyewall (corneosclera) does not have a full-thickness wound
Contusion	Closed-globe injury resulting from a blunt object; injury can occur at the site of impact or at a distant site secondary to changes in globe configuration or momentary intraocular pressure elevation
Rupture	Full-thickness wound caused by a blunt object
Open globe	The eyewall (corneosclera) has a full-thickness wound
Laceration	Full-thickness corneal and/or sclera wound caused by a sharp object
Lamellar laceration	Closed globe injury of the eyewall (corneosclera) or bulbar conjunctiva usually caused by a sharp object; the wound occurs at the impact site
Penetrating injury	Single full-thickness wound of the eyewall (corneosclera), usually caused by a sharp object
Perforating injury	Two full-thickness wounds (entrance and exit) of the eyewall (corneosclera) usually caused by a missile
Intraocular foreign body	The retained foreign object causes a single entrance wound
Superficial foreign body	Closed globe injury resulting from a projectile; the foreign body becomes lodged into the conjunctiva and/or eyewall (corneosclera) but does not result in a full-thickness eyewall defect

Based on data from Pieramici et al. 1997.[2]

Vision-limiting factors in open-globe injuries are numerous, and may occur immediately, or develop months to years following the injury. These potential limiting factors include corneal scarring or decompensation, hyphema formation with glaucomatous complications, cataract formation or subluxation of the lens, vitreous hemorrhage, retinal tear, dialysis, and detachment, development of proliferative vitreoretinopathy (PVR), choroidal hemorrhage, macular and optic nerve contusive damage, ciliary body dysfunction with phthisis bulbi formation, and sympathetic ophthalmia. While many of these conditions can be surgically repaired, numerous eyes are lost to recurrent retinal detachment with PVR, or ciliary body shutdown. The personal impact of the injuries is difficult to define, though millions of dollars are spent in hospitalization costs, treatment, and in lost working revenue.

Over the last several decades, the prognosis for patients with open-globe injuries has significantly improved. This has been attributed to the advent of enhanced microsurgical techniques and instrumentation, along with an improved understanding of the pathophysiology of ocular trauma along with the wound-healing response in injured eyes.[3]

SURGICAL TECHNIQUE

Preoperative evaluation

Before the ocular examination for an eye injury is performed, it is imperative to obtain a detailed and complete clinical history. This is critical in terms of performing excellent patient care, and it is also very important in light of potential medicolegal considerations

TABLE 8.2 Ocular injury classification scheme

	Description
Open-globe injury	
A	Rupture
B	Penetrating
C	Intraocular foreign body
D	Perforating
E	Mixed
Visual acuity grade	
1	>20/40
2	20/50 to 20/100
3	19/100 to 5/200
4	4/200 to light perception
5	No light perception
Pupil	
Positive	Relative afferent pupillary defect present in affected eye
Negative	Relative afferent pupillary defect absent in affected eye
Zone	
I	Isolated to cornea (including the corneoscleral limbus)
II	Corneoscleral limbus to a point 5 mm posterior into the sclera
III	Posterior to the anterior 5 mm of sclera
Closed-globe injury	
A	Contusion
B	Lamellar laceration
C	Superficial foreign body
D	Mixed
Visual acuity grade	
1	>20/40
2	20/50 to 20/100
3	19/100 to 5/200
4	4/200 to light perception
5	No light perception
Pupil	
Positive	Relative afferent papillary defect present in affected eye
Negative	Relative afferent papillary defect absent in affected eye
Zone	
I	External (limited to bulbar conjunctiva, sclera, cornea)
II	Anterior segment (involving structures in anterior segment internal to the cornea and including the posterior lens capsule: also include pars plicata but not pars plana)
III	Posterior segment (all internal structures posterior to the posterior lens capsule)

Based on data from Pieramici et al. 1997.[2]

which may arise at a later date. It is also absolutely essential to check visual function at the start of the examination process, since on rare occasions there is the concern that the examination process may potentially alter the findings and adversely affect the outcome. Vision at presentation is a critical determinant of final visual outcome, as patients with initial vision of 5/200 or better have a 28 times greater chance of salvaging acuity at this level.[4] Conversely, documentation of no light perception is an extremely poor prognostic finding, with only rare isolated cases recovering functional vision. While it is imperative to fully assess the extent of the injury, it must be accomplished without causing any further damage to the injured eye. If one is unable to do so secondary to inadequate patient cooperation or because of the young age of the patient, the examination can be completed in the operating room environment under anesthesia.[5]

Imaging studies

Radiologic studies and/or echography should be obtained in all cases of open-globe injuries, or whenever a ruptured globe or an IOFB is suspected, particularly when opaque media precludes a view of the posterior segment. It is difficult to defend an undiagnosed retained IOFB, especially if a possible IOFB was not looked for. While conventional x-rays are perhaps the simplest and most readily available method for IOFB identification, they are of limited use. Computerized tomography (CT) scanning has become the standard method for imaging ruptured globes and detecting and localizing IOFBs (Fig. 8.1) because of its sensitivity and inherent advantages, yet it is not perfect in terms of detecting an occult rupture of the globe.[6] Magnetic resonance imaging (MRI) has also been used to identify and localize IOFBs but magnetic IOFBs have been shown to move on exposure to the magnetic field and visual loss and vitreous hemorrhage have been attributed to the movement of an occult IOFB and MRI.

Echography, particularly high-frequency echography, is more effective than plain films in the detection of IOFBs and, dependent upon the echographer's skill, appears to be as effective as CT scanning. Echography may actually be more effective than CT scanning when an IOFB is non-metallic.[7]

MANAGEMENT OF OPEN-GLOBE INJURIES (NON-IOFB CASES)

General principles of management

The emergent management of open-globe trauma is guided by a few simple tenets. After a complete ocular examination confirming the diagnosis, and pending surgical repair, the eye should be shielded to avoid any further damage. Infection prophylaxis should be considered, especially if there will be a delay in repairing the globe beyond 24 hours, and the patient's tetanus status should be checked and updated. While most open-globe injuries are repaired as soon as the patient is medically cleared for surgery, it appears that in the absence of infection, even a delay up to 36 hours may not significantly adversely affect the outcome.[8]

The first goal of surgery is to restore the integrity of the globe, and this is accomplished by meticulous wound identification and closure. It is critical to determine the full extent

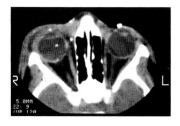

FIGURE 8.1 CT scan demonstrating several intraocular and adnexal BB gun pellets.

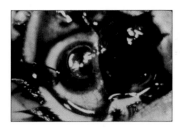

■ **FIGURE 8.2** Assault with a broken glass bottle virtually bisected the globe. Prolapsed intraocular contents are seen, and air has spontaneously entered the eye. The full posterior extent of the injury could not be appreciated until the patient underwent surgical exploration of the globe. The laceration extended an additional 12 mm posteriorly in the inferior direction. While the injury was repaired, and the integrity of the globe restored, the patient did not recover functional vision.

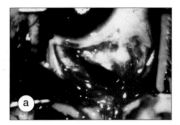 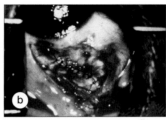

■ **FIGURE 8.3** (**a**) Scleral laceration secondary to a knife stab wound. Following a complete ocular assessment, which documented vitreous hemorrhage but no retinal detachment, the wound was meticulously cleaned, and then (**b**) closed with interrupted 9-0 nylon sutures.

of the injury. If a corneal laceration extends to or beyond the limbus, a conjunctival peritomy should be performed to fully identify the laceration in its entirety (Fig. 8.2).

Corneal, corneoscleral, and scleral lacerations

Principles guiding repair of lacerations or ruptures of the globe are in general the same, whether in the form of a straightforward corneal laceration, or a complex rupture with prolapse of intraocular contents. The primary goal is restoration of the integrity of the globe, with return of the intraocular pressure back into the normal range. A simple corneal laceration without tissue loss can be closed with interrupted 10-0 nylon sutures. Prolapsed iris/uvea or other intraocular contents should be reposited unless necrotic or obviously infected. Incarcerated tissues may be swept from the wound with the aid of a cyclodialysis spatula.

While corneal or corneoscleral lacerations are generally quite obvious (Fig. 8.3), detection of scleral lacerations may require exploration. If there is a high degree of suspicion for a ruptured globe, the conjunctiva should be opened in all four quadrants. The regions of the muscle insertions should be closely inspected, as this is often the site of an occult rupture. If a scleral laceration is found and it extends toward or beneath a muscle insertion, the muscle may be gently lifted upward away from the surface of the globe with a muscle hook.

Uveal tissue that may have prolapsed through the scleral laceration site is generally reposited as the wound is being closed, unless appearing necrotic or infected. When there is extruded vitreous, it is generally cut flush with the scleral surface with sharp scissors. Instruments should never be blindly inserted into the vitreous cavity. If there is apparent prolapse of retina, every attempt should be made to reposit the tissue back into the eye, and then the damaged retina should be carefully assessed and repaired (see below in the sections on *Vitreous hemorrhage and proliferation* and also in the *Retinal detachment* section).

Timing of surgery

Timing of surgical repair of a retinal problem following an open-globe injury has never been optimally determined. While the integrity of the globe is generally restored within 24 hours of the initial injury, the preferred timing of vitrectomy repair remains controversial. Experimental surgical models have shown the relatively rapid development of intra-ocular proliferation and organization,[9–15] yet have not provided clear guidelines regarding the most appropriate timing of surgical intervention.

Various authors have advocated early intervention, though the studies were not rigidly controlled. Some surgeons have advocated immediate or early vitrectomy in cases of penetrating or perforating ocular trauma,[16,17] though this issue remains quite controversial.[18,19] Immediate surgical repair is suggested in an effort to prevent severe inflammatory changes that may occur after injury, and to prevent or lessen the risk of intraocular proliferation which may lead to retinal detachment with PVR. In addition, performing all surgical procedures in one setting eliminates the need for multiple procedures.

Conversely, there may be advantages to delaying vitreous surgery. It allows more time for further diagnostic evaluation, and permits repair in a more controlled atmosphere.[1] Most importantly, delaying vitreous surgery may allow for spontaneous separation of the posterior hyaloid from the retina, thus facilitating more complete and less hazardous vitreous removal. Additionally, if there was anterior segment hemorrhage associated with the initial injury, a delay in the surgery may allow for spontaneous clearing of the hemorrhage, thereby lessening the need for removal of the lens. Delaying repair beyond 14 days, however, is not recommended due to concerns of sympathetic ophthalmia (see section on *Sympathetic ophthalmia* below).

As noted above, however, the timing of surgical repair issue is still not fully resolved, and in the absence of endophthalmitis or a retained IOFB, timing is left up to the discretion of the individual surgeon.[18,19] Most commonly, the vitrectomy repair is scheduled 5–10 days following the initial ocular injury.

Cataract, subluxed, and dislocated lenses

A contusive injury to the eye can impart enough energy into the lens to cause opacification, or it may lead to subluxation or dislocation (Fig. 8.4). Alternatively, an open-globe injury that violates the lens capsule will generally also lead to either cataract formation or lens subluxation. Surgical extraction of a subluxated or cataractous lens should be considered when the cataract leads to significant visual impairment, or if removal will aid in the visualization and management of associated posterior segment damage. Dependent upon the degree of lens damage, and the stability of the lens itself, it can be removed via routine anterior segment approaches (limbal or clear cornea), though oftentimes it is removed via a pars plana approach. A pars plana approach often offers significant advantages, including the ability to repair associated posterior segment damage (Fig. 8.5). If lens particles are displaced posteriorly, it is imperative to remove the particles via a vitrectomy approach; otherwise, untoward vitreous traction will be exerted upon the retina and vitreous base. Following removal of the lens, the peripheral retina should be carefully inspected, as should all sclerotomy sites, checking for retinal tears, dialyses, and/or detachment. Even in the absence of trauma, the risk of retinal detachment is substantial (approximately 15%) in the setting of a subluxed or dislocated lens.[20]

Management of the patient's monocular aphakic status is controversial. Posterior chamber intraocular lens placement may be difficult due to compromised zonular support, though lenses can be sutured in the ciliary sulcus utilizing a variety of techniques.[21] Anterior chamber lens implants may be utilized, as long as there is no significant compromise of angle structures from the effects of the injury[22] and the cornea is healthy.

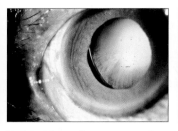

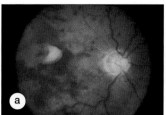

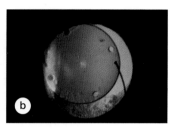

■ **FIGURE 8.4** Blunt trauma to the eye resulted in a partially subluxated and mildly cataractous lens. The lens was removed via a pars plana approach and an anterior chamber lens was inserted through the limbus.

■ **FIGURE 8.5** (**a**) A ruptured globe resulted in damage to the lens, displacing fragments onto the retinal surface. Retinal hemorrhages were also seen, though there was no retinal detachment. The lens remnants were removed via pars plana lensectomy/vitrectomy surgery, and (**b**) an intraocular lens was sutured in place in the ciliary sulcus.

Vitreous hemorrhage and proliferation

Vitreous hemorrhage may develop secondary to damage to the ciliary body, retinal, and/or choroidal vessels. In the presence of an open-globe injury, scleral indentation should be avoided at least until all corneoscleral wounds are closed, and a possible occult rupture of the sclera has been ruled out.

In the setting of vitreous hemorrhage following closed-globe injury, and in the absence of associated ocular abnormalities, a period of observation for a month or two is warranted to allow for spontaneous clearing of the hemorrhage. Echography is essential to rule out the possibility of an underlying retinal tear, retinal detachment, and/or choroidal detachment. In contrast, hemorrhage occurring in association with an open-globe injury is generally surgically evacuated 7–10 days following injury, due to the close link between an open-globe injury, retinal detachment, hemorrhage, and the fibrovascular proliferative response.

The overall prognosis for eyes with vitreous hemorrhage following closed-globe ocular injury is associated primarily with vision-limiting factors such as macular damage from contusive effects of the injury, including commotio retinae, macular hole formation, and choroidal rupture. Impaired vision may also result from retinal tears, detachment, and dialyses, along with choroidal hemorrhages. The vitreous hemorrhage itself is generally not a major concern, as it either clears spontaneously or can be successfully surgically removed.

Retinal detachment

It is relatively uncommon for a patient to develop an acute rhegmatogenous retinal detachment following blunt ocular trauma. In cases where a detachment does occur, however, the patient tends to be quite young, with more organized vitreous. This oftentimes provides internal tamponade even in the setting of a retinal tear or dialysis. In spite of the above-noted relative protective factor, atypical retinal tears are encountered, with the tears tending to be quite large and more posterior in location (Fig. 8.6). Treatment of these abnormalities is quite complex, often requiring a vitrectomy approach, with an array of retinopexy, scleral buckling techniques, possible creation of a retinotomy or retinectomy, and the use of temporary intraoperative agents (perfluorocarbon liquids, intraocular air or gas) and/or permanent postoperative internal tamponade agents (silicone oil) (Fig. 8.7).

A particular problem seen with perforating ocular injuries is that of retinal or vitreous incarceration in the scleral laceration sites. If occurring anteriorly, the tissue can generally be cleared with vitrectomy techniques, excised with a retinotomy (if needed), and the site

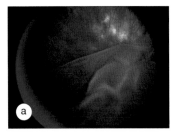
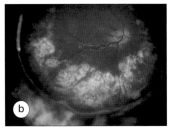

FIGURE 8.6 (**a**) A 270° giant retinal tear following blunt ocular trauma. (**b**) Successful surgical repair ensued via pars plana lensectomy/vitrectomy, with intraoperative use of perfluorocarbon liquid, use of intraoperative photocoagulation, placement of a peripheral scleral buckle, and use of silicone oil.

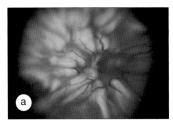
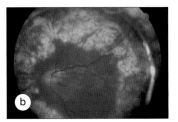

FIGURE 8.7 (**a**) Recurrent retinal detachment with advanced PVR following repair of an open-globe injury 6 weeks earlier. (**b**) The retinal detachment was repaired via a vitrectomy approach with extensive retinal membrane dissection and removal, intraoperative use of liquid perfluorocarbon, use of photocoagulation, placement of a peripheral scleral buckle, and use of silicone oil.

is often supported with a scleral buckle. More posteriorly located sites generally require use of a retinotomy to clear the tissue, the site is demarcated with laser, and internally supported with either a long-acting gas or silicone oil tamponade.[23–25] These sites are still oftentimes prone to development of recurrent proliferation (Fig. 8.8).

In cases of open-globe injuries, when it is not certain if retinal damage has occurred, it is unclear if placement of a prophylactic scleral buckle is warranted. Such a buckle may support the vitreous base and guard against later contraction of the vitreous base. Additionally, it may also provide support of a scleral laceration site where vitreous and/or retina may be incarcerated. However, it is still unclear as to the true benefit of a prophylactic scleral buckle.[26–29] If definite retinal tears are documented, however, they are treated with retinopexy, and generally supported with a scleral buckle and/or internal tamponade agents.

Retinopexy and prophylactic retinopexy

Retinopexy must be considered whenever retinal injury has occurred in association with an open-globe injury. In the setting of a scleral laceration without definite evidence of retinal tear formation, the intent of retinopexy treatment is to form a retinal adhesion at the site of injury in an effort to limit or prevent possible retinal detachment formation. The use of prophylactic retinopexy may be counterproductive, however, in that it may actually stimulate fibrovascular proliferation, and worsen the scenario.[30–35] In general, we only recommend laser retinopexy or cryotherapy when definite retinal holes or tears are documented.

Retinal tamponade

Management of complex retinal detachment associated with open-globe injury often requires either long-acting intraocular gas or silicone oil tamponade. If retinal breaks, retinotomy, or retinectomy are inferiorly located, then silicone oil is particularly useful,[36–40]

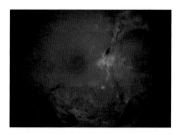

■ **FIGURE 8.8** This patient had been treated for a perforating ocular injury sustained via a gunshot injury. Recurrent proliferation has developed at the posterior perforation site, leading to recurrent retinal detachment.

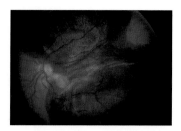

■ **FIGURE 8.9** Limited suprachoroidal/subretinal hemorrhage in a patient who sustained a localized rupture of the globe when struck with a wooden bat. The hemorrhage spontaneously resorbed over a 6-week timeframe.

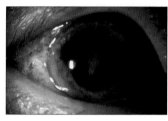

■ **FIGURE 8.10** Postoperative appositional suprachoroidal hemorrhage in a patient who had previously sustained an open-globe injury. The patient had spontaneously lost his lens, and had undergone surgical closure of a large scleral laceration.

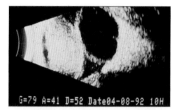

G=79 A=41 D=52 Date04-08-92 10H

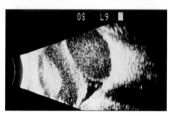

OS L9

■ **FIGURE 8.11** Echographic appearance of appositional suprachoroidal hemorrhage. Bottom: Acute hemorrhagic clot. Top: Liquefaction of the hemorrhage 10 days later. The patient then underwent successful drainage of the suprachoroidal hemorrhage.

although its use generally necessitates at least one additional surgical procedure to remove the oil 3–6 months after placement. One should not extrapolate the findings from the Silicone Oil Study into a traumatic setting.[41–44] In general, silicone oil is employed more frequently in the setting of trauma, especially with inferiorly located pathology.

Suprachoroidal hemorrhage

Suprachoroidal hemorrhage is an occasional complication of open-globe injuries. Hemorrhages can occur in limited extent (Fig. 8.9), or can be appositional or 'kissing'. The appositional hemorrhages are particularly problematic, as they may cause angle closure with flattening of the anterior chamber, elevated uncontrolled intraocular pressure, and are often associated with concurrent overlying retinal detachment (Fig. 8.10). Surgical drainage is often required, generally after the hemorrhagic choroidal detachment has liquefied sufficiently to allow for easier removal.[45,46] Liquefaction of the hemorrhage generally occurs at an average of 10–14 days after occurrence. Even following surgical evacuation, visual recovery is often limited at less than 20/200, and a significant number of eyes will have persistent postoperative hypotony, or will have no light perception vision.[45–49]

When confronted with massive suprachoroidal hemorrhage with controlled intraocular pressure, a serial echographic examination to monitor for liquefaction of the hemorrhage has been shown to be beneficial (Fig. 8.11). Once liquefaction occurs, sclerotomy drainage

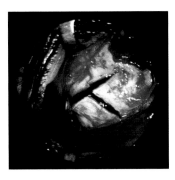

■ **FIGURE 8.12** T-shaped sclerotomy overlying the quadrant with the most prominent degree of suprachoroidal hemorrhage.

can proceed, and the chance of success is markedly improved. A radial or T-shaped scleral incision measuring several millimeters in length is made at or anterior to the equator in the quadrant(s) with the greatest extent of hemorrhage (Fig. 8.12). The suprachoroidal space is entered with a sharp myringotomy blade or needle, and gentle pressure is placed on the globe. An anterior chamber infusion with either fluid or air (dependent upon the status of the lens) is used to maintain intraocular pressure, and help push the hemorrhage out of the suprachoroidal space, through the sclerotomy site, and out of the eye. Often-times, this approach is then combined with pars plana vitrectomy surgery, so that any internal damage can be repaired once the majority of the suprachoroidal hemorrhage has been cleared.

Postoperative care

The majority of patients who undergo surgery for repair of an open-globe injury are treated as outpatients. The one key concern is the higher risk of infection associated with open-globe injuries (and this will be discussed in greater detail within the *Surgical management of retained intraocular foreign bodies* section under *Endophthalmitis*). The majority of patients are sent home on topical cycloplegics, corticosteroids, and antibiotics, and some of them will also have a short course of systemic antibiotics (oral or possibly intravenous to be administered by a home nurse). Many of them will also have an intraocular air or gas bubble, thus they may be instructed to position themselves in a particular fashion for a period of time, dependent upon the specific location of the trauma within the eye.

The patients are seen quite frequently early in the postoperative timeframe, generally on day 1, then again between days 5 and 7, and in most cases about 2 weeks later. The frequent checks are necessary to rule out development of infection, to assess the overall healing process, and also to monitor for possible elevated intraocular pressure (IOP). The IOP may rise due to the direct effects of the trauma, and possibly be exacerbated by the use of intraocular tamponade agents. Follow-up continues indefinitely, as there are numer-ous late sequelae of trauma which may develop long after the initial trauma and associated surgical repair.

Prognosis and outcome

Approximately 3000 open-globe injuries occur annually in the United States. A number of factors have been identified as correlating with long-term visual prognosis. These factors include the level of vision at presentation,[50] type of injury, location and extent of injury, lenticular involvement, presence of an afferent papillary defect, presence of retinal detach-ment, presence or absence of an IOFB, development of endophthalmitis and virulence of the offending organism(s), and possibly the presence of vitreous hemorrhage.[50–56]

The prognosis for eyes with open-globe injuries has steadily improved over the past 25 years, though it still remains a significant and sometimes devastating cause of ocular morbidity. In 1983, visual results of 5/200 or better were achieved in 31% of cases,[51] while this improved to 57% by 1996.[52] The results continue to slowly improve, recognizing that it is difficult to directly compare case series. Macular abnormalities remain the most common cause of limited visual function, and are more commonly seen in the closed-globe injury group.

SURGICAL MANAGEMENT OF RETAINED INTRAOCULAR FOREIGN BODIES (IOFBs)

As described above, the advent of vitreous microsurgical techniques has revolutionized the treatment of open-globe injuries. This also applies to management of eyes with retained IOFBs. In general, the prognosis for ocular injuries with retained IOFBs is much more favorable than penetrating or perforating injuries,[57] with almost 60% of cases achieving a final level of vision at 20/40 or better, and 80% being >5/200. In cases where there is trauma to the optic nerve or macula, even with currently available microsurgical techniques, visual recovery may still be limited however.

There are a variety of surgical techniques available to remove IOFBs, and these include vitrectomy removal with forceps, internal and/or external magnets, scleral cutdown, or removal via an anterior segment approach. Factors such as size, shape, location, number, and magnetic properties of the IOFB help determine the method and route of removal. A vitrectomy approach allows for controlled removal of IOFBs, repair of the concurrent intraocular damage, and possibly also reduces the risk of endophthalmitis.[58] It is virtually impossible to determine which method of removal is best, and selection is generally determined on a case-by-case basis. One must also be cognizant of the high risk of endophthalmitis that is seen with retained IOFBs, and there is also long-term concern of toxicity from the material of which the foreign body is comprised. General guidelines for management of IOFBs are listed in Table 8.3 and will be discussed in greater detail in following sections of this chapter.

Mechanism of injury and type of foreign body

In a series of 105 eyes with intraocular foreign bodies,[57] 72% of patients were injured as a result of hammering metal on metal, 11 eyes (10%) were injured by shotgun or BBs, 7

TABLE 8.3 Guidelines for management of intraocular foreign bodies

Location and type	Clear media	Poorly visualized
Intravitreal		
Magnetic	External magnet	Vitrectomy, with either rare earth magnet or forceps
Non-magnetic	Vitrectomy with forceps	Vitrectomy with forceps
Intraretinal		
Magnetic	Scleral cutdown (anterior) or vitrectomy with rare earth magnet or forceps	Vitrectomy with either rare earth magnet or forceps
Non-magnetic	Scleral cutdown (anterior) or vitrectomy with forceps	Vitrectomy with forceps
Intraocular		
Large size (>5 mm)	Vitrectomy with forceps	Vitrectomy with forceps
	Delivery through either pars plana or limbus	Delivery through either pars plana or limbus

(7%) by an explosion, and 11 (10%) by other mechanisms. In other studies, 70–80% of IOFBs occurred in relationship with hammering metal on metal, and 80–90% of IOFBs were metallic.[59–61] The most commonly encountered metals are iron and lead, though IOFBs composed of copper, zinc, silver, gold, platinum, and nickel have been noted. From 55 to 80% of metallic IOFBs are magnetic. Wound location varies dependent on the mechanism of injury, though approximately 65% of IOFBs enter through the cornea, 25% through the sclera, and at the corneoscleral junction in 10%. Wound size varied from less than 1 mm to 12 mm in length. Most eyes contained only one foreign body; however, about 8% of eyes harbored at least two. Sixty-one percent of IOFBs were located in the vitreous, 14% were intraretinal, and 5% were subretinal. The remainder was located in the anterior chamber (15%) or lens (8%).

Methods of IOFB extraction
Magnetic extraction

External electromagnets and internal rare earth magnets can be used to remove magnetic foreign bodies from the posterior segment via a direct or indirect approach.[57,62] The direct approach refers to placement of the electromagnet over a scleral cutdown adjacent to the magnetic IOFB.[62] The IOFB should be situated at or anterior to the equator of the eye, and be either intraretinal or subretinal in location. Visualization and localization by indirect ophthalmoscopy are essential. A scleral cutdown is made over the site of the IOFB, generally in a T-shaped configuration, and diathermy is applied to the uveal bed. The external electromagnet is then utilized, bringing the IOFB through the uvea, where it is either removed directly or grasped with a forceps. The sclerotomy site is then sutured closed. In select situations, especially in the presence of a retinal tear, the IOFB site is treated with either cryotherapy or photocoagulation, and supported with a scleral buckle.

The indirect approach involves removal of the IOFB through the pars plana, as close as possible to the location of the IOFB.[57,62] The sclerotomy site is opened with a myringotomy blade, and diathermy is also applied to the uveal bed. The magnet should be directed toward the IOFB, so that when the magnetic field is applied, the IOFB will not cause any inadvertent damage to surrounding intraocular structures. With the external electromagnet, there may be arcing of the magnetic field, thus as the IOFB is extracted from the eye, it could strike either the anterior retina or the posterior surface of the lens. This approach is used primarily for small, magnetic, intravitreal IOFBs (Fig. 8.13), or even for IOFBs on the retinal surface that are not encapsulated. Good surgical results have been reported with these methods.[62–65]

Extraction with vitrectomy

There is no statistically significant difference in visual outcome between the different routes of extraction[57] when the method chosen is appropriate for the type of IOFB and associated ocular abnormalities. Pars plana vitrectomy with forceps removal of the IOFB (Table 8.3) should be used in all cases with non-magnetic foreign bodies (Fig. 8.14), posterior, incarcerated foreign bodies, media opacities precluding view of the IOFB or fundus,

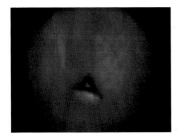

FIGURE 8.13 Intravitreal, metallic, magnetic IOFB entered the eye while the patient was hammering metal on metal. It was suspended in the vitreous cavity, free of retinal tissue, and there was only a small amount of associated vitreous hemorrhage. The IOFB was removed with the external magnet, which was placed over the pars plana. No complications were encountered.

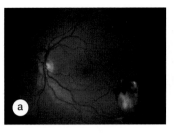 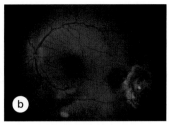

FIGURE 8.14 (**a**) Intraretinal glass IOFB with associated localized retinal detachment and hemorrhage. The glass IOFB entered the eye when an overhanging light fixture fell onto the patient's face, and it lodged in the retina. (**b**) The IOFB was removed via a vitrectomy approach and a retinotomy. Photocoagulation was applied around the edges of the retinotomy, and intravitreal air tamponade was employed, The vision recovered to 20/20.

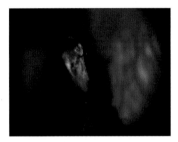 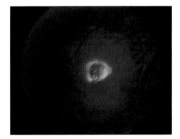

FIGURE 8.15 Very large metallic IOFB, located intraretinally with associated retinal tear and hemorrhage. The IOFB was removed via a vitrectomy approach. Once the hemorrhage was removed around the IOFB, along with associated encapsulated tissue, the IOFB was brought into the mid-vitreous cavity with an internal magnet, transferred to a forceps, and removed from the eye.

FIGURE 8.16 Intraretinal IOFB with localized retinal detachment. Also note the sheathed retinal vessels, which were indicative of early endophthalmitis. The IOFB was removed with an internal vitrectomy approach and a forceps. Intravitreal antibiotics were employed to treat the associated *Staphylococcus epidermidis* endophthalmitis, and the patient recovered vision to 20/25.

associated ocular injuries requiring vitrectomy, lensectomy, or other manipulations (Fig. 8.15), and in cases with signs and symptoms of endophthalmitis (Fig. 8.16). Even with clear media and an adequate view of the IOFB, a pars plana vitrectomy approach may be beneficial by irrigating fluid through the eye, thus diluting any possible bacterial load and reducing the risk of endophthalmitis.[57]

When the IOFB is poorly visualized due to cataract or vitreous hemorrhage, vitrectomy and lensectomy are necessary. If the IOFB is not incarcerated or encapsulated, an intraocular rare earth magnet may be used to secure a magnetic foreign body, and either pass it off to a forceps in the mid-vitreous cavity, or in the case of a large IOFB (>5 mm), possibly bring it into the anterior chamber, for removal through a limbal incision. If the IOFB is non-magnetic, intraocular forceps or gentle aspiration with a soft-tipped instrument may be used to secure the IOFB.

Removal of intraretinal foreign bodies is more difficult, and may require careful dissection of a fibrous capsule and segmentation of any adhesions that might induce retinal traction (Figs 8.14–8.16). Visual prognosis depends largely on the impaction site, with macular involvement portending a poorer visual prognosis. Still, up to 49% of cases can attain a visual acuity of 20/40 or better.[60]

Comparison of the treatment methods

Accurate comparison of the treatment methods is difficult because no controlled, prospective, randomized study has been performed, and each case needs to be dealt with individually dependent upon numerous features of the IOFB. When used appropriately, either primary external magnetic extraction or vitrectomy with internal IOFB removal can provide excellent visual and anatomic results, with at least 60% of patients achieving a final visual acuity of 20/40 or better.[57] In addition, vitrectomy has been associated with a lower incidence of enucleation after penetrating trauma.[57]

Retinal detachment and retinopexy

A slight degree of controversy exists regarding application of retinopexy at the site of an intraretinal foreign body. In the majority of cases where an IOFB has impacted the retina, or the IOFB has been removed from an intraretinal location, retinopexy is applied to the site. However, it has been questioned as to whether retinopexy and even removal of the posterior hyaloids is necessary for IOFBs that are located posteriorly.[60] It was felt that spontaneous retinopexy occurred at the foreign body impact site, and that further treatment with either laser photocoagulation or cryotherapy would possibly stimulate fibrous proliferation, retinal breaks, or hemorrhage, thus potentially worsening the situation.

Endophthalmitis

Trauma accounts for approximately 25% of cases of culture-proven endophthalmitis, with infection occurring in 2–7% of open-globe injuries,[62,66] and up to 30% of retained IOFBs.[67] Cases of suspected infection should have an aqueous paracentesis performed, followed by a vitreous tap for culture purposes. The vitreous specimen is best obtained through the vitrectomy cutter, as then there is no traction placed on the vitreous base or retina. Approximately 0.2–0.3 cc of undiluted vitreous provides an adequate sample for culture purposes, and then the entire vitreous washings can also be collected at the end of the case, and sent for culture purposes.

Trauma-related endophthalmitis has a spectrum of causative organisms similar to other types of exogenous endophthalmitis, although the incidence of *Bacillus* species infection is much higher, ranging between 25 and 50%. *Staphylococcus* coagulase negative organisms account for approximately 24% of infections, followed by *Streptococcus* species in 13%, *Staphylococcus aureus* in 8%, and Gram-negative organisms in 7%. The setting of trauma also carries the risk of polymicrobial infections.

In the majority of cases, the intravitreal injections most commonly employed consist of vancomycin (1 mg/0.1 cc) with ceftazidime (2.25 mg/0.1 cc) or, alternatively, amikacin (200–400 mcg/0.1 cc). Intravitreal antibiotics provide the main defense in the treatment of proven infection. Subconjunctival, topical, and systemic antibiotics are also generally employed, with the usual medications and dosages outlined in Box 8.1. The treatment of postoperative endophthalmitis has changed considerably over the past 5 years, as there are better antimicrobials, particularly the fourth generation fluoroquinolones,[68,69] which readily penetrate into even non-inflamed eyes, even when administered orally.

Vancomycin is still the intravitreal antibiotic of choice for Gram-positive coverage, including *Bacillus* species and *Propionibacterium acnes*. Cephalosporins, including cefazolin and ceftazidime, provide good broad-spectrum coverage for Gram-positive and some Gram-negative organisms, though are relatively ineffective against *Enterococcus* and methicillin-resistant staphylococcal organisms. The aminoglycosides, including gentamicin and amikacin, are chosen for Gram-negative coverage; however, as there is a definite risk of retinal toxicity[70] (Fig. 8.17), this class of antibiotic is rarely employed today. The quinolones, in particular the new fourth generation agents moxifloxacin and gatifloxacin, provide excellent coverage against the bacterial species most frequently involved in cases of traumatic endophthalmitis, though they do lack coverage against *Streptococcus* and *Pseudomonas* species.[68,69] While moxifloxacin appears to be safe to utilize intravitreally, it is not

---

BOX 8.1 Antibiotics and corticosteroids in the management of bacterial endophthalmitis

Intravitreal

1. Vancomycin (1 mg) with ceftazidime (2.25 mg) or amikacin (200–400 mcg)
2. Dexamethasone (400 mcg) (controversial)

Periocular (subconjunctival)

1. Vancomycin (25–50 mg) with ceftazidime (100 mg)
2. Occasionally use dexamethasone (4–12 mg)

Topical

1. Over-the-counter fourth generation fluoroquinolones (Vigamox or Zymar)
2. Occasionally use fortified vancomycin (50 mg/cc) or ceftazidime (50 mg/cc)
3. Topical corticosteroid and cycloplegic

Systemic

1. Moxifloxacin 400 mg daily (orally) for 3–5 days
2. Occasionally use vancomycin (1 g q 12 h IV), ceftazidime (1 g q 8 h IV), cefazolin (1 g q 8 h IV), or ciprofloxacin (400 mg q 12 h IV, or 750 mg q 12 h orally) for 1–3 days
3. Occasionally use prednisone (0.7–1 mg/kg/day) for 3–5 days

---

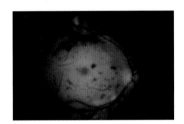

■ **FIGURE 8.17** Appearance of the retina 2 days following intravitreal surgery for postoperative endophthalmitis. Intravitreal vancomycin and gentamicin were administered. The appearance is that of macular infarction, typical of gentamicin toxicity. The patient inadvertently received a higher than anticipated dose of medication, resulting in the problem. Vision only recovered to hand motions.

yet commonly employed. As can be seen, the combination of intravitreal vancomycin with either ceftazidime or amikacin provides excellent broad-spectrum coverage against the majority of organisms that are associated with traumatic endophthalmitis.

Regarding systemic antibiotics, the true extent of the need has not yet been determined, though it is common to employ some form of coverage for at least a few days. The results of the Endophthalmitis Vitrectomy Study (EVS)[71] in the treatment of postoperative endophthalmitis suggested that intravenous antibiotics did not play a significant role. The antibiotics employed were aminoglycosides and cephalosporins. Penetration into the eye is quite limited with these classes of antibiotic. Additionally, it is not suggested to extrapolate these results into the setting of open-globe injuries, as different organisms are encountered, which oftentimes have much greater virulence. Organisms such as *Bacillus* species are also often associated with toxins. Therefore, it is presently recommended that patients suffering open-globe injuries, with or without retained IOFBs, receive some form of supplemental systemic antibiotic for at least 1–3 days (Box 8.1). It is becoming much more common to employ oral moxifloxacin 400 mg daily for 3–5 days, as this can readily be done as an outpatient, and the antibiotic has been shown to penetrate the eye very readily when administered orally.[69] Alternatively, intravenous vancomycin (1 g q 12 h), ceftazidime (1 g q 8 h), or intravenous or oral ciprofloxacin (400 mg or 750 mg q 12 h, respectively) for 1–3 days, can be utilized (Box 8.1).

Prophylactic antibiotics

The role of prophylactic intravitreal antibiotics is unclear, especially given the reports of antibiotic toxicity with the aminoglycosides. In contrast, prophylactic use of intravitreal vancomycin and even ceftazidime is quite safe, and can be employed. The question is whether or not it is truly needed in most cases.

In a series of retained IOFBs,[58] bacterial cultures of removed IOFBs or vitreous were positive in 7 of 25 cases (28%), even in the absence of the usual signs of clinical infection. Prompt surgical intervention with vitrectomy (and no intravitreal antibiotics), even in high-risk cases associated with organic matter contamination, resulted in excellent anatomic and visual outcomes, without development of endophthalmitis. All patients recovered vision to 20/70 or better, despite potentially virulent growth of organisms including several cases involving *Bacillus* species. However, it should be pointed out that a delay in primary repair of more than 24 hours can lead to a fourfold increased risk (from 3.5 to 13.4%) for the development of infectious endophthalmitis.[72] Thus the role and/or need of prophylactic antibiotics remain unclear, especially in the setting of prompt surgical care.

Corticosteroids

The proper use of intravitreal corticosteroids in the setting of endophthalmitis remains unknown and controversial.[73–76] Due to uncertainty regarding their potential benefit versus harm, they were not employed in the Endophthalmitis Vitrectomy Study (EVS). While corticosteroids may be beneficial for suppressing inflammation and potentially limiting ocular damage, they can also potentiate an infection. Their effect may truly be dependent upon the timing of administration, and may be organism specific. If employed, the following dosages are commonly utilized: intravitreal (dexamethasone 400 mcg/0.1 cc, or triamcinolone 4 mg/0.1 cc), periocular (dexamethasone 4–12 mg), and systemic (prednisone 0.7–1 mg/kg/day).

Postoperative care

Similar to the discussion in the *Management of open-globe injuries (non-IOFB cases)* under the *Postoperative care* section of this chapter, the majority of patients who undergo surgery for repair of a retained IOFB are treated as outpatients. As was described previously, the key concern is the high degree of associated endophthalmitis, which typically runs between 7 and 13%,[57] to as high as 30% for patients with IOFBs associated with organic matter contamination.[67] All recommendations that were discussed previously, apply equally well here to patients with retained IOFBs. Regarding recommended antibiotic regimens and routes of administration, please refer to Box 8.1.

One final concern pertains to the rare case where it may be elected to leave a foreign body in place (or possibly there was an undetected IOFB). Not only is it necessary to monitor the patient closely for possible infection, one also needs to watch for possible toxicity from the IOFB itself (siderosis, chelosis, etc.).

Prognosis and outcome

Findings predictive of a final visual acuity of 20/40 or better after ocular injuries with retained IOFBs are: (1) an initial visual acuity of 20/40 or better; and (2) the need for only one or two operations for anatomic stabilization of the injury and its complications.[57] The size of the entrance wound and the size of the IOFB have also been associated with outcome. Additionally, the association of vitreous hemorrhage with IOFBs, and IOFB location within the retina have been associated with a worsened prognosis.

As noted at the start of this section on retained IOFBs, patients with foreign bodies carry a quite good prognosis for anatomic and visual outcomes, as approximately 60% achieve a final outcome of 20/40 or better, and 80% are >5/200.[57] These results are much more favorable than patients with open-globe injuries in general. It is important to remember, however, that IOFBs comprised of BBs almost uniformly carry a very poor prognosis and tend to occur in children.[77]

LATE COMPLICATIONS

Despite excellent repair of open-globe injuries, numerous late complications may still arise. Many of these complications are amenable to further surgical repair. Anterior segment complications include corneal decompensation that may arise from the trauma itself, or may occur due to gradual corneal thickening if significant endothelial cell loss occurred from the trauma or secondary to the surgical repair. Penetrating keratoplasty surgery is often indicated. Numerous glaucoma complications can arise, once again as a direct result of the trauma, or secondary to the subsequent surgery or adjuncts employed in the course of surgical repair of the retina.

Late posterior segment complications include macular epiretinal membrane formation, which is quite common (Fig. 8.18). Tractional and rhegmatogenous retinal detachment may also occur, especially since most scleral lacerations have at least some degree of vitreous (and possible retinal) incarceration. This alters the normal vitreoretinal relationship, increasing traction on the vitreous base. The majority of these complications are amenable to further vitrectomy surgery, though some eyes will succumb to uncontrolled intraocular proliferation with recurrent retinal detachment, or to hypotony from ciliary body shutdown.

SYMPATHETIC OPHTHALMIA

Sympathetic ophthalmia is a bilateral inflammatory condition of the uveal tract, characterized by nodular or diffuse infiltration with epithelioid cells and lymphocytes. It may have a very insidious onset, and its course may vary extensively, with periods of remission and exacerbation. Although the precise cause is unknown, the majority of cases follow open-globe injuries or less commonly following intraocular surgery. The incidence has been estimated to be approximately 1 in 1000 cases of open-globe injury. The inflammation appears in the injured (excited) eye usually within 1–2 months, and is then followed shortly thereafter by similar inflammation in the sympathizing eye.

The injured eye exhibits low-grade uveitis, iris thickening, and the pupil is unresponsive to light. The patient may develop iris nodules at the pupillary margin, along with corneal endothelial precipitates. The sympathizing eye generally develops a low-grade uveitis with keratic precipitates, photophobia, and ocular pain. The iris may become thickened and unresponsive, leading to a vascularized pupillary membrane, and possible secondary glaucoma. The posterior segment will have retinal and choroidal swelling, whitish spots indicative of Dalen–Fuchs nodules, and possibly an exudative retinal detachment (Fig. 8.19).

Evidence points toward an extremely small risk of sympathetic ophthalmia if the injured eye is enucleated within 2 weeks of the date of the injury. Therefore, all surgical repair

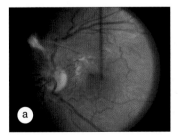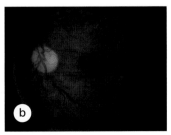

FIGURE 8.18 (a) Appearance of a patient who underwent removal of an IOFB 2 months earlier. The posterior hyaloid was not removed at the time of the initial surgery, and subsequent proliferation developed along the retinal surface. (b) Postoperative appearance following removal of the epiretinal membrane. Vision recovered from 20/400 to 20/50.

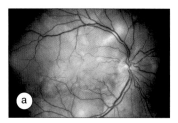 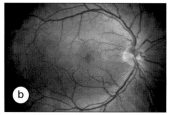

FIGURE 8.19 (**a**) Fellow eye of a patient 2 months following an open-globe injury. The patient developed sympathetic ophthalmia, with extensive intraocular inflammation and diffuse chorioretinal swelling with multiple pigment epithelial detachments. The visual acuity is 20/80. (**b**) Follow-up of the patient 3 months later, following institution of systemic corticosteroids. Vision has returned to 20/20, with resolution of the posterior segment abnormalities. The corticosteroids were slowly tapered over a 12-month course.

attempts should be planned within this timeframe. However, isolated cases of sympathetic ophthalmia have been reported as early as 5 days following trauma, and as late as 60 years following the inciting event.[78–82]

Once the diagnosis of sympathetic ophthalmia has been established, enucleation of the exciting eye is generally not recommended, as it will not arrest the process, and the exciting eye could end up offering the better vision of the two eyes. However, if there is little or no vision, enucleation may still be recommended.

Corticosteroids are the mainstay of therapy for sympathetic ophthalmia. The sympathizing eye has an approximate 60% chance of recovering 20/50 or better vision (Fig. 8.19b). High-dose corticosteroids may need to be employed initially, along with a tapering dose of medication for a year or two. Using corticosteroids from the time of injury does not prevent the development of sympathetic ophthalmia.

PREVENTION OF OCULAR INJURY

Ocular trauma causes tremendous morbidity, especially among young male patients and otherwise healthy individuals. A significant portion of ocular injury could be avoided with the proper use of eye protection and education. This certainly holds true in the realm of sports-related injuries[83] and in many work-related injuries as well.

CONCLUSION

Substantial ocular trauma continues to occur via both closed-globe as well as open-globe etiologies. Both types of injury may lead to significant visual compromise via a variety of mechanisms. Visual prognosis most closely correlates with the severity of the initial injury, and with the level of vision at presentation. Numerous acute issues such as intraocular hemorrhage, retinal tears and detachment need to be addressed in a timely fashion, and then there is the concern regarding numerous long-term sequelae. The two most significant long-term concerns are retinal detachment with PVR and ciliary body shutdown, especially following open-globe injuries. These two problems account for the majority of cases of irreversible visual impairment.

There is no doubt that there have been significant advances in vitreoretinal surgical techniques and instrumentation over the past 20 years. The pathophysiology of both closed-globe and open-globe trauma is also much better understood. Still, not every eye can be salvaged from the effects of trauma, as recurrent intraocular proliferation and ciliary body shutdown cannot be fully prevented or adequately treated. Additionally, numerous questions remain regarding optimal management of these injuries, ranging from timing of vitrectomy intervention, to proper use of antibiotics, to the type of surgical approach which is employed. Many of these issues will never be fully resolved in a controlled clinical trial format. However, in spite of that potential limitation, we should continue to see substantial improvement in the upcoming years, to the point of being able to successfully manage the majority of trauma-related ocular injuries.

REFERENCES

1. Sternberg P Jr. Trauma: principles and techniques of treatment. In: Ryan SJ, ed. Retina. St Louis: Mosby; 1994:2351–2378.
2. Pieramici DJ, Sternberg P, Aaberg TM Sr, et al. A system for classifying mechanical injuries of the eye (globe). Am J Ophthalmol 1997; 123:820–831.
3. Ryan SJ. Traction retinal detachment. XLIX Edward Jackson Memorial Lecture. Am J Ophthalmol 1993; 115:1–20.
4. Gilbert CM, Soong HK, Hirst LW. A two year prospective study of penetrating ocular trauma at the Wilmer Ophthalmological Institute. Ann Ophthalmol 1987; 19:104–106.
5. Harlan JB Jr, Pieramici DJ. Evaluation of patients with ocular trauma. Ophthalmology Clin North Am 2002; 15:153–161.
6. Joseph DP, Pieramici DJ, Beauchamp NJ Jr. Computed tomography in the diagnosis and prognosis of open-globe injuries. Ophthalmology 2000; 107:1899–1906.
7. Bryden FM, Pyott AA, Bailey M, McGhee CN. Real time ultrasound in the assessment of intraocular foreign bodies. Eye 1990; 4:727–731.
8. Barr CC. Prognostic factors in corneoscleral lacerations. Arch Ophthalmol 1983; 101:919–924.
9. Cleary PE, Ryan SJ. Method of production and natural history of experimental posterior penetrating eye injury in the rhesus monkey. Am J Ophthalmol 1979; 88:212–220.
10. Topping TM, Abrams GW, Machemer R. Experimental double perforating injury of the posterior segment in rabbit eyes. The natural history of intraocular proliferation. Arch Ophthalmol 1979; 97:735–742.
11. Abrams GW, Topping TM, Machemer R. Vitrectomy for injury. The effect on intraocular proliferation following perforation of the posterior segment of the rabbit eye. Arch Ophthalmol 1979; 97:743–746.
12. Winthrop SR, Cleary PE, Minckler DS, Ryan SJ. Penetrating eye injuries. A histopathological review. Br J Ophthalmol 1980; 64:809–817.
13. Cleary PE, Ryan SJ. Vitrectomy in penetrating eye injury: results of a controlled trial of vitrectomy in an experimental posterior penetrating eye injury in the rhesus monkey. Arch Ophthalmol 1981; 99:287–292.
14. Gregor Z, Ryan SJ. Complete and core vitrectomies in the treatment of experimental posterior penetrating eye injury in the Rhesus monkey. I. Clinical features. Arch Ophthalmol 1983; 101:441–445.
15. Gregor Z, Ryan SJ. Complete and core vitrectomies in the treatment of experimental posterior penetrating eye injury in the Rhesus monkey. II. Histologic features. Arch Ophthalmol 1983; 101:446–450.
16. Coleman DJ. Early vitrectomy in the management of the severely traumatized eye. Am J Ophthalmol 1982; 93:543–551.
17. de Juan E Jr, Sternberg P Jr, Michels RG. Timing of vitrectomy after penetrating ocular injuries. Ophthalmology 1984; 91:1072–1074.
18. Mieler WF, Mittra RA. The role and timing of pars plana vitrectomy in penetrating ocular trauma [editorial]. Arch Ophthalmol 1997; 113:1191–1192.
19. Mittra RA, Mieler WF. Controversies in the management of open-globe injuries involving the posterior segment. SUV Ophthalmol 1999; 44:215–225.
20. Scott IU, Flynn HW Jr, Middy WE, et al. Clinical features and outcomes of pars plana vitrectomy in patients with retained lens fragments. Ophthalmology 2003; 110:1567–1572.
21. Chan CK. An improved technique for management of dislocated posterior chamber implants. Ophthalmology 1992; 99:51–57.
22. Malinowski SM, Mieler WF, Koenig SB, Han DP, Pulido JS. Combined pars plana vitrectomy–lensectomy and open-loop anterior chamber lens implantation. Ophthalmology 1995; 102:211–215.
23. Han DP, Rychwalski PJ, Mieler WF, Abrams GW. Management of complex retinal detachment with combined relaxing retinotomy and intravitreal perfluoro-n-octane injection. Am J Ophthalmol 1994; 118:24–32.
24. Han DP, Pulido JS, Mieler WF, Johnson MW. Vitrectomy for proliferative diabetic retinopathy with severe equatorial

fibrovascular proliferation. Am J Ophthalmol 1995; 119:563–570.

25. Zhang MN, Jiang CH. 360-Degree retinectomy for severe ocular rupture. Chin J Traumatol 2005; 8(6):323–327.

26. Chang TS, McGill E, Hay DA, et al. Prophylactic scleral buckle for prevention of retinal detachment following vitrectomy for macular hole. Br J Ophthalmol 1999; 83:944–948.

27. Stone TW, Siddiqui N, Arroyo JG, McCuen BW, Postel EA. Primary scleral buckling in open-globe injury involving the posterior segment. Ophthalmology 2000; 107:1923–1926.

28. Arroyo JG, Postel EA, Stone T, McCuen BW, Egan KM. A matched study of primary scleral buckle placement during repair of posterior segment open globe injuries. Br J Ophthalmol 2003; 87:75–78.

29. Warrasak S, Euswas A, Hongsakorn S. Posterior segment trauma: types of injuries, result of vitreoretinal surgery and prophylactic encircling scleral buckle. J Med Assoc Thai 2005; 88:1916–1930.

30. Jaccoma EH, Conway BP, Campochiaro PA. Cryotherapy causes extensive breakdown of the blood–retinal barrier. A comparison with argon laser photocoagulation. Arch Ophthalmol 1985; 103:1728–1730.

31. Campochiaro PA, Kaden IH, Vidaurri-Leal J, et al. Cryotherapy enhances intravitreal dispersion of viable retinal pigment epithelial cells. Arch Ophthalmol 1985; 103:434–436.

32. Hsu HT, Ryan SJ. Experimental retinal detachment in the rabbit. Retina 1986; 6:66–69.

33. Campochiaro PA, Bryan JA, Conway BP, Jaccoma EH. Intravitreal chemotactic and mitogenic activity. Implication of blood–retinal barrier breakdown. Arch Ophthalmol 1986; 104:1685–1687.

34. Campochiaro PA, Gaskin HC, Vinores SA. Retinal cryopexy stimulates traction retinal detachment formation in the presence of an ocular wound. Arch Ophthalmol 1987; 105:1567–1570.

35. Steel DHW, West J, Campbell WG. A randomized controlled study of the use of transscleral diode laser and cryotherapy in the management of rhegmatogenous retinal detachment. Retina 2000; 20:346–357.

36. Chang S, Reppucci V, Zimmerman NJ, Heinemann MH, Coleman DJ. Perfluorocarbon liquids in the management of traumatic retinal detachments. Ophthalmology 1989; 96:785–791.

37. Antoszyk AN, McCuen BW II, deJuan E, Machemer R. Silicone oil injection after failed primary vitreous surgery in severe ocular trauma. Am J Ophthalmol 1989; 107:537–543.

38. Alexandridis E. Silicone oil tamponade in the management of severe hemorrhagic detachment of the choroids and ciliary body after surgical trauma. Ophthalmologica 1990; 100:189–193.

39. Spiegel D, Nasemann J, Nawrocki J, Gabel VP. Severe ocular trauma managed with primary pars plana vitrectomy and silicone oil. Retina 1997; 17:275–285.

40. Cekic O, Hatman C. Severe ocular trauma managed with primary pars plana vitrectomy and silicone oil [letter; comment]. Retina 1998; 18:287–288.

41. The Silicone Study Group. Vitrectomy with silicone oil or sulfur hexafluoride gas in eyes with severe proliferative vitreoretinopathy: results of a randomized clinical trial. Silicone Study Report 1. Arch Ophthalmol 1992; 110:770–779.

42. The Silicone Study Group. Vitrectomy with silicone oil or perfluoropropane gas in eyes with severe proliferative vitreoretinopathy: Results of a randomized clinical trial. Silicone Study Report 2. Arch Ophthalmol 1992; 110:780–792.

43. McCuen BW II, Azen SP, Stern W, et al. Vitrectomy with silicone oil or perfluoropropane gas in eyes with severe proliferative vitreoretinopathy. Results in Group 1 versus Group 2 (Silicone Study Report #3). Retina 1993; 13:279–284.

44. Blumenkranz MS, Azen SP, Aaberg TM, et al. Relaxing retinotomy with silicone oil or long-acting gas in eyes with severe proliferative vitreoretinopathy (Silicone Study Report #5). Am J Ophthalmol 1993; 116:557–564.

45. Wirostko WJ, Han DP, Mieler WF, Pulido JS, Connor TB Jr, Kuhn E. Suprachoroidal hemorrhage: outcome of surgical management according to hemorrhage severity. Ophthalmology 1998; 105:2271–2275.

46. Scott IU, Flynn HW Jr, Schiffman J, Smiddy WE, Murray TG, Ehlies F. Visual acuity outcomes among patients with appositional suprachoroidal hemorrhage. Ophthalmology 1997; 104:39–46.

47. Meier P, Wiedemann P. Massive suprachoroidal hemorrhage: secondary treatment and outcome. Graefes Arch Clin Exp Ophthalmol 2000; 238:28–32.

48. Moshfeghi DM, Kim BY, Kaiser PK, Sears JE, Smith SD. Appositional suprachoroidal hemorrhage: a case-control study. Am J Ophthalmol 2004; 138:959–963.

49. Feretis E, Mourtzoukos S, Mangouritsas G, Kabanarou SA, Inoba K, Xirou T. Secondary management and outcomes of massive

suprachoroidal hemorrhage. Eur J Ophthalmol 2006; 16:835–840.

50. Sternberg P Jr, deJuan E Jr, Michels RG, Auer C. Multivariate analysis of prognostic factors in penetrating ocular injuries. Am J Ophthalmol 1984; 98:467–472.

51. de Juan E, Sternberg P, Michels RG. Penetrating injuries, types of injuries and visual results. Ophthalmology 1983; 90:1318–1323.

52. Pieramici DJ, MacCumber MW, Humayun MU, Marsh MJ, de Juan E Jr. Open-globe injury. Update on types of injuries and visual results. Ophthalmology 1996; 103:1798–1803.

53. Lieb DF, Scott IU, Flynn HW Jr, Miller D, Feuer WJ. Open globe injuries with positive intraocular cultures: factors influencing final visual acuity outcomes. Ophthalmology 2003; 110:1560–1566.

54. Cruvinel Issac DL, Ghanem VC, Nascimento MA, Torigoe M, Kara-Jose N. Prognostic factors in open globe injuries. Ophthalmologica 2003; 217:431–435.

55. Rahman I, Maino A, Devadason D, Leatherbarrow B. Open globe injuries: factors predictive of poor outcome. Eye 2006; 20:1336–1341.

56. Entezari M, Rabel HM, Badalabadi MM, Mohebbi M. Visual outcome and ocular survival in open-globe injuries. Injury 2006; 37:633–637.

57. Williams DF, Mieler WF, Abrams GW, Lewis H. Results and prognostic factors in penetrating ocular injuries with retained intraocular foreign bodies. Ophthalmology 1988; 95:911–916.

58. Mieler WF, Ellis MK, Williams DF, Han DP. Retained intraocular foreign bodies and endophthalmitis. Ophthalmology 1990; 97:1532–1538.

59. DeBustros S. Posterior segment intraocular foreign bodies. In: Shingleton BJ, Hersh PS, Kenyon KR, eds. Eye trauma. St Louis: Mosby-Year Book; 1991.

60. Ahmadieh H, Sajjadi H, Azarmina M, Soheilian M, Mahavrivand N. Surgical management of intraretinal foreign bodies. Retina 1994; 14:397–403.

61. Ambler JS, Sanford MM. Management of intraretinal foreign bodies without retinopexy in the absence of retinal detachment. Ophthalmology 1991; 98:391–394.

62. Chow DR, Garretson BR, Kuczynski B, et al. External versus internal approach to the removal of metallic intraocular foreign bodies. Retina 2000; 20:364–369.

63. Greven CM, Engelbrecht NE, Slusher MM, Nagy SS. Intraocular foreign bodies: management, prognostic factors, and visual outcomes. Ophthalmology 2000; 107:823–828.

64. Wani VB, Al-Ajmi M, Thalib L, et al. Vitrectomy for posterior segment intraocular foreign bodies: visual results and prognostic factors. Retina 2003; 23:654–660.

65. Soheilian M, Feghi M, Yazdani S, et al. Surgical management of non-metallic and metallic intraocular foreign bodies. Ophthalmic Surg Lasers Imaging 2005; 36:189–196.

66. Brinton GS, Topping TM, Hyndiuk RA, Aaberg TM, Reeser FH, Abrams GW. Post-traumatic endophthalmitis. Arch Ophthalmol 1984; 102:547–550.

67. Boldt HC, Pulido JS, Blodi CF, Folk JC, Weingeist TA. Rural endophthalmitis. Ophthalmology 1989; 96:1722–1726.

68. Hariprasad SM, Mieler WF. Vitreous and aqueous penetration of orally administered gatifloxacin in humans. Arch Ophthalmol 2003; 121:345–350.

69. Hariprasad SM, Shah GK, Mieler WF, et al. Vitreous and aqueous penetration of orally administered moxifloxacin in humans. Arch Ophthalmol 2006; 124:178–182.

70. Campochiaro PA, Conway BP. Aminoglycoside toxicity—a survey of retinal specialists. Implications for ocular use. Arch Ophthalmol 1991; 109:946–950.

71. Endophthalmitis Vitrectomy Study Group. Results of the Endophthalmitis Vitrectomy Study. A randomized trial of immediate vitrectomy and of intravenous antibiotics for the treatment of post-operative bacterial endophthalmitis. Arch Ophthalmol 1995; 113:1479–1496.

72. Thompson JT, Parver LM, Enger CL, Mieler WF, Liggett PE. Infectious endophthalmitis after penetrating injuries with retained intraocular foreign bodies. National Eye Trauma System. Ophthalmology 1993; 100:1468–1474.

73. Dev S, Han DP, Mieler WF, et al. The role of dexamethasone as an adjunct in the management of postoperative bacterial endophthalmitis. EVRS 2004; 1:13–20.

74. Gan IM, Ugahary LC, van Dissel JT, van Meurs JC. Effect of intravitreal dexamethasone on vitreous vancomycin concentrations in patients with suspected postoperative bacterial endophthalmitis. Graefes Arch Clin Exp Ophthalmol 2005; 243:1186–1189.

75. Gan IM, Ugahary LC, van Dissel JT, et al. Intravitreal dexamethasone as adjuvant in the treatment of postoperative endophthalmitis: a prospective randomized trial. Graefes Arch Clin Exp Ophthalmol 2005; 243:1200–1205.

76. Falk NS, Beer PM, Peters GB 3rd. Role of intravitreal triamcinolone acetonide in the treatment of postoperative endophthalmitis. Retina 2006; 26:545–548.

77. Williams DF, Mieler WF, Abrams GW. Intraocular foreign bodies in young people. Retina 1990; 10(S):545–549.

78. Chan CC, Roberge RG, Whitcup SM, Nussenblatt RB. 32 cases of sympathetic ophthalmia. A retrospective study at the National Eye Institute, Bethesda, MD, from 1982 to 1992. Arch Ophthalmol 1995; 113:597–600.

79. Ramadan A, Nussenblatt RB. Visual prognosis and sympathetic ophthalmia. Curr Opin Ophthalmol 1996; 7:39–45.

80. Kilmartin DJ, Dick AD, Forrester JV. Sympathetic ophthalmia risk following vitrectomy: should we counsel patients? Br J Ophthalmol 2000; 84:448–449.

81. Gurdal C, Erdener U, Irkec M, Orhan M. Incidence of sympathetic ophthalmia after penetrating eye injury and choice of treatment. Ocul Immunol Inflamm 2002; 10:223–227.

82. Damico FM, Kiss S, Young LH. Sympathetic ophthalmia. Semin Ophthalmol 2005; 20:191–197.

83. Rubin MP, Alexandrou TJ, Vinger PF, Mieler WF. Sports injuries. In: Albert DM, Jakobiec FA, eds. Principles and practice of ophthalmology, 3rd edn. Philadelphia: Saunders; 2007: Chapter 379.

9 Surgery for proliferative vitreoretinopathy

Allan E. Kreiger

Reattachment rates for retinal detachment surgery steadily improved after Gonin convincingly demonstrated that closure of retinal breaks was the essential element governing success. Surgical methods changed and results improved with the introduction of new technology that allowed the surgeon to locate and close the breaks with scleral buckling techniques. The major cause of failure occurred when a phenomenon termed massive vitreous retraction (MVR) occurred. It was recognized that scarring and fibrosis within the vitreous rendered closure of retinal breaks impossible by scleral buckling alone.

When vitreous surgery became available, it was hoped that removal of this vitreous traction would improve success rates in these inoperable cases. Although some improvement did occur, it became evident that removing the vitreous alone was not enough. Thus, greater attention was given to the MVR process and why it caused operations, including vitrectomy, to fail.

MVR was renamed massive periretinal proliferation (MPP) as clinicians realized that cells proliferating on the surface of the retina led to contractile membranes that prevented anatomic closure of retinal breaks. Basic research led to better understanding of the origin of these cells (retinal pigment epithelial [RPE] cells, glial cells, fibroblasts) and prompted efforts to moderate or limit cell proliferation. Furthermore, the tendency for MPP to recur was explained by this knowledge. MPP was renamed proliferative vitreoretinopathy (PVR) officially to represent more accurately the pathologic process.[1-4]

Surgeons, struggling to improve success rates,[5-11] realized that scarring behaved differently posterior to versus within the vitreous base, and PVR was subdivided into anterior and posterior PVR[12-17] (Fig. 9.1). Surgical technique recognizes this difference and addresses it directly.

It is essential that the vitreoretinal surgeon realizes the pathologic anatomy of PVR, especially the difference between anterior PVR and posterior PVR when attempting surgical repair. Understanding the anatomy of the vitreous base and the relationships of the vitreous to all normal and abnormal structures in the ciliary region is key[18] (Fig. 9.2).

It is well established that PVR exists in a spectrum of severity. Pathologic study of epiretinal membranes indicates that they can exist from single cell membranes without any clinical importance, through more organized membranes leading to retinal puckering, up to more severe forms involving marked retinal distortion and detachment. Most clinical classifications are based on the appearance of the retina ophthalmoscopically. From a surgical standpoint, the most useful classification remains anterior and posterior PVR since the methods of repair are different in each instance.[15] In the simplest form of posterior PVR, the procedure for macular pucker, namely vitrectomy, and membrane peeling is the treatment of choice (see Chapter 5, *Epiretinal membrane surgery*, by George A. Williams, M.D.). As posterior PVR becomes more severe and contributes to retinal detachment, peeling of epiretinal membranes causing starfolds or puckering of the retina becomes essential to mobilize the retina enough to allow the breaks to close and the retina to fit back against the pigment epithelium.

With anterior PVR, the situation becomes more complex because of the anatomy of the vitreous base and its relationship to the ciliary structures of the eye. Most importantly, because of the adherence of the vitreous and retina within the vitreous base it is impossible to remove the vitreous from the retinal surface or to remove scar from the surface in this

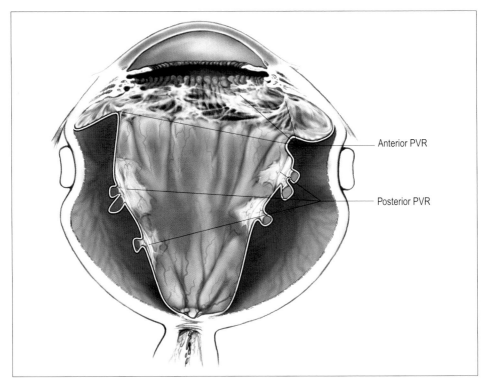

FIGURE 9.1 Anterior and posterior PVR. Anterior PVR is defined by scarring within the vitreous base and anterior vitreous. Posterior PVR is defined by scarring on the retinal surface posterior to the posterior border of the vitreous base.

region. Therefore, tractional forces cannot be eliminated completely in this zone without removing retina as well as vitreous. Furthermore, traction within the vitreous base occurs in multiple directions (Fig. 9.3). Fibrosis within the vitreous base pulls the retina centrally and moves the basal retina forward, foreshortening it. Circumferential contraction within the base draws the retina together like a 'purse-string'. Most often, these findings are more marked inferiorly, particularly after previous vitrectomy, probably because RPE cells and inflammatory cells settle there because of gravity or are concentrated there because of intraocular gas or silicone oil.

Finally, in many cases of retinal detachment that have had multiple operations, the retina itself becomes atrophic and foreshortened, thus creating an intraretinal force that prevents reattachment. It is also important to realize that vitreous connection to previous pars plana incisions or fibrous proliferation from these wounds needs to be addressed and eliminated during surgical repair.

The surgical approach to PVR should take all the above into consideration. Elimination of tractional forces is the key to success and should be the goal of all operations. The likelihood of recurrent proliferation should be recognized and planned for. Antiproliferative drugs have been tried with varying success and improvements in this area may prove to be important in the future. Currently, however, our efforts are limited to what we can do mechanically to alter the pathologic anatomy.

Surgical strategy begins with thorough analysis of this anatomy. Intervention should be titrated to eliminate the important forces present. With posterior PVR, epiretinal membranes that prevent hole closure may be managed by vitrectomy and membrane peeling

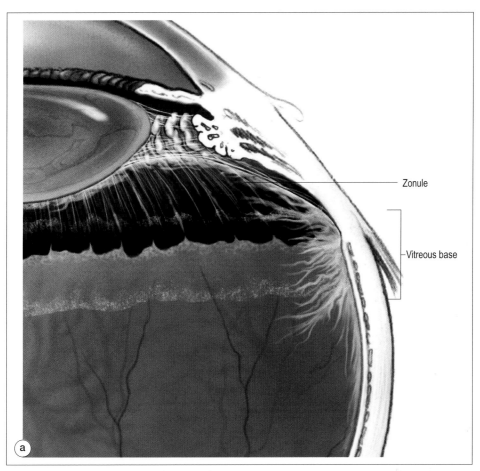

■ FIGURE 9.2 Pars plana anatomy. (**a**) The vitreous base and the ciliary portion of the zonule along the ciliary body. (**b**) The relationship of the anterior hyaloid to the vitreous base, the entire zonule, and the lens.

alone, along with an encircling scleral buckle to support the vitreous base. As anterior PVR becomes more of a problem, removal of the anterior vitreous and more aggressive scleral buckling may be necessary. In cases with established anterior PVR, more radical measures are indicated.

Currently, most cases of PVR fall into this latter category. Many have had multiple operations including pneumatic retinopexy, scleral buckling, vitrectomy, gas or silicone oil injection, and retinotomy with severe anterior PVR. The surgical technique will take this into consideration.

INSTRUMENTS AND DEVICES

- The standard vitrectomy instrument capable of fast cutting rate
- Fragmatome
- Instruments necessary to do a scleral buckle
- Instruments for removal of a polymethyl methacrylate (PMMA) or foldable intraocular lens (anterior segment tray)
- Iris retractors and/or intraocular adrenaline (epinephrine) $1:10\,000$

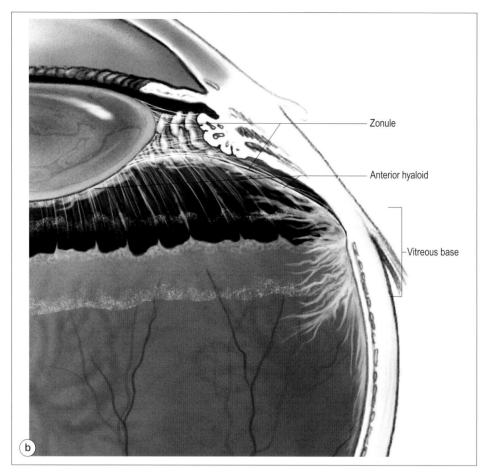

FIGURE 9.2 Cont'd

- Epiretinal membrane forceps
- Vertical cutting intraocular scissors
- Triamcinolone acetonide (Kenalog)
- Intraocular bipolar coagulation
- Extendable and flexible subretinal cannula
- Intraocular photocoagulator (endolaser probe)
- Long-acting intraocular gas, e.g. perfluoropropane (C_3F_8)
- Silicone oil

INDICATIONS AND CONTRAINDICATIONS

The decision whether or not to operate on a patient with PVR is based on the risk for and benefit to the patient. While vision is often limited even with reattachment of the retina, blindness in that eye is inevitable if there is no intervention. The health and visual needs of the patient are important factors. The condition of the fellow eye should be taken into consideration, knowing that threats to the vision of that eye are frequent in patients with rhegmatogenous disease. Having a 'spare tire' is a benefit some patients desire. On the other hand, the prognosis for reattachment with any useful vision decreases as more and

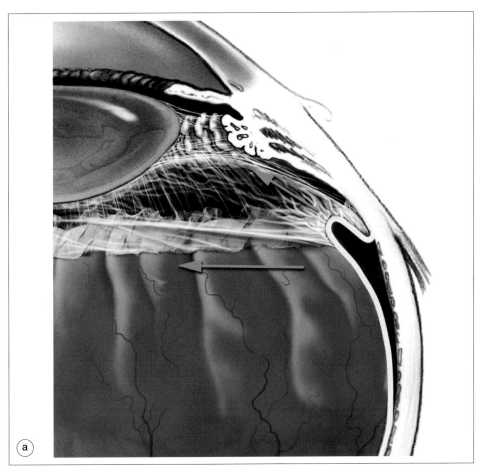

FIGURE 9.3 Tractional forces in anterior PVR. (**a**) Circumferential traction foreshortening the circumference of the vitreous base like a 'purse-string'. (**b**) Contraction of the basal vitreous gel creating anterior folding of the basal retina toward the ciliary body. (**c**) Contraction of the anterior vitreous centrally, pulling the basal retina centrally and anteriorly toward the lens capsule.

more operations are done, and there is a point where the risk and morbidity of the operation are not justified. The views of the patient are especially important in determining this point, and a candid discussion with the patient is essential in making the proper decision with them.[19–21]

SURGICAL TECHNIQUE

1. In order to adequately access the anterior vitreous and manage anterior PVR effectively, the conjunctiva must be opened widely for 360° at the limbus and undermined so that a scleral depressor can be inserted and scleral depression can be done correctly. Without this, exposure is limited and it is impossible to do a proper anterior base dissection. Furthermore, if a good 360° encircling buckle is not already present, opening the conjunctiva is necessary to do that.
2. In severe cases of anterior PVR the crystalline lens or an intraocular lens must be removed. This allows for complete removal of the posterior lenticular vitreous and

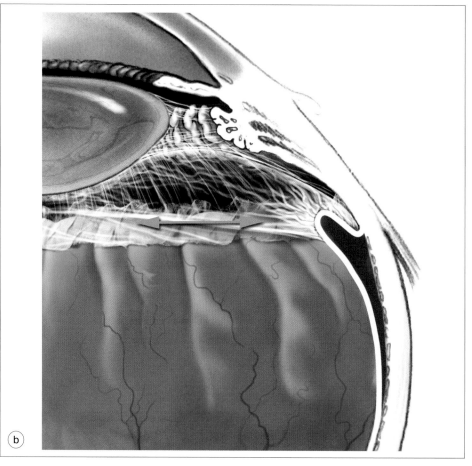

FIGURE 9.3 Cont'd

lysis of adhesions to the posterior capsule and iris. It is important to remove the entire capsule as adhesions commonly exist there. PMMA lenses require a large 5–6 mm incision for removal whereas foldable lenses can be removed through a smaller incision after being cut in half in the anterior chamber.

3. Iris retractors are placed if pupillary dilation is not good. Occasionally, adrenaline 1:10 000 will suffice.

4. Residual posterior vitreous is removed and epiretinal membranes are peeled. The macula or within the funnel of the detachment is often the best place to begin. A small amount of Kenalog dusted on the surface of the retina often facilitates this and makes the membranes more visible.

5. If the retina is sufficiently mobilized at this juncture and if the vitreous base is supported by a scleral buckle, then the retina can be reattached with perfluorocarbon liquid (PFL), or with a combination of fluid–air exchange coupled with internal drainage of subretinal fluid through a preexisting retinal break with a flexible cannula. Posterior retinotomy is rarely necessary. The retinal breaks are surrounded by endophotocoagulation and either long-acting gas or silicone oil is injected. If silicone oil is used, an inferior iridectomy is carried out with the vitreous cutter.

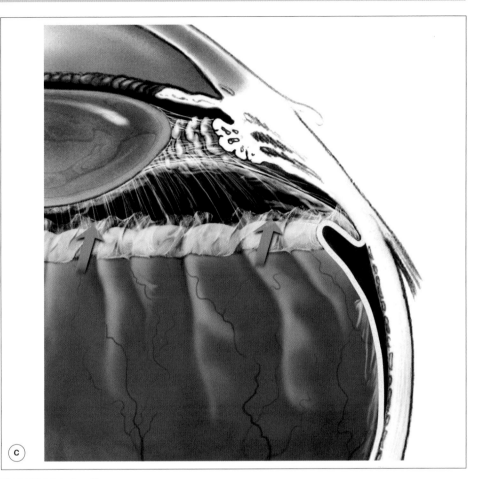

■ **FIGURE 9.3** Cont'd

6. In cases with significant anterior PVR the anterior pathology must be addressed. Using scleral depression, the anterior structures are exposed and adhesions and traction are minimized. The surgeon holds a cotton-tipped applicator in one hand as a scleral depressor and the vitreous cutter in the other. The depressor should be placed well posteriorly (near the equator) in order to rotate the anterior retina and ciliary region into view. Considerable depression is often needed to accomplish this. With the assistant shining a light pipe through the pupil, the dissection can be undertaken. The goal is to remove all the vitreous anteriorly down to the surface of the basal retina and to remove adhesions between the vitreous and the lens capsule, old sclerotomy adhesions, and the ciliary body. Thus, it is essential that the lens capsule be removed in these severe cases. If the retina is sufficiently mobilized at this point, one can proceed as in number 5 above.

7. Most often, however, at this point there is sufficient contraction within the base to prevent lasting reattachment, and one must remove the anterior basal retina to accomplish one's goals. The zone of greatest contraction is usually inferiorly, so this is the region that is removed. If retinectomy becomes necessary (a decision that requires critical clinical judgment) one should do it for at least 180°. Recurrences are most

likely to occur inferiorly and smaller retinectomies do not prevent recurrence as well as those that are 180°.

8. The inferior retinectomy is performed after first outlining the posterior vitreous base with diathermy between the 3 o'clock and 9 o'clock positions inferiorly. One can use the vitreous cutter or vertical cutting scissors to make the incision anterior to this line, but the retina from the posterior base to the ora serrata should be removed. Intraocular diathermy is used to coagulate any bleeding vessels.

9. Infrequently, subretinal scarring prevents the retina from conforming and must be removed. Access to the subretinal space is easy through the inferior retinectomy. Forceps with larger gripping surfaces, such as pyramidal forceps, grasp the membranes better than forceps with a smaller grasping surface, such as Chang forceps. Smaller posterior retinotomies may be required to access the membranes in the absence of an inferior retinectomy. They can be performed with a blade, the diathermy probe or the vitreous cutter, and should be limited to a size that just allows the forceps to be inserted.

10. The retina is then reattached. Fluid–air exchange and internal drainage with an extendable soft-tipped cannula is often successful; however, perfluorocarbon liquid may be used. Rarely, does the edge of the retina slip posteriorly.

11. Endophotocoagulation is then carried out to surround the retinotomy and any other breaks. An encircling buckle is done if not already present.

12. An inferior iridectomy is performed and silicone oil injected up to the level of the iris.

13. Postoperatively, the patient is kept face down for 24 hours and then advised not to lie on their back.

14. Silicone oil is removed 2–3 months postoperatively if the retina is completely flat.

OUTCOME

The outcome depends in most part on the severity of PVR, especially anterior PVR. Our most recent experience with severe anterior PVR cases requiring 180° retinectomy demonstrated that there was a final reattachment rate of 93%. Reoperations were required in 40%. Visual acuity ranged from 20/40 to light perception, and was improved or stabilized in 70% of eyes.[18]

COMPLICATIONS

The main complications include endophthalmitis, retinal tears, retinal detachment, potential toxicity from tPA and cataract. The complications associated with vitrectomy are also covered in Chapter 2, *Vitrectomy surgery* by Abdhish R. Bhavsar, MD.

POSTOPERATIVE CARE

The main portions of postoperative care pertain to postoperative positioning and most surgeons recommend at least one day of upright positioning after surgery to allow the gas bubble to squeegee the subretinal hemorrhage out of the macular region and then perhaps 1–5 days of face down positioning to allow the macula to become attached and to close the 39-gauge retinotomy sites. The typical postoperative medications include topical steroid and cycloplegic drops. A topical antibiotic may also be used per the surgeon's preference. Follow up is typically scheduled for the day after surgery, one week later, 3–4 weeks later and then 4–8 weeks later. Additional treatment for exudative AMD is then administered as needed.

REFERENCES

1. Machemer R, Aaberg TM, Freeman HM, Irvine AR, Lean JS, Michels RM. An updated classification of retinal detachment with proliferative vitreoretinopathy. Am J Ophthalmol 1991; 112(2):159–165.
2. Schepens CL. Proliferative vitreoretinopathy (PVR). Ophthalmology 1987; 94(2):201.
3. Ryan SJ. The pathophysiology of proliferative vitreoretinopathy in its management. Am J Ophthalmol 1985;100(1):188–193.
4. Michels RG. Surgery of retinal detachment with proliferative vitreoretinopathy. Retina 1984; 4(2):63–83.
5. Abrams GW, Azen SP, McCuen BW 2nd, Flynn HW Jr, Lai MY, Ryan SJ. Vitrectomy with silicone oil or long-acting gas in eyes with severe proliferative vitreoretinopathy: results of additional and long-term follow-up. Silicone Study Report 11. Arch Ophthalmol 1997; 115(3):335–344.
6. Charteris DG. Proliferative vitreoretinopathy: pathobiology, surgical management, and adjunctive treatment. Br J Ophthalmol 1995; 79(10):953–960.
7. McCuen BW 2nd, Azen SP, Stern W, Lai MY, Lean JS, Linton KL, Ryan SJ. Vitrectomy with silicone oil or perfluoropropane gas in eyes with severe proliferative vitreoretinopathy. Silicone Study Report 3. Retina 1993; 13(4):279–284.
8. Lewis H, Aaberg TM, Abrams GW. Causes of failure after initial vitreoretinal surgery for severe proliferative vitreoretinopathy. Am J Ophthalmol 1991; 111(1):8–14.
9. Lewis H, Burke JM, Abrams GW, Aaberg TM. Perisilicone proliferation after vitrectomy for proliferative vitreoretinopathy. Ophthalmology 1988;95(5):583–591.
10. Gonvers M. Temporary silicone oil tamponade in the management of retinal detachment with proliferative vitreoretinopathy. Am J Ophthalmol 1985; 100(2):239–245.
11. Sternberg P Jr, Machemer R. Results of conventional vitreous surgery for proliferative vitreoretinopathy. Am J Ophthalmol 1985; 100(1):141–146.
12. Diddie KR, Azen SP, Freeman HM, et al. Anterior proliferative vitreoretinopathy in the silicone study. Silicone Study Report 10. Ophthalmology 1996; 103(7):1092–1099.
13. Lopez PF, Grossniklaus HE, Aaberg TM, Sternberg P Jr, Capone A Jr, Lambert HM. Pathogenetic mechanisms in anterior proliferative vitreoretinopathy. Am J Ophthalmol 1992; 114(3):257–279.
14. Lean JS, Stern WH, Irvine AR, Azen SP. Classification of proliferative vitreoretinopathy used in the silicone study. The Silicone Study Group. Ophthalmology 1989; 96(6):765–771.
15. Aaberg TM. Management of anterior and posterior proliferative vitreoretinopathy. XLV. Edward Jackson memorial lecture. Am J Ophthalmol 1988; 106(5):519–532.
16. Elner SG, Elner VM, Diaz-Rohena R, Freeman HM, Tolentino FI, Albert DM. Anterior proliferative vitreoretinopathy. Clinicopathologic, light microscopic, and ultrastructural findings. Ophthalmology 1988; 95(10):1349–1357.
17. Lewis H, Aaberg TM. Anterior proliferative vitreoretinopathy. Am J Ophthalmol 1988; 105(3):277–284.
18. Quiram PA, Gonzales CG, Hu W, Gupta A, Yoshizumi MO, Kreiger AE, Schwartz SD. Outcomes of vitrectomy with inferior retinectomy in patients with recurrent rhegmatogenous retinal detachments and proliferative vitreoretinopathy. Ophthalmology 2006; 113(11):2041–2047.
19. Brown GC, Brown MM, Sharma S, Busbee B, Landy J. A cost–utility analysis of interventions for severe proliferative vitreoretinopathy. Am J Ophthalmol 2002; 133(3):365–372.
20. Schwartz SD, Kreiger AE. Proliferative vitreoretinopathy: a natural history of the fellow eye. Ophthalmology 1998; 105(5):785–788.
21. McCormack P, Simcock PR, Charteris D, Lavin MJ. Is surgery for proliferative vitreoretinopathy justifiable? Eye 1994; 8(Pt 1):75–76.

Surgery for submacular hemorrhage

Keye L. Wong

INSTRUMENTS

The main instrument needed is a 39-gauge (or 41-gauge) flexible translocation cannula which creates a self-sealing retinotomy. Vitrectomy surgery with wide-field viewing systems and use of a wide-field light pipe are helpful. Cathflo Activase (Alteplase, Genentech, San Francisco, California) is a recombinant tissue plasminogen activator (tPA) which is Food and Drug Administration approved for the restoration of function to central venous access devices when they have become clotted and blood is unable to be withdrawn. The use of tPA for ocular disorders is therefore off-label. tPA comes in a 2 mg vial (Cathflo Activase) used for clearing central venous lines and costs about $60, whereas a 50 mg vial used for treatment of acute myocardial infarctions (Tenecteplase) costs $1924 to the pharmacy and $9330 billed to insurance. 2 mg Alteplase is reconstituted with 8 cc of sterile water (not bacteriostatic) to provide a concentration of 25 mcg/0.1 cc.

INDICATIONS AND CONTRAINDICATIONS

Subretinal hemorrhage may result from multiple etiologies. Although age-related macular degeneration (AMD) may be the most common etiology, other causes include high myopia, trauma, angioid streaks, diabetic retinopathy, macroaneurysms, Valsalva maneuver, idiopathic, presumed ocular histoplasmosis syndrome, and other inflammatory diseases affecting the retina and choroid (acute posterior multifocal placoid pigment epitheliopathy [APMPPE], birdshot, etc.).

Animal models suggest that the presence of whole blood between the neurosensory retina and the retinal pigment epithelium (RPE) is sufficient to cause permanent and irreversible damage to the photoreceptors. When whole blood was injected into the subretinal space of rabbits, irreversible damage to the photoreceptors was observed in as little as 24 hours.[1] Three theoretical mechanisms were proposed to cause this photoreceptor damage: (1) toxic effects of iron released from hemoglobin; (2) a nutritional deficit created by the physical barrier of the hemorrhage between the retina and RPE; and (3) mechanical damage to the photoreceptors created by clot retraction. The theoretical damage created by clot retraction was supported by experimental studies in a holangiotic cat model in which autologous blood was injected into the subretinal space.[2] Within 1 hour fibrin was associated with tearing of photoreceptor outer segments. Within 2–3 days the blood clot had become organized with secondary degeneration of the photoreceptor outer segments observed.

Despite the evidence demonstrated in these animal models suggesting irreversible damage to the photoreceptors within 1–3 days, the natural history of subretinal hemorrhage is not necessarily ominous and may vary depending upon the etiology and the thickness of the hemorrhage. In a multicenter retrospective review of subretinal hemorrhages due to ruptured macroaneurysms managed by observation alone, a final visual acuity of 20/40 was observed in 37%.[3] This favorable outcome was noted even though the mean time for clearance of subretinal hemorrhage was 4.6 months. Other case series suggest that submacular hemorrhages from causes other than AMD and choroidal neovascularization may have a relatively benign natural history.[4,5]

In contrast, several retrospective chart reviews propose that subretinal hemorrhages secondary to AMD have a much poorer prognosis.[6-8] The Submacular Surgery Group B Trial[9] evaluated subfoveal choroidal neovascular lesions greater than 3.5 disc areas in which at least 50% of the lesion was composed of blood. Eligible subjects were randomized to either surgical extraction or observation. In the observation arm, only 11% of patients maintained a vision of 20/200 at 24 months as compared to 38% at baseline, and 40% of patients lost vision to 20/800 at 24 months.

Given the generally poor natural history of subretinal hemorrhages secondary to AMD, and the variable natural history of non-AMD subretinal hemorrhages, it seems reasonable to restrict potential surgical interventions to the AMD subgroup. Pars plana vitrectomy with internal drainage and/or mechanical extraction of the subretinal clot can be technically challenging and complicated. Using such a surgical technique on patients with 'massive' subretinal hemorrhage and initial vision of 20/400, Vander et al. reported that 4 of 11 patients developed retinal detachment secondary to proliferative vitreoretinopathy.[10] Larger series also demonstrate a high complication rate of mechanical extraction of subfoveal neovascular complexes. At 24 months of follow-up the Submacular Surgery Trial did not find a visual acuity benefit for surgical removal of subfoveal choroidal neovascularization in AMD either with or without blood. Without blood there was a 5% retinal detachment rate among 226 eyes[11] whereas removal of hemorrhagic subfoveal choroidal neovascular lesions resulted in a 16% retinal detachment rate in 168 eyes. Half of these retinal detachments in the hemorrhagic group were complicated by PVR.[9] The results of the Submacular Surgery Trial therefore suggest that mechanical extraction of hemorrhagic choroidal neovascular membranes has a higher retinal detachment and PVR rate. My personal experience has been similarly challenging and supportive of the poor results reported in the literature. I have therefore abandoned this approach.

I have adopted the technique of tPA-assisted pneumatic hemodisplacement.[12] Indications for this surgical technique are acute or subacute loss of vision due to subfoveal hemorrhage secondary to AMD. The mechanical goal of surgery is to effect displacement of hemorrhage away from the subfoveal photoreceptors. The patient should be advised that subsequent management of the presumed underlying choroidal neovascularization is necessary.

This technique was initially reported by Carl Awh at the 2001 Vitreous Society Annual Meeting and conceptualized following the observation of an iatrogenic subfoveal hemorrhage occurring at the time of limited macular translocation surgery. In spite of this complication the surgery was successfully completed with subsequent fluid–air exchange and postoperative upright positioning to facilitate inferior displacement of the macula. On the first postoperative day the hemorrhage had migrated completely to the far inferior periphery of the subretinal space. Dr Awh hypothesized that the rapid movement of hemorrhage was facilitated by the temporary retinal detachment. Further investigation of the literature suggested that tPA retinal toxicity was concentration and not volume dependent, for which he subsequently began in 1999 to investigate the use of a dilute solution of tPA to facilitate pneumatic displacement of thick submacular hemorrhages (C Awh, personal communication).

Tissue plasminogen activator is a thrombolytic enzyme which has limited enzymatic effect in the absence of fibrin. However, in the presence of fibrin within a thrombus, tPA binds to fibrin and converts the entrapped plasminogen to plasmin. This plasmin then initiates local fibrinolysis. Because fibrin may be responsible for mechanical tearing of the photoreceptors, the adjunctive use of this agent in management of subretinal hemorrhage may be helpful. Toxicity studies in rabbits[13] and cats[14] show no toxic effects of intravitreal tPA at 25 mcg but increasing toxicity at doses of 50–100 mcg. When injected into the subretinal space of cats at concentrations of 0.0125–100 mcg/0.1 cc,[15] toxic effects were not seen at 20 mcg/0.1 mL but were seen at 100 mcg/0.1 mL.

SURGICAL TECHNIQUE

10.1

A standard three-port pars plana vitrectomy is performed with removal of the posterior hyaloid. Tissue plasminogen activator (25 mcg/0.1 cc of sterile water) is injected into the subretinal space via a 39-gauge flexible cannula initially designed for use during retinal translocation surgery. This infusion can be performed either with surgeon control by using the viscous fluid injector or with assistant control using flexible tubing connected to a tuberculin syringe containing the tPA solution. If under surgeon control the infusion pressure should be adjusted such that the drip rate is 1–2 drops per second. If the tPA solution is injected under assistant control the assistant should be alerted that the tactile resistance to infusion is high due to the small gauge of the infusion needle. The assistant should be warned that if a tuberculin syringe without a Luer-lock connection is utilized, a high infusion pressure may cause the tubing to spontaneously disconnect from the syringe with subsequent loss of the tPA solution from the syringe. Insertion of the cannula into the eye should be done with direct visualization under microscope illumination to prevent bending of the flexible cannula upon entry through the sclerotomy. Translocation cannulas are available for 25-gauge vitrectomy systems.

I prefer a wide-angle viewing system with a wide-field illumination in order that the entire posterior pole can be visualized and illuminated during the surgery. Since my depth perception is not as acute with the wide-field viewing system I utilize the visual clue of the tip of the flexible translocation cannula 'touching' its shadow as a determination of when the cannula is about to penetrate the retina (Fig. 10.1). Infusion is initiated just prior to touching the retina. There will often be centrifugal displacement of the subretinal hemorrhage as the cannula initially touches the retina but prior to penetration (Fig. 10.2). Penetration of the retina is identified primarily by the development of a subretinal bleb, at which time further advancement of the translocation cannula is halted. With a constant infusion rate, the centrifugal advancing edge of the subretinal bleb is initially easily visible. The first 0.1 cc of infusion will create a bleb of approximately one disc diameter (Fig. 10.3). The subsequent injection of an additional 0.1 cc of fluid will only increase the bleb's diameter by about 20% (Fig. 10.4). It may therefore appear that continued infusion is not penetrating the subretinal space whereas, in reality, the incremental increase in the diameter of the subretinal bleb becomes more difficult to recognize. To therefore create a large subretinal bleb, patience by the surgeon will often be advisable rather than resorting to a second or third infusion site.

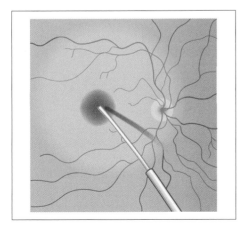

■ **FIGURE 10.1** The translocation cannula is advanced until the tip of the cannula 'touches' the tip of its shadow.

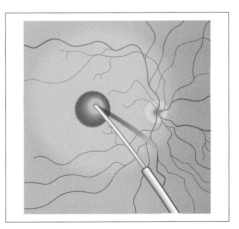

■ **FIGURE 10.2** As the translocation cannula penetrates the retina there will often be a slight peripheral displacement of the subretinal hemorrhage.

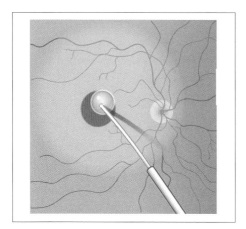

FIGURE 10.3 0.1 cc of subretinal fluid infusion will typically cause a bleb of about one disc diameter in size.

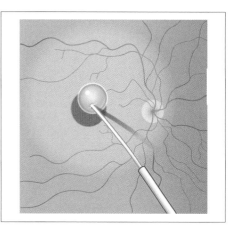

FIGURE 10.4 Subsequent subretinal infusion of an additional 0.1 cc will only increase the bleb diameter by 20%.

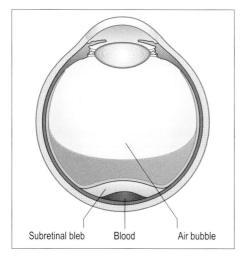

Subretinal bleb   Blood   Air bubble

FIGURE 10.5 With the patient supine, a partial gas bubble has no effect on the macula.

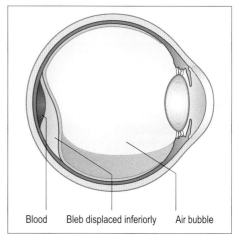

Blood   Bleb displaced inferiorly   Air bubble

FIGURE 10.6 With the patient head up, a partial gas bubble will displace the subretinal fluid inferiorly and thus create a larger potential space for displacement of the 'liquefied' hemorrhage.

The surgical goal of the subretinal infusion is twofold. The first is to deliver tPA to beyond the margins of the blood clot to effect liquefaction. The second goal is to create a potential space for the liquefied blood to migrate away from the subfoveal area. A volume of 0.2–0.3 mL is typically sufficient to create a bleb which extends anterior to the temporal arcades. There may be an asymmetric migration of the subretinal bleb. Since the blood seems to migrate inferiorly I attempt to continue infusion until I create a subretinal bleb which extends beyond the inferotemporal arcade and also encompasses the boundaries of hemorrhage. A 75% air exchange is performed and a postoperative head-up position is recommended. In my opinion the purpose of this air bubble is primarily to effect inferior displacement of fluid from the induced subretinal bleb. By maintaining a head-up position, a partial gas fill creates a larger potential space inferiorly to which the hemorrhage can subsequently migrate (Figs 10.5 and 10.6).

In the recovery area the patient is instructed to maintain a supine position for 15 min such that the tPA can induce its enzymatic effect on the submacular blood clot. After discharge from the recovery room the patient is instructed to maintain postoperative positioning in a head-up position during waking hours and to sleep with the operated eye down to allow migration of the blood either inferiorly or temporally.

Postoperative fluorescein angiography or imaging studies are performed with treatment of choroidal neovascularization as indicated.

OUTCOME

In 29 eyes of 28 patients reported by Olivier et al.,[12] total displacement of submacular hemorrhage was achieved in 25 eyes and subtotal displacement was achieved in the other 4 eyes. At 3 months of follow-up, 17 of 29 eyes had gained two lines of visual acuity whereas 2 of 29 eyes had lost two lines of visual acuity.

The first 50 procedures which I performed were between June 2002 and January 2005. The average age of these patients was 80 ± 7 years, with 30 being female. All of these subfoveal hemorrhages were related to AMD. The typical indications were acute loss of vision related to the subfoveal hemorrhage with a history of preceding better vision. The majority (60%) of patients had preoperative vision of 20/200–20/400.

Preoperative visions were as shown in Table 10.1; best postoperative visions were as shown in Table 10.2.

Of the 24 patients who achieved best postoperative vision of 20/100, several of these patients were 20/40 (Table 10.3). Although best postoperative vision is often not as good as 'final' postoperative vision or postoperative vision at 1 year, this may still be a reasonable way to evaluate efficacy of this procedure in light of the advent of more potent pharmacologic therapy (i.e. bevacizumab or ranibizumab) which has a greater anti-angiogenic effect than prior therapies.

One of the factors relating to visual success may be the timing of surgery. When comparing the lines of improved vision (best postoperative vision minus preoperative vision) as related to the time between reported onset of symptoms and surgery, there appears to be a better chance of vision recovery with earlier surgery (Table 10.4).

TABLE 10.1

Preoperative visual acuity	≥20/100	20/200	20/400	20/800	CF	HM
No. of patients	5	15	15	2	10	3

TABLE 10.2

Best postoperative visual acuity	≥20/100	20/200	20/400	20/800	CF	HM
No. of patients	24	16	5	0	4	1

TABLE 10.3

Best postoperative visual acuity	≥20/40	20/50–20/60	20/70–20/80	20/100
No. of patients	10	5	5	4

TABLE 10.4

Time from onset to surgery	1–2 days	3–4 days	5–7 days	1–2 weeks	3–4 weeks	>4 weeks
No. of lines of vision improved	6.2 ± 4.0	3.9 ± 2.8	2.8 ± 2.7	1.5 ± 1.5	2.2 ± 2.9	1.6 ± 1.4

TABLE 10.5

Time from onset to surgery	1–2 days	3–4 days	5–7 days	1–2 weeks	3–4 weeks	≥4 weeks
No. achieving visual acuity ≥20/40	3/6	3/7	1/8	0/8	3/9	0/12

In spite of a trend for patients that underwent early surgery to have a better visual outcome, there were some patients that underwent surgery 3–4 weeks after onset of symptoms and still obtained a best postoperative vision of 20/40 (Table 10.5).

Two rhegmatogenous retinal detachments occurred in this group of 50 patients. One of the detachments was from a macular hole in a highly myopic individual.

COMPLICATIONS

The main complications include endophthalmitis, retinal tears, retinal detachment, potential toxicity from tPA and cataract. The complications associated with vitrectomy are also covered in Chapter 2, *Vitrectomy surgery* by Abdhish R. Bhavsar, MD.

POSTOPERATIVE CARE

The main portions of postoperative care pertain to postoperative positioning and most surgeons recommend at least one day of upright positioning after surgery to allow the gas bubble to squeegee the subretinal hemorrhage out of the macular region and then perhaps 1–5 days of face down positioning to allow the macula to become attached and to close the 39-gauge retinotomy sites. The typical postoperative medications include topical steroid and cycloplegic drops. A topical antibiotic may also be used per the surgeon's preference. Follow up is typically scheduled for the day after surgery, one week later, 3–4 weeks later and then 4–8 weeks later. Additional treatment for exudative AMD is then administered as needed.

REFERENCES

1. Glatt H, Machemer R. Experimental subretinal hemorrhage in rabbits. Am J Ophthalmol 1982; 94:762– 773.
2. Toth CA, Morse LS, Hjelmeland LM, et al. Fibrin directs early retinal damage after experimental subretinal hemorrhage. Arch Ophthalmol 1991; 109:723–729.
3. McCabe CM, Flynn HW Jr, McLean WC, et al. Nonsurgical management of macular hemorrhage secondary to retinal macroaneurysms. Arch Ophthalmol 2000; 118:780–785.
4. Berrocal MH, Lewis ML, Flynn HW Jr. Variations in the clinical course of

submacular hemorrhage. Am J Ophthalmol 1996; 122:486–493.

5. Uyama M, Matsubara T, Fukushima I, et al. Idiopathic polypoidal choroidal vasculopathy in Japanese patients. Arch Ophthalmol 1999; 117:1035–1042.

6. Bennett SR, Folk JC, Blodi CF, et al. Factors prognostic of visual outcome in patients with subretinal hemorrhage. Am J Ophthalmol 1990; 109:33–37.

7. Avery RL, Fekrat S, Hawkins BS, et al. Natural history of subfoveal subretinal hemorrhage in age-related macular degeneration. Retina 1996; 16:183–189.

8. Scupola A, Coscas G, Soubrane G, et al. Natural history of subretinal hemorrhage in age-related macular degeneration. Ophthalmologica 1999; 213:97–102.

9. SST Research Group. Surgery for hemorrhagic choroidal neovascular lesions of age-related macular degeneration: ophthalmic findings. SST Report No. 13. Ophthalmology 2004; 111:1993–2006.

10. Vander JF, Federman JL, Greven C, et al. Surgical removal of massive subretinal hemorrhage associated with age-related macular degeneration. Ophthalmology 1991; 98:23–27.

11. SST Research Group. Surgery for subfoveal choroidal neovascularization in age-related macular degeneration: ophthalmic findings. SST Report No. 11. Ophthalmology 2004; 111:1967–1980.

12. Olivier S, Chow DR, Packo KH, et al. Subretinal recombinant tissue plasminogen activator injection and pneumatic displacement of thick submacular hemorrhage in age-related macular degeneration. Ophthalmology 2004; 111:1201–1208.

13. Johnson MW, Olsen KR, Hernandez E, et al. Retinal toxicity of recombinant tissue plasminogen activator in the rabbit. Arch Ophthalmol 1990; 108:259–263.

14. Hrach CJ, Johnson MW, Hassan AS, et al. Retinal toxicity of commercial intravitreal tissue plasminogen activator solution in cat eyes. Arch Ophthalmol 2000; 118:659–663.

15. Benner JD, Morse LS, Toth CA, et al. Evaluation of a commercial recombinant tissue-type plasminogen activator preparation in the subretinal space of the cat. Arch Ophthalmol 1991; 109:1731–1736.

11 Intravitreal injections

Abdhish R. Bhavsar

INSTRUMENTATION

- Topical medications (dilating drops)
  - Tropicamide 1%
  - Phenylephrine 2.5%
- Topical anesthetic, e.g. proparacaine hydrochloride or tetracaine (Bausch & Lomb)
- Povidone iodine 5%
- Medication to be administered by intravitreal injection
- Calipers
- Lid speculum, sterile
- Cotton-tipped applicators, sterile
- Gauze eye patch (used only if there is excessive subconjunctival hemorrhage post injection)
- 30-gauge, 5/8 inch needle for intravitreal injection
- Appropriate needles, filter needles, and syringes if needed for dilution or other preparation of the medicine for injection
- 1 cc syringe and 30-gauge, 5/8 inch needle for potential anterior chamber paracentesis
- Tissue, i.e. Kleenex

INDICATIONS

Intravitreal injections are performed in order to deliver medication into the vitreous cavity for the treatment of a variety of retinal conditions and diseases. The indications range broadly from the treatment of endophthalmitis to macular degeneration and from macular edema due to diseases such as diabetic retinopathy and uveitis to vitreous hemorrhage. A number of current indications for intravitreal injections are listed in Box 11.1.

BACKGROUND

Intravitreal injection as a method of administering substances into the vitreous cavity has been present for almost a century. In 1911 Ohm described a method of injecting air into the vitreous cavity to achieve tamponade of the retina for repair of retinal detachment.[1] Injection of pharmacotherapeutic agents into the vitreous cavity began in the 1940s with intravitreal injection of penicillin for experimental endophthalmitis.[2] However, the use of intravitreal injections was not common. In the 1970s the discovery of additional antibiotic agents led to further use of intravitreal injections including kanamycin and gentamicin, which were used in experimental models of endophthalmitis.[3,4] Over the next two decades, additional support for the clinical use of intravitreal injections for endophthalmitis came with the publication of additional case series.[5–8]

The use of other pharmacotherapeutics administered by intravitreal injection was delayed until the 1980s and 1990s. 5-Fluorouracil was administered by intravitreal injection in vitreoretinal surgery to decrease fibroblast proliferation.[9] Intravitreal injection of ganciclovir was then used to treat a patient with cytomegalovirus (CMV) retinitis.[10] Intravitreal dexamethasone phosphate was then studied in a randomized trial and was injected

BOX 11.1 Potential indications for intravitreal injections[a]

Endophthalmitis

- Antibiotics (e.g. vancomycin, ceftazidime, clindamycin, amikacin)

Exudative macular degeneration

- Triamcinolone acetonide (typically as an adjunct to verteporfin [Visudyne])
- Pegaptanib sodium[b]
- Ranibizumab[b]
- Bevacizumab

Macular edema related to diabetic retinopathy, pseudophakia, retinal vein occlusions, or uveitis

- Triamcinolone acetonide
- Bevacizumab
- Ranibizumab
- Pegaptanib

Neovascular glaucoma

- Bevacizumab
- Triamcinolone acetonide

Rubeosis

- Bevacizumab
- Triamcinolone acetonide

Uveitis or vasculitis

- Triamcinolone acetonide

Vitreous hemorrhage

- Ovine hyaluronidase

[a]*The indications listed are potential indications at this time for intravitreal injection of a variety of medications, which may or may not be approved by the FDA for intravitreal use.*
[b]*These medications are approved by the FDA for intravitreal injection for the treatment of specific diseases.*

after vitrectomy surgery for diabetic retinopathy.[11] Another steroid, triamcinolone acetonide, was administered intravitreally in exudative age-related macular degeneration (AMD) patients as part of a pilot study.[12] Intravitreal injection of tissue plasminogen activator (tPA) and expansile gas was used to help dissolve and displace submacular hemorrhage in a retrospective series of patients.[13]

The first pharmacotherapy approved by the Food and Drug Administration (FDA) for intravitreal injection was fomivirsen sodium (Vitravene, Isis Pharmaceuticals, Carlsbad, California) for CMV retinitis.[14] This was followed by anti-VEGF (vascular endothelial growth factor) intravitreal agents for exudative AMD: pegaptanib sodium (Macugen, OSI-Eyetech-Pfizer Pharmaceuticals, New York, New York, and Gilead Sciences, San Dimas, California), which gained FDA approval in 2004,[15,16] and ranibizumab (Lucentis, Genentech, Inc., San Francisco, California) which gained approval in 2006.[17] Although ovine hyaluronidase (Vitrase, Ista Pharmaceuticals, Irvine, California) has been shown to have safety and modest efficacy for the clearance of severe vitreous hemorrhage in phase III clinical trials,[18,19] it has not received FDA approval for intravitreal use for the clearance of vitreous hemorrhage. However, it is currently approved by the FDA as an adjunct to help with the dispersion of other drugs.[20]

There are a number of pharmacotherapies that have not been approved by the FDA, but that are currently used for the treatment of retinal diseases by intravitreal injection, including, but not limited to:

- antibiotics (i.e. vancomycin, ceftazidime, clindamycin) for endophthalmitis
- triamcinolone acetonide (Kenalog, Bristol Meyers Squibb, New York, New York) for macular edema due to diabetic retinopathy,[21,22] pseudophakia,[23] retinal vein occlusion[24,25]
- triamcirolone acetonide for exudative age-related macular degeneration, typically as an adjunct to verteporfin,[26–29] for rubeosis and neovascular glaucoma[30]
- bevacizumab (Avastin, Genentech, Inc., San Francisco, California) for exudative AMD,[31,32] macular edema due to pseudophakia,[33] retinal vein occlusion,[34,35] diabetic retinopathy,[36] and rubeosis or neovascular glaucoma.[37]

There has been a tremendous increase in the number of intravitreal injections performed by retina specialists over the past few years and there are a number of agents under development that may be administered by intravitreal injection in the future. Knowledge of appropriate injection techniques and methods of minimizing potential risks of the injection procedure are essential.

PREOPERATIVE PREPARATION

The preparation of the patient prior to intravitreal injection includes a discussion of the risks, benefits, and alternatives to the injection. The surgeon performing the injection should initiate this discussion prior to the preparation of the eye. The author prefers to include family members in this discussion as well, provided that the patient would like them to be part of the discussion. After appropriate informed consent is obtained, the preparation of the eye is carried out.

The preparation of the eye and ocular surface is critical.[38–40] After dilation of the pupil with tropicamide and phenylephrine, the author: (1) confirms the pathology to be treated and the eye to be treated with slit lamp biomicroscopy and fundus examination; and (2) confirms verbally with the patient the eye to be treated and the medication to be injected.

PROCEDURE

The preparation of the patient and family members prior the injection is essential. The patient and family are counseled by the physician prior to each injection about the medication to be injected; about treatment options, risks, benefits, and alternatives; and about the injection procedure itself. The author then marks the correct eye to be injected with a piece of paper tape containing the notation 'OD' or 'OS' and the name of the medication to be injected. The author has also trained his staff members to review with the patient and their family members the injection procedure, medications, side effects and risks, so that the information can be repeated for patient retention. The staff also obtains the written confirmation of the treatment eye and the patient completes the consent form. The author has also instituted a separate 'Patient Responsibility' form containing the signs and symptoms that the patient is responsible for noticing and containing an acknowledgement that it is the patient's responsibility for contacting the physician under those circumstances (Box 11.2).

The physical setup for intravitreal injections in the office is important. Since the procedure of intravitreal injections is frequently utilized today, and will likely be more frequently utilized in the near future, it is critical to organize the injection-related equipment and materials in an efficient and reproducible manner. When the setup is the same time after time, then the chance of missing a step is minimized. For example, the staff places the speculum, calipers, povidone iodine, topical anesthetic, needles, syringes, and medicine to be injected in the same general location on the table just prior to each injection procedure (Fig. 11.1a). The author has started to use a stainless steel injection tray in his primary office locations for placement of all of the injection-related materials, including

BOX 11.2 Patient responsibility form

This particular form also has some specific language pertaining to Avastin. This form can be tailored to specific medications or it can be altered for general use for all intravitreal injections. Adapted from OMIC (Ophthalmic Mutual Insurance Company) web site: http://www.omic.com

Patient responsibility/consent form

Patient responsibilities

I will immediately contact my ophthalmologist if any of the following signs of infection or other complications develop: pain, blurry or decreased vision, sensitivity to light, redness of the eye, or discharge from the eye. I have been instructed NOT to rub my eyes or swim for 3 days after the injection. I will keep all post-injection appointments or scheduled phone calls so my doctor can check for complications. _____ **Patient's initials**

Although the likelihood of serious complications affecting other organs of my body is low, I will immediately contact my primary care physician or go to the Emergency Room if I experience abdominal pain associated with constipation and vomiting, abdominal bleeding, chest pain, severe headache, slurred speech, or weakness on one side of my body. As soon as possible, I will also notify my ophthalmologist of these problems. _____ **Patient's initials**

I will inform my ophthalmologist if I need to have any surgery, and I will inform any other surgeons, including dentists, that I am on medication that needs to be stopped before I can have surgery. _____ **Patient's initials**

Patient consent

The above explanation has been read by/to me. The nature of my eye condition has been explained to me and the proposed treatment has been described. The risks, benefits, alternatives, and limitations of the treatment have been discussed with me. All my questions have been answered.

I understand that Avastin was approved by the Food and Drug Administration for the treatment of metastatic colorectal cancer, and has not been approved for the treatment of eye conditions. Nevertheless, I wish to be treated with Avastin, and I am willing to accept the potential risks. _____ **Patient's initials**

I hereby authorize Dr. _____/Dr. _____ to administer the intravitreal injection of Avastin in my **right/left** eye at regular intervals as needed. This consent will be valid until I revoke it or my condition changes to the point that the risks and benefits of this medication for me are significantly different.

_____   _____
Patient's signature   Date

_____   _____
Witness's signature   Date

the medication to be injected (Fig. 11.1b). The tray can be prepared in advance with all the appropriate items, such as needles, syringes, speculum, and calipers. Multiple trays can be prepared at the beginning of the clinic. The staff typically prepares six trays at the start of the clinic and places them neatly on a side counter. The only item absent from the tray is the medication to be injected which is chosen just prior to bringing the injection tray into the room. This improves office efficiency and also improves the presentation of the injection materials in front of the patient. The trays are wiped clean with a sterilizing solution after each use and are prepared once again for an upcoming injection. The author has approximately 20 sets of sterilized calipers and specula in each office that are sterilized at the end of the prior clinic day, so that staff time for sterilization procedures during the middle of the clinic day can be minimized.

After the eye has been dilated, and after confirmation of the correct eye and correct medication for injection, several drops of topical anesthetic (proparacaine or tetracaine) are placed on the ocular surface. The author marks the correct eye for injection by placing

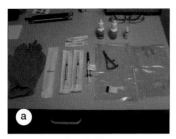
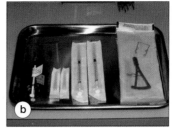

■ **FIGURE 11.1** (**a**) Example of equipment organization and setup for intravitreal injection, including topical anesthetic, povidone–iodine, sterile calipers, sterile lid speculum, 1-cc syringes and 30-gauge needles for intravitreal injection and for potential paracentesis, and gloves. (**b**) Example of a stainless steel 'injection' tray containing syringes, needles, speculum and caliper.

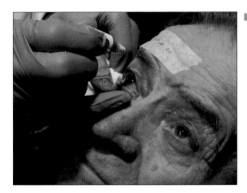

■ **FIGURE 11.2** Example of marking the eye for injection with paper tape containing notation of medicine and eye for injection and placement of povidone–iodine on the conjunctival surface.

a piece of paper tape with a notation of the medicine and eye to be injected (Fig. 11.2). Several drops of topical povidone iodine 5% are then placed on the ocular surface and lids. There has been no study that has proven that any medication reduces the risk of endophthalmitis after intravitreal injections. However, povidone iodine is the only substance proven to reduce the risk of endophthalmitis after intraocular surgery.[41] Although there may be a synergistic effect of topical antibiotics and topical povidone iodine in reducing the culture-positive rate of the preoperative conjunctival surface, topical antibiotics have not been shown to reduce the risk of endophthalmitis.[42] (Topical antibiotics may be placed on the ocular surface as an option; however, the author does not typically use such antibiotics since there is no evidence to support their use to reduce the risk of infection after intraocular surgery or intravitreal injections.) There is some evidence from case series that topical povidone iodine 5% pre- and post-injection is sufficient to reduce the risk of endophthalmitis, and that antibiotic prophylaxis is not necessary for intravitreal injections.[44] The excess anesthetic and povidone iodine are blotted away from the periocular region with a clean tissue. Care is taken to avoid placing pressure on the lids or lid margins in order to avoid expressing bacteria from within the glands in the eyelids onto the ocular surface.

For endophthalmitis patients, the typical anesthetic procedure is slightly altered, in that the author recommends using a subconjunctival injection of lidocaine 2% in the quadrant of the anticipated vitreous tap and injections. For specific management of endophthalmitis, please refer to Chapter 16, *Vitreous biopsy for endophthalmitis or cytology*, by Robert G. Josephberg, M.D.

The patient is instructed on the next steps of the procedure, including placement of the speculum and the injection itself. The author prepares the patient by telling them that he will be counting down to the injection time and be counting the seconds during the injection itself. The patient is instructed that the actual injection itself (the time that the needle is in the eye) will take less than 3 seconds. The patient is instructed to keep both hands down and to avoid moving during the procedure. A lid speculum is then placed and care is taken to avoid excess manipulation or pressure on the eyelids. The patient is instructed to look superonasally in order to expose the inferotemporal quadrant.

Sterile calipers are used to measure 3.0–3.5 mm posterior to the limbus in aphakic or pseudophakic patients and 3.5–4.0 mm posterior to the limbus in phakic patients (Fig. 11.3). The author typically makes an episcleral mark at a slightly different meridian from the intended injection site to avoid any possible contamination of the injection site itself (Fig. 11.4).

The cap is removed from the needle of the injection syringe and held in one hand, such that the end of the injection plunger is in contact with the index finger (Fig. 11.5). A cotton-tipped applicator is held with the other hand and placed near the ocular surface to guard against movement of the eyelids toward the injection site. If there is excess fluid pooling in the inferior conjunctival fornix, then the cotton-tipped applicator can also be used to sequester this fluid (Fig. 11.6).

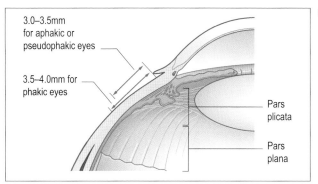

3.0–3.5mm for aphakic or pseudophakic eyes

3.5–4.0mm for phakic eyes

Pars plicata

Pars plana

■ **FIGURE 11.3** Pars plicata, pars plana and appropriate locations for intravitreal injections for aphakic/pseudophakic and phakic eyes.

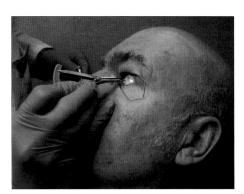

■ **FIGURE 11.4** Marking the injection site with sterile calipers.

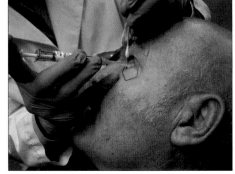

■ **FIGURE 11.5** Injection technique with one hand holding the syringe and the index finger of the same hand on the plunger performing the injection.

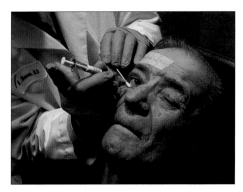

FIGURE 11.6 Injection technique of using a cotton-tipped applicator to guard against lid movement during the injection and also to absorb excess fluid pooling in the inferior fornix during the injection.

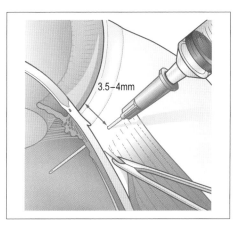

3.5–4mm

FIGURE 11.7 Intravitreal injection demonstrating needle entry through the sclera, pars plana, and into the vitreous.

FIGURE 11.8 Injection technique demonstrating appropriate positioning and angle of needle toward center of the vitreous cavity.

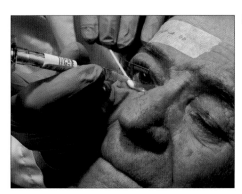

The author prepares the patient by counting 'three, two, one' and then the injection is performed by placing the needle perpendicular to the scleral surface and then penetrating the sclera with the needle traversing approximately 4 mm toward the center of the vitreous cavity (Fig. 11.7). The medicine is injected over approximately 3 seconds with the same index finger and hand that is already holding the syringe. While the injection is performed, the author counts 'one thousand one, one thousand two, one thousand three', by which time the injection is completed and the needle is removed from the eye. Care is taken during the injection to avoid anterior placement of the needle in order to prevent lens damage (Fig. 11.8).

The speculum is removed from the eye. The author places at least one drop of povidone iodine 5% on the ocular surface of the eye to reduce the chance of any bacteria remaining viable which may have been expressed onto the ocular surface or injection site during the removal of the speculum. A drop of povidone iodine 5% placed on the ocular surface at the conclusion of intraocular surgery has been demonstrated to be effective at minimizing the number of bacterial colony-forming units and species for the first postoperative day compared to a broad-spectrum antibiotic.[43] In addition, the antimicrobial effect of a drop of povidone iodine 5% has been shown to last at least 24 hours after intraocular surgery, which was not the case for the antibiotic studied.[43] (*Optional*: A drop of topical antibiotic can be placed on the ocular surface, but this has not been proven to be as effective as povidone iodine with respect to reduction of bacterial colonies cultured from the ocular surface.)

The author typically checks the intraocular pressure (IOP) within 5 min after the injection to be certain that the IOP is physiologic or at least less than 35 mmHg. If the IOP is over 35 mmHg, then another IOP measurement is obtained 5 min later. If the IOP remains over 35 mmHg, then an anterior chamber paracentesis is performed to remove 0.05cc–1.0cc, depending on the injection volume, with a 30-gauge needle through the limbus. If the IOP is less than 35 mmHg, then the patient is discharged home.

POSTOPERATIVE CARE

There is typically no need for a surgical dressing after intravitreal injection. However, if there is excessive subconjunctival hemorrhage, then a sterile gauze eye patch can be placed over the eyelids after the injection and kept in place for 2 hours.

There is typically no need for postoperative medications, unless there is some particular underlying disease that requires treatment (e.g. uveitis) which may require a topical cycloplegic medication and topical prednisolone acetate to prevent posterior synechiae.

The use of topical antibiotics is controversial. The author does not recommend and does not routinely use topical antibiotics after intravitreal injection at this time, since there is no evidence that the use of antibiotics reduces the risk of endophthalmitis after intravitreal injection. In addition, there is a concern that frequent use of topical antibiotics over time, as in the case of patients receiving multiple intravitreal injections of ranibizumab, pegaptanib or bevacizumab every 4–6 weeks, may increase the chances of bacterial resistance. However, many retinal specialists do use topical antibiotics and this is left to your discretion.

The most important aspect of care after intravitreal injection is to inform and warn the patient of potential severe side effects or risks of injection, which include endophthalmitis, retinal tear or detachment, severe inflammatory response (which can occur after triamcinolone acetonide injection) or secondary glaucoma.

Patients should be instructed to contact you immediately if they notice:

- pain,
- increase in floaters compared to immediately post injection,
- flashing lights,
- decreased vision,
- increased redness,
- yellow or green discharge,
- nausea or vomiting,
- shadow or curtain obscuring vision.

Typical and expected side effects immediately after injection include: tearing, redness and burning from the povidone iodine used to prepare the ocular surface and limited subconjunctival hemorrhage at the injection site. Floaters can occur from the injection, especially when triamcinolone is injected. Occasionally air bubbles injected during the procedure can also cause floaters. The floaters related to triamcinolone injection typically resolve with a few weeks; floaters due to air bubbles typically resolve within a few days.

Patients should be warned not to rub the eye after injection, since they can create a corneal abrasion. The author suggests instructing patients to gently blot the periocular region and lids with a clean tissue if they experience tearing.

COMPLICATIONS

Possible postoperative complications may include: endophthalmitis (1% or less), retinal tear or detachment (1% or less), ocular hypertension or secondary glaucoma (approximately 30–40% for triamcinolone acetonide), severe inflammatory response (1% or less), cataract, retinal or vitreous hemorrhage, retinal vein occlusion, optic disc atrophy, hypotony or rarely anaphylaxis.[16,19,39]

PROGNOSIS

The prognosis for the intravitreal injection procedure itself is generally very good. The prognosis for each individual patient will depend on the underlying disease process that is being treated. For self-limited conditions such as pseudophakic cystoid macular edema, a single intravitreal injection of triamcinolone acetonide is typically curative. In the case of exudative macular degeneration patients, repetitive injections of medication are typically needed over a longer period of time and in many cases over several years. The prognosis for these patients is more guarded over the long run. However, it is the case now, more than ever before, that patients have a higher chance of maintaining and improving their visual acuity, even in the case of exudative macular degeneration.

REFERENCES

1. Ohm J. Uber die behandlung der netzhautablosung durch operative entleerung der subretinalen flussigkeit und einspritzung von luft in den glaskorper. Albrecht von Graefes Arch Ophthalmol 1911; 79:442–450.
2. von Stallman L, Meyer K, DiGrandi J. Experimental study on penicillin treatment of ectogenous infection of vitreous. Arch Ophthalmol 1944; 32:179–189.
3. Peyman GA, Nelson P, Bennett TO. Intravitreal injection of kanamycin in experimentally induced endophthalmitis. Can J Ophthalmol 1974; 9:322–327.
4. Peyman GA, Paque JT, Meisels HI, Bennett TO. Postoperative endophthalmitis: a comparison of methods for treatment and prophylaxis with gentamicin. Ophthalmic Surg 1975; 6:45–55.
5. Forster RK, Zachary IG, Cottingham AJ Jr, Norton EWD. Further observations on the diagnosis, cause, and treatment of endophthalmitis. Am J Ophthalmol 1976; 81:52–56.
6. Peyman GA, Vastine DW, Raichand M. Experimental aspects and their clinical application. Ophthalmology 1978; 85:374–385.
7. Baum J, Peyman GA, Barza M. Intravitreal administration of antibiotic in the treatment of bacterial endophthalmitis. III. Consensus. Surv Ophthalmol 1982; 26:204–206.
8. Pavan PR, Brinser JH. Exogenous bacterial endophthalmitis treated without systemic antibiotics. Am J Ophthalmol 1987; 104:121–126.
9. Blumenkrantz MS, Hernandez E, Ophir A, Norton EWD. 5-Fluorouracil: a new application in complicated retinal detachment for an established antimetabolite. Ophthalmology 1984; 91:122–130.
10. Henry K, Cantrill H, Fletcher C, et al. Use of intravitreal ganciclovir (dihydroxy propoxymethyl guanine) for cytomegalovirus retinitis in a patient with AIDS. Am J Ophthalmol 1987; 103:17–23.
11. Blankenship GW. Evaluation of a single intravitreal injection of dexamethasone phosphate in vitrectomy surgery for diabetic retinopathy complications. Graefes Arch Clin Exp Ophthalmol 1991; 229:62–65.
12. Penfold PL, Gyory JF, Hunyor AB, Billson FA. Exudative macular degeneration and intravitreal triamcinolone. A pilot study. Aust N Z J Ophthalmol 1995; 23:293–298.
13. Hassan AS, Johnson MW, Schneiderman TE, et al. Management of submacular hemorrhage with intravitreous tissue plasminogen activator injection and pneumatic displacement. Ophthalmology 1999; 106(10):1900–1907.
14. Vitravene. Online. Available: www.fda.gov/cder/consumerinfo/druginfo/vitravene.HTM.
15. Macugen. Online. Available: www.fda.gov/bbs/topics/news/2004/new01146.html.
16. Gragoudas ES, Adamis AP, Cunningham ET Jr, et al. A prospective, randomized controlled clinical trial of pegaptanib, an anti-VEGF aptamer, for neovascular age-related macular degeneration. N Engl J Med 2004; 351:2805–2816.
17. Lucentis. Online. Available: www.fda.gov/bbs/topics/NEWS/2006/NEW01405.html.
18. Kuppermann BD, Thomas EL, De Smet MD, Grillone LR. Pooled efficacy results from two multinational randomized controlled clinical trials of a single intravitreous injection of highly purified ovine hyaluronidase (Vitrase®) for the

management of vitreous hemorrhage. Am J Ophthalmol 2005; 104(4):573–584.

19. Kuppermann BD, Thomas EL, De Smet MD, Grillone LR. Safety results of two phase III trials of an intravitreous injection of highly purified ovine hyaluronidase for the management of vitreous hemorrhage. Am J Ophthalmol 2005; 104(4):585–597.

20. Vitrase. Online. Available: www.fda.gov/bbs/topics/ANSWERS/2004/ANS01287.html.

21. Bhavsar AR. Diabetic retinopathy: the latest in current management. Retina 2006; 26(6 Suppl):S71–S79.

22. Martidis A, Duker JS, Greenberg PB, et al. Intravitreal triamcinolone for refractory diabetic macular edema. Ophthalmology 2002; 109(5):920–927.

23. Conway MD, Canakis C, Livir-Rallatos C, Peyman GA. Intravitreal triamcinolone acetonide for refractory chronic pseudophakic cystoid macular edema. J Cataract Refract Surg 2003; 29(1):27–33.

24. Greenberg PB, Martidis A, Rogers AH, Duker JS, Reichel E. Intravitreal triamcinolone acetonide for macular oedema due to central retinal vein occlusion. Br J Ophthalmol 2002; 86(2):247–248.

25. Ip MS, Kumar KS. Intravitreous triamcinolone acetonide as treatment for macular edema from central retinal vein occlusion. Arch Ophthalmol 2002; 120(9):1217–1219.

26. Spaide RF, Sorenson J, Maranan L. Combined photodynamic therapy with verteporfin and intravitreal triamcinolone acetonide for choroidal neovascularization. Ophthalmology 2003; 110(8):1517–1525.

27. Augustin AJ, Schmidt-Erfurth U. Verteporfin and intravitreal triamcinolone acetonide combination therapy for occult choroidal neovascularization in age-related macular degeneration. Am J Ophthalmol 2006; 141(4):638–645.

28. Bhavsar AR. Combined intravitreal triamcinolone and PDT in the treatment of minimally classic subfoveal CNV with or without RAP lesions. Poster presented at the Annual Meeting of the American Academy of Ophthalmology, New Orleans, October 24, 2004.

29. Bhavsar AR. The Insight Registry Study Group. Patients treated with verteporfin therapy combined with intravitreal triamcinolone acetonide for CNV due to AMD: The Patient Insight Registry. Poster presented at the Annual Meeting of the American Academy of Ophthalmology, Chicago, October 15–16, 2005.

30. Jonas JB, Hayler JK, Sofker A, Panda-Jonas S. Regression of neovascular iris vessels by intravitreal injection of crystalline cortisone. J Glaucoma 2001; 10(4):284–287.

31. Rosenfeld PJ, Moshfeghi AA, Puliafito CA, Michels S, Marcus EN, Venkatraman AS. Systemic bevacizumab (Avastin) therapy for neovascular age-related macular degeneration (SANA) study: 12 week outcomes. Presented at the American Society of Retina Specialists Annual Meeting, Montreal, Canada, July 18, 2005.

32. Avery RL, Pieramici DJ, Rabena MD, Castellarin AA, Nasir MA, Giust MJ. Intravitreal bevacizumab (Avastin) for neovascular age-related macular degeneration. Ophthalmology 2006; 113(3):363–372.

33. Mason JO 3rd, Albert MA Jr, Vail R. Intravitreal bevacizumab (Avastin) for refractory pseudophakic cystoid macular edema. Retina 2006; 26(3):356–357.

34. Rosenfeld PJ, Fung AE, Puliafito CA. Optical coherence tomography findings after an intravitreal injection of bevacizumab (Avastin) for macular edema from central retinal vein occlusion. Ophthal Surg Lasers Imaging 2005; 36(4):336–339.

35. Iturralde D, Spaide RF, Meyerle CB, et al. Intravitreal bevacizumab (Avastin) treatment of macular edema in central retinal vein occlusion: a short-term study. Retina 2006; 26(3):279–284.

36. Spaide RF, Fisher YL. Intravitreal bevacizumab (Avastin) treatment of proliferative diabetic retinopathy complicated by vitreous hemorrhage. Retina 2006; 26(3):275–278.

37. Avery RL. Regression of retinal and iris neovascularization after intravitreal bevacizumab (Avastin) treatment. Retina 2006; 26(3):352–354.

38 Aiello LP, Brucker AJ, Chang S, et al. Evolving guidelines for intravitreous injections. Retina 2004; 24(5 Suppl): S3–S19.

39. Jager RD, Aiello LP, Patel SC, Cunningham ET. Risks of intravitreous injection: a comprehensive review. Retina 2004; 24(5):676–698.

40. Ta CN. Minimizing the risk of endophthalmitis following intravitreous injections. Retina 2004; 24(5):699–713.

41. Speaker MG, Menikoff JA. Prophylaxis of endophthalmitis with topical povidone iodine. Ophthalmology 1991; 98:1769–1775.

42. Isenberg S, Apt L, Yoshimori R, Khwarg S. Chemical preparation of the eye in

ophthalmic surgery IV: comparison of povidone–iodine on the conjunctiva with a prophylactic antibiotic. Arch Ophthalmol 1985; 103:1340–1342.

43. Apt L, Isenberg SJ, Yoshimori R, et al. The effect of povidone–iodine solution applied at the conclusion of ophthalmic surgery. Am J Ophthalmol 1995; 119(6):701–705.

44. Bhavsar AR. A consecutive series of 1,000 intravitreous injections without topical antibiotic prophylaxis. Poster presented at the Annual Meeting of the American Academy of Ophthalmology, Las Vegas, November 12–13, 2006.

Pneumatic retinopexy

W. Sanderson Grizzard and Mark E. Hammer

INSTRUMENTS AND DEVICES

Pneumatic retinopexy is an innovative, minimally invasive technique for reattaching the retina. Since its independent development by Professor Dominquez[1] in Spain and by Dr Hilton[2] in San Francisco, there has been controversy about its success rate and its appropriate use. Hopefully this chapter will put pneumatic retinopexy in its proper place in the armamentarium of retinal procedures.

The surgeon required for pneumatic retinopexy is likely to be creative and innovative. He or she must be good at finding retinal tears and have sufficient self-confidence to try an office operation that has a slightly higher failure rate in order to offer the patient a superior overall result. The surgeon must also be willing to explain the procedure to patients so that the patient will do their part.

Patients must be cooperative and be able to maintain position well. They must either understand the need for positioning or be willing to follow instructions without understanding. In this surgery, like no other, the patient and their family are really co-surgeons and must take responsibility for the surgery's outcome. The greatest cause of poor results is poor patient compliance. Gender appears to have an effect on how easily patients can be educated. In their paper on failures, Grizzard et al.[3] found that women had a much higher success rate than men. This was thought to be due to the fact that women naturally follow directions better. Subsequently, when male patients were given additional education and family members were actively involved, this gender difference disappeared.

The equipment needed for pneumatic retinopexy is inexpensive and available in most retinal surgeons' offices (Box 12.1). Surgeons predominantly use sulfur hexafluoride (SF_6) gas for pneumatic retinopexy. Most detachments can be treated with an injection of 0.45 mL of gas and this can be injected safely following anterior chamber paracentesis. SF_6 doubles in size after being injected and persists for 7–10 days. This is long enough for the retinopexy to cause adherence. Perfluoropropane (C_3F_8) is also used but is reserved for special situations where a larger or longer lasting bubble is desired. C_3F_8 quadruples in size and lasts for 3–6 weeks. Three-tenths of a milliliter can be injected safely, usually without paracentesis. C_3F_8 is used for pneumatic reoperations, cases of multiple tears, and occasionally for inferior breaks. The main problem with C_3F_8 is that it lasts too long and this leads to a longer period of no air travel. The longer lasting gas, however, has not been documented to cause any particular complication. Air can also be used but requires a larger volume of gas, about 0.6 mL, and occasionally requires reinjection. It does not increase in size at all and is gone within 3–5 days.[4]

Depending on the ocular pathology, both laser and cryopexy are used for retinopexy. Laser causes more rapid adherence than cryopexy and is less inflammatory. Still, for small peripheral tears that are not elevated, cryopexy is the preferred treatment. The advantage of cryopexy is that the treatment is carried out in detached retina and small peripheral tears are easier to find. Once the retina is reattached by the gas bubble, these peripheral tears can be hard to locate for laser treatment. It is also easier on the patient and surgeon to do the operation in one sitting.

For larger tears, multiple tears, or tears in a highly elevated retina, a gas bubble is injected first and the retina is allowed to reattach. Laser is then performed on the second

---

BOX 12.1 Equipment needed for pneumatic retinopexy

- Sterile gloves
- Sterile drape
- Lid speculum
- Single dose sterile tetracaine
- 10% single use povidone iodine solution
- Balanced salt solution for dilution of povidone iodine solution
- Sterile container (urinalysis cup) for preparation of dilute povidone iodine
- 0.22 μm Millipore filter
- Two 1.0 mL tuberculin syringes
- Two 30-gauge, ½ inch needles (may have one 27-gauge for paracentesis)
- Six to eight sterile cotton-tipped applicators
- Calipers
- 20-diopter indirect ophthalmoscopy lens
- Tissue forceps with teeth
- Antibiotic drops
- Eye patch
- Gas tank (C_3F_8 or SF_6)
- Warning bracelet for intraocular gas
- Cryopexy unit and probe
- Laser with indirect ophthalmoscope attachment

---

day. The indirect ophthalmoscope delivery system for laser and a surgical table that tilts the patient to the head-down position greatly facilitate the use of second-day laser. It is difficult to perform laser at the slit lamp because the gas bubble interferes with treatment of a superior tear. A superior bullous detachment is a definite, positive indication for pneumatic retinopexy. If laser is planned but cannot be carried out because of peripheral cataract or residual cortex, cryopexy can always be applied the next day in the newly attached retina.

INDICATIONS AND CONTRAINDICATIONS

Indications

When considering a patient for pneumatic retinopexy it is important to consider both the eye and the patient. The eye must have a detachment that has pathology and characteristics that are amenable to the pneumatic approach. In addition to the eye, the patient must have physical, social, intellectual, and attitudinal attributes that will assure compliance with the rigid positional requirements necessary to make pneumatic retinopexy work. The lens status, natural or pseudophakic, has absolutely no impact on whether or not a patient should be a candidate for pneumatic retinopexy.

The original criteria established by George Hilton are the best eyes for pneumatic retinopexy. The original criteria were superior tears (superior eight clock hours), single tears or multiple tears in less than one clock hour, absence of grade 3 proliferative vitreoretinopathy (PVR), and a good view of the entire peripheral retina.[2] These are the ideal eyes for pneumatic retinopexy and will give the greatest success. These are also the best criteria for starting surgeons to use so they can learn the subtleties of the operation.

Criteria have now expanded to include all eyes that have a reasonable chance of success without definite contraindications. Eyes have been successfully treated with multiple tears, inferior tears, PVR as long as the membranes were away from the tear, in eyes where the tear could not be located, and in eyes with giant tears. Multiple tears in multiple quadrants usually are not a problem. Other patients with more challenging retinal pathology can also be repaired with pneumatic retinopexy, but often these patients are best served by a vitrectomy, buckle, or both.

Contraindications

Eye contraindications have evolved over the 20 years of pneumatic experience. Some are relative and some are nearly absolute. Patients with limited lattice degeneration and an already detached vitreous do well. Patients with extensive lattice and adherent vitreous probably should not be treated with pneumatic retinopexy. Most patients with lattice fall somewhere in between and many do well with the procedure.

Inferior tears were originally excluded from treatment but subsequent experience and publications have demonstrated that it is possible to treat some of these patients.[5] Patients should be agile and highly motivated. Inferior chronic detachments do not work well because of the viscous subretinal fluid. Recent acute detachments and recurrences following vitrectomy can be treated with face-down and head-down positioning.

Proliferative vitreoretinopathy is a contraindication because pneumatic retinopexy is not a good operation for detachments with significant epiretinal membrane formation. These eyes need membrane peeling and scleral buckling to deal with the tractional component of the detachment. Occasionally patients with superior tears and inferior starfolds can be successfully treated, but be sure to prepare yourself and your patient for the possibility of more surgery.

In eyes where the periphery cannot be seen for 360° because of residual cortex, cataract or hemorrhage, caution is advised. If the entire extent of the detachment can be seen and the causative break identified, then it may be worth a try. If there is extensive detachment and some of the periphery of the detachment is obscured, it may still be worth a try but missed breaks are likely.

Retinoschisis is a contraindication. These chronic detachments with viscous fluid do not respond well to pneumatic retinopexy. In addition to the problem of chronic viscous fluid, the vitreous is usually attached and the inner wall of the schisis cavity keeps the outer wall break from being closed by the bubble.

Chronic detachments in general and inferior chronic detachments specifically are poor candidates. The fluid is viscous and is not absorbed quickly. In addition, it does not shift easily away from the tears so that the retinopexy can form a scar between the pigment layer and the neurosensory retina. Longstanding detachments are also those that develop the problem of chronic inferior fluid that can take over a year to absorb.

Selection of the patient is more difficult and more important than selection of the eye. In the original papers on pneumatic retinopexy, not enough attention was paid to the patient and how important proper patient selection was to the success of the technique. Poor patient selection and poor patient education are the main reasons pneumatic retinopexy fails.

The ideal patient for pneumatic retinopexy is someone who is cooperative and responsible, and has some degree of trust for the medical profession. Irresponsible people who don't have jobs or families to care for them are not good candidates. Following the positioning regimen for pneumatic retinopexy requires discipline.

It is very important for the surgeon to have an educational plan as an integral part of the pneumatic retinopexy procedure. Video presentations, prepared written instructions or brochures are a must in preparing the patient and their family for the operation. The Tornambe leveler is helpful in educating patients and in simplifying instructions for others. If the patient is instructed to 'put the bubble at 3 o'clock in the leveler', the patient has a clear understanding of what to do (Fig. 12.1).

Patients who are male, macho, and not good listeners are unlikely to follow instructions. It is important to educate other family members about the importance of positioning and make it a team project. If only the patient is privy to the instruction the chance of failure is much greater. It is also important to stress that if the patient doesn't comply they will

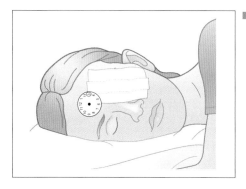

■ **FIGURE 12.1** Use of the Tornambe leveler. The patient is on her right side for a tear at the 3 o'clock position. A patch has been placed on her eye and the Tornambe leveler on her forehead. The bubble is at 3 o'clock, showing the patient how they must position their head so that the bubble in the eye will close the retinal tear.

have to go to the expensive hospital and have painful surgery that includes putting a silicone buckle around their eye that will change their refraction so that they will need glasses—a particularly useful encouragement if the eye is emmetropic from laser-assisted in situ keratomileusis (LASIK) or after cataract surgery.

SURGICAL TECHNIQUE

12.1

The surgical procedure begins with a good fundus examination. It is often necessary to examine the patient with indirect ophthalmoscopy and scleral depression and also slit lamp using a corneal contact lens. If the patient cannot tolerate a careful fundus examination they are not good candidates. Inferior or unseen tears will always lead to failure. It is important to do a careful drawing that includes each retinal break and each break's relationship to the larger retinal vessels. Once the retina is attached, these breaks may be impossible to locate and the fundus drawing will be helpful for postoperative laser.

Next, discuss with the patient and their family the options for treatment that include scleral buckling, vitrectomy, or pneumatic retinopexy. The American Academy of Ophthalmology patient education brochure is well written and has good illustrations. Stress that if they cannot or will not follow positioning instructions, pneumatic retinopexy is a waste of time. Also review the slightly lower initial results and prepare for the possibility of failure. Assure them that this is just a first step that is often successful, but that further surgery in the hospital is sometimes necessary. Mention that, for the most part, the operation that will be needed if the procedure fails is the same operation that would be done if we went straight to surgery, and often a buckle and the hospital can be avoided by using the pneumatic approach.

Set the stage so that the patient and family are enthusiastic about the procedure and about being able to stay out of the hospital. They should also have a firm understanding and commitment to make it work. Tell them from the beginning that the success or failure is more in their hands than those of the surgeon. This first step of education is often the most neglected.

For anesthesia, use a subconjunctival injection over the area of the tear if cryopexy is to be used and also inject anesthesia where the gas injection is planned. After topical conjunctival anesthesia, inject 0.4–0.5 mL of 2% lidocaine with a 30-gauge needle. Inject into the fornix where the cryopexy is going to be done and inject so the anesthetic dissects posteriorly. Wait about 10 min before beginning treatment. Be sure to dispose of the syringe with the anesthetic at this time. It is possible to grab this syringe inadvertently during the pneumatic procedure and inject anesthetic into the eye by mistake.

After obtaining adequate anesthesia, do the cryopexy if that is the strategy being used. Use the indirect ophthalmoscope to locate the tears, indent the sclera with the cryoprobe,

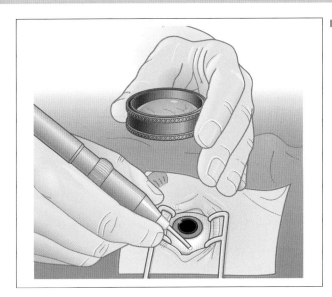

FIGURE 12.2 Cryoretinopexy. The tear is visualized with indirect ophthalmoscopy and the cryoprobe is placed outside the conjunctiva. The cryoprobe's indentation can be seen in relationship to the tear and treatment can be performed in an attached or a detached retina.

locate it over the tear, and then activate the probe with the foot pedal (Fig. 12.2). Treat until there is a white, retinal freeze. Some surgeons use a lid speculum and others use an assistant's finger. If it is difficult to reach the posterior aspect of a tear, rather than rip the conjunctiva, do laser at a later date.

If more than 10 applications of cryopexy are to be used, it may be better to use laser. There is a little evidence and a lot of strong feeling that cryopexy causes PVR.[6] Not everyone agrees,[7] and many retinal detachments have been cured with cryopexy.

Next, the gas syringe is prepared by filling a tuberculin syringe with the required amount of gas. A stepdown valve (or regulator) is necessary to lower the pressure from the gas cylinder. A 0.22 μm Millipore gas filter is placed on the tuberculin syringe and the gas is allowed to fill the syringe. The syringe should fill passively from the pressure in the system rather than from pulling on the plunger. This reduces the risk of dilution with air. Fill the syringe twice: expel all the gas the first time in order to flush the air out of the system; the second time, fill the syringe to 0.8 or 0.9 mL. Place a 30-gauge needle on the syringe and expel the excess gas so that the syringe holds the amount of gas you want to inject. Then lay it aside. Next, prepare a paracentesis syringe by placing a 27- or 30-gauge needle on a tuberculin syringe and remove the plunger.

Now prepare the eye for injection. Irrigate the conjunctiva with 5% povidone iodine solution, apply an eye drape, and use a lid speculum to open the lids. (The use of a lid speculum for this part of the operation is important in preventing endophthalmitis.) Apply an undiluted, 10% solution of povidone iodine to the conjunctiva and allow it to work for 60–90 seconds. Next, dry the limbus and injection site with a cotton-tipped applicator. Anterior chamber paracentesis is then carried out with a 27- or 30-gauge needle on a tuberculin syringe with the plunger removed. Using the prepared paracentesis syringe, place a cotton-tipped applicator next to the injection site to provide counter traction for the injection and to stabilize the eye. Position the paracentesis needle so that it is parallel to the iris and enter the anterior chamber. After the needle enters the anterior chamber, position the cotton-tipped applicator on the corneal center and gently press on the cornea (Fig. 12.3). This allows the aqueous to egress passively through the needle into the syringe. Keep the applicator on the cornea until 0.2 or 0.25 mL of aqueous is in the syringe. Then remove the needle and gently lift the applicator off the cornea. This technique keeps the

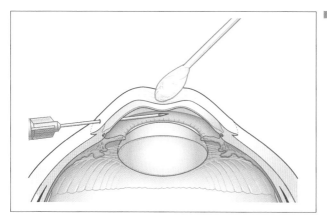

FIGURE 12.3 Anterior chamber paracentesis. Paracentesis is performed by inserting a 30- or 27-gauge needle into the anterior chamber attached to a tuberculin syringe that has had its plunger removed. Pressure is then placed on the central cornea and the aqueous will passively leave the eye and the iris and lens will not come forward and inadvertently hit the needle.

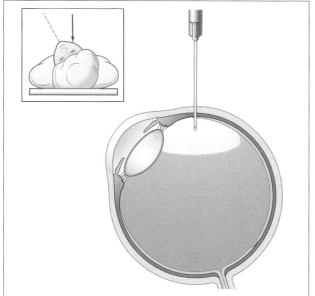

FIGURE 12.4 Injection of gas bubble. The patient and eye must be positioned correctly such that the needle is directed toward the center of the earth and the center of the eye at the same time. The injection point should be at the highest point of the eye. The needle is then withdrawn so that approximately 2 mm of needle remains in the eye. The gas is then injected into the eye with a single, smooth motion. A single bubble should then form around the needle tip.

lens and iris away from the needle tip and a large amount fluid can be safely removed. The anterior chamber is then noticeably shallow.

Next, take the gas syringe and inject 0.4–0.5 mL of SF_6 gas through the conjunctiva, sclera, and pars plana at a location 4 mm posterior to the limbus. The key to getting a single bubble is to position the eye so that the needle is directed to the center of the eye and the center of the earth at the same time. Insert the needle for 5 or 6 mm and retract the needle so that about 2–3 mm of the needle is inside the eye. Since the bubble will seek the highest point in the eye, this permits the bubble to form around the needle tip and a single bubble will result (Fig. 12.4). Inject firmly, but not violently. Very fast and very slow injection is more likely to get multiple bubbles. Next, inspect the eye with indirect ophthalmoscopy to check for central retinal artery flow and to see if a single, mobile bubble was obtained.

In order to prevent macular detachment or to do a steamroller maneuver, instruct the patient to look down to position the bubble over the macula. This allows for displacement of fluid away from the macula. This is important for superior detachments where the macula is not already detached and keeps the bubble from displacing fluid posteriorly and causing macula detachment. Macula detachment can happen but as was learned from doing macular/retinal translocation surgery, it is more difficult to detach a macula than you think. If it does happen, there will probably be no visual consequence.

This controversial and very useful maneuver that displaces subretinal fluid back into the vitreous cavity is what George Hilton popularized as the 'steamroller' technique. He named it after the piece of road-building equipment that is used to flatten and spread asphalt that has been laid for a roadbed. It is useful in patients with bullous detachments and larger holes. It is difficult to push much fluid through a small hole, but with bullous detachments and larger tears it can be very useful. Do the maneuver by having the patient lie face down and look at the floor. Then have the patient gradually lift up their head in the direction of the tear if the tear is superior or have the patient roll to their side if the tear is lateral. Some of the subretinal fluid is then pushed back into the vitreous cavity. This is a slow maneuver and usually takes several minutes.

A single bubble is important if the tear is larger than a disc diameter. For smaller tears it is not critical. The problem with trying to get a single bubble is that sometimes you can inject into the space of Petit and have the bubble get trapped anteriorly. These anteriorly trapped bubbles are usually not a serious problem and by placing the patient face down they will break through into the posterior vitreous cavity after expansion of the bubble.

If there are multiple small bubbles and a large tear, particularly with some traction, be careful. Dr Hilton liked to flick the eye with a cotton-tipped applicator. This causes the multiple bubbles to coalesce. Alternatively, position the patient so that the bubble is away from the tear overnight and see the patient the next day. Because a single bubble is the lowest entropy state, the bubbles will coalesce over time. If the tear is superior it may not be possible to keep the bubbles away from the tear. If this is the case, try to get the subretinal fluid to go back through the hole by the 'steamroller' maneuver so that the hole will be flat against the pigment epithelium and gas will not be able to go through the hole.

If you are sending someone home with a large superior tear and small bubbles, be sure to test the eye by examining the patient in the upright position before they leave the office. Small bubbles that enter the subretinal space can usually be moved back into the vitreous cavity by having the patient lie flat with the hole at the highest point. The bubble will appear in the hole, and it can be coaxed into the vitreous cavity with scleral depression. Scleral depression increases the pressure in the subretinal space and the bubble will pop through the retinal tear back into the vitreous cavity. If the bubble is allowed to expand in the subretinal space, removal becomes a problem. If the subretinal bubble is not too large and you cannot get it out, simply position the patient as you usually would. The smaller, subretinal bubble will dissipate first and you can close the hole as well from the subretinal space as from the vitreous cavity. This problem is best dealt with by avoiding it.

If the central retinal artery is closed, wait about 5 min before taking action. If it is still closed at that time, do another paracentesis using the above described technique of passive removal of the aqueous with pressure on the cornea. This keeps the lens away from the needle. Be sure the patient has at least light perception vision prior to leaving the hospital or office.

If cryopexy was performed, then the procedure is finished. If you elected to do laser on the second day, then you have one more step. Always use second-day laser for bullous detachments and also for those cases where the pneumatic retinopexy procedure has a lower chance of success. In those cases, it is reasonable to inject a bubble and see what happens. Sometimes the retina flattens and laser can be performed the next day. If the retina doesn't flatten, then surgery can be performed the next day and the eye hasn't been inflamed with cryopexy.

In order to undertake postoperative laser, it is best to use the indirect laser. It is also critical to do a careful fundus drawing at the initial visit and locate all the tears relative to the retinal vasculature. When the retina reattaches, it is sometimes impossible to see the tears. This is particularly true for smaller tears, but even larger tears can be hard to find. It is important not to treat through a bubble because the bubble can unpredictably focus the laser and cause hemorrhage from the choroid. For superior tears, use a table that tilts in the Trendelenburg position or use an examination chair with the patient's head extended over the back of the chair. By placing the patient in a head-down position, the bubble is displaced inferiorly and the superior tears are easily treated (Fig. 12.5). Scleral depression is usually needed for anterior tears. Use three to four rows of laser around the tear or lattice, being sure to get the anterior margin as well as the posterior margin.

If the media are hazy because of peripheral cataract or residual cortex, and this prevents you from doing laser, then treat the tears with cryopexy instead. The caution about displacing the bubble away from the tear for laser does not apply to cryopexy.

On the first postoperative visit, check for signs of infection in the anterior chamber, check the eye pressure, and see if the retina is attached or mostly reattached. If the retina is completely reattached or if the subretinal fluid is markedly decreased, then the operation will usually succeed. Praise the patient and encourage positioning for two more days until they are seen again. Urge them to call if their vision worsens or pain develops.

For eyes that are not reattached, try to establish why. Is the patient positioning correctly? Is there a new or missed break? Is there PVR? The most common cause of first-day failure is poor patient compliance. If a break cannot be found to explain the failure, don't panic, but reinforce positioning instructions in front of the whole family. Painstakingly review the need for the co-surgeons (whole family) to do their job and threaten that they will have to head to the dreaded and expensive hospital. Amazingly, many of these patients will be doing fine when they return the third day.

If a previously undetected break is seen and it can be addressed by the pneumatic approach, change the positioning instructions to cover that break. Sometimes an injection of more gas may be helpful. If there is an inferior tear, then it is time for the operating room.

If the patient is doing well on the fourth day, relax positioning requirements. If the retina remains detached after repeated emphasis on positioning, and even if a causative new break cannot be found, then it is time for the operating room. Most often there will be a missed break found at surgery.

If 360° laser is planned, this is the time to start. Again the indirect laser works best. Dr Tornambe has been the main enthusiast for this technique and it does offer some

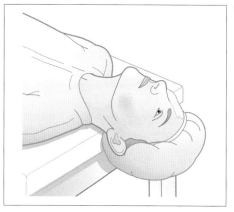

FIGURE 12.5 Positioning for the treatment of a superior tears with indirect laser. The patient's head is placed over the edge of the treatment table or the examination chair so that the bubble will move away from the tear.

advantage, particularly if the peripheral retina looks thin, if there are multiple tears, or if there is peripheral lattice or other peripheral abnormalities.

COMPLICATIONS

The main complications that appear postoperatively are new or missed breaks, endophthalmitis, subretinal gas, hemorrhage, and PVR.

New or missed break is a controversial subject. New breaks definitely occur but most new breaks are really missed breaks. If "new" breaks occur more often than 10% of the time, then you probably need to do another retinal fellowship. It is not surprising that new breaks occur following retinal reattachment. Retinal detachment releases the vitreoretinal forces that lead to retinal tears. A detached retina doesn't tear. When the retina is reattached, these forces reappear and new tears can develop. There is another mechanism of new tear formation caused by epiretinal membrane formation. These are the tears of PVR and usually occur later and are not typical horseshoe tears.

When new breaks or missed breaks are discovered, treat them as you would the initial break. If it is amenable to pneumatic retinopexy, then try it again. If it looks like PVR is developing, then go to the operating room to do a vitrectomy, scleral buckle, or both. For scleral buckle surgery, please refer to Chapter 1, Scleral buckling surgery by Charles P. Wilkinson, MD and Abdhish R. Bhavsar, MD. For vitrectomy surgery with or without scleral buckle surgery, please refer to Chapter 2, Vitrectomy surgery by Abdhish R. Bhavsar, MD.

For endophthalmitis, be aggressive and do a vitrectomy with culture and injection of antibiotics. Do a culture and Gram stain at the beginning of the vitrectomy. If the retina is attached, do a vitrectomy and injection of antibiotics, leaving some gas in the eye. Use full doses of antibiotics and then do a partial fluid–gas exchange. If the retina is detached, do a vitrectomy, add antibiotics, and then a complete fluid–gas exchange. Also inject periocular antibiotics and sometimes use systemic antibiotics. The results of the Endophthalmitis Vitrectomy Study do not apply to endophthalmitis from pneumatic retinopexy.

For subretinal gas, do not do anything if the retina is attaching. The subretinal gas will go away first as it is in contact with the choroid and is smaller than the bubble in the vitreous cavity. If there is a large amount of subretinal gas that has expanded and cannot be pushed out of the subretinal space and the retina remains detached, then vitrectomy or external drainage may be necessary.

For external drainage, position your sclerotomy so it is 1–2 mm behind the pars plana and at a place where it is at the highest point of the eye. As you cut down over the bubble, the gas will leave as you penetrate the choroid. You can also use a small needle for the sclerotomy. If you are going to remove the gas internally, be careful when doing your sclerotomy for vitrectomy because the subretinal gas will push the retina anteriorly over the pars plana and your knife may go through the retina as well. Position the eye so that the bubble is on the opposite side of the eye and do your sclerotomy. Then take a silicone-tipped needle and go across the eye and remove the gas. You do not have to get it all out because the small bubble that remains can usually be worked out by scleral depression.

If the patient develops a postoperative vitreous hemorrhage, it is usually because a bridging vessel broke. If the hemorrhage is significant, be aggressive in this situation. Blood and retinal detachment are a recipe for PVR. Do a vitrectomy to remove the blood and reattach the retina if it is not already attached. Interestingly, the retina is usually attached because the bridging vessel gets torn as the retina reattaches. It is necessary to be aggressive because new tears may also be the cause of the bleeding.

Postoperative PVR usually means it was there beforehand and you missed it. Pneumatic retinopexy doesn't cause PVR, but pneumatic retinopexy is a bad operation for PVR. The difference in first operation success rates between pneumatic retinopexy and scleral buckle, or vitrectomy with a buckle, is that a buckle treats early PVR pretty well. Before vitrectomy, the only treatment for PVR was a high scleral buckle without vitrectomy and this was successful in reattaching the retina 34.7% of the time.[7] If the operation is failing because of PVR, do a vitrectomy with encircling buckle. Often that will be adequate treatment for success. The PVR seen in pneumatic retinopexy failure is not as severe as the PVR seen in buckle failures.

OUTCOME

In the original report by Hilton and Grizzard, there was success in 18 of 20 cases or a first operation success rate of 90%.[2] A subsequent review of 27 different reported series showed a range of first operation success from 53 to 100%.[3] The most definitive study on pneumatic retinopexy was the randomized controlled trial of pneumatic retinopexy versus scleral buckling. Using the same entrance criteria as in the original report, the prospective controlled trial had an initial single operation success rate of 81% when additional laser or cryopexy was not counted as a second operation. This number was not statistically different from a similarly calculated success rate for scleral buckling that was 84%. The ultimate anatomic success rate was 99% for pneumatic retinopexy and 98% for scleral buckling.[8,9] Most pneumatic studies show that even if the original procedure fails, the ultimate success rate remains high. An initial attempt with pneumatic retinopexy does not disadvantage the eye for subsequent success.

Tornambe reported his experience of 302 cases with expanded entry criteria. His initial success rate was only 68%. He noted a higher failure rate in eyes that were pseudophakic and had more extensive detachments. The failure rate also increased with number of breaks. He noted increased success in eyes that had laser retinopexy for 360° between the vitreous base and ora serrata.[10]

The most exciting point about pneumatic retinopexy is that visual results are better when compared to scleral buckling. In the prospective randomized trial, eyes with macula-on detachments have good visual outcome in both groups. However, in eyes with macula-off detachments of less than 2 weeks, there was markedly better vision in the pneumatic group. Eighty percent of the pneumatic group saw 20/50 compared to only 56% in the scleral buckle group.[8] At 2 years, 89% of the same group were seeing 20/50 or better.[9]

Pneumatic retinopexy has also been shown not to cause lens changes as have been noted in phakic patients who have had vitrectomy. In a study using Scheimpflug photography to assess lens changes, there was no evidence of lens changes in 2 years after pneumatic retinopexy.[11] Vitrectomy alone has not to my knowledge been compared to pneumatic retinopexy in a prospective evaluation.

Another interesting question is how should the surgeon approach a patient with a retinal detachment and, depending on the surgeon's prejudice, what percent of cases are amenable to office surgery? We analyzed 37 consecutive cases of retinal detachment seen in our practice from June 2004 to January 2005. We performed laser photocoagulation on 5% and pneumatic retinopexy on 51%. Only 44% were taken primarily to the surgical suite. Our initial success rate for pneumatic retinopexy using this aggressive pneumatic approach was 74%.

SOCIOECONOMIC CONSIDERATIONS

It has become evident that in order for pneumatic retinopexy to reach its optimum use, the health care system must be friendly toward innovation and reward the physician for new surgical advances and increases in productivity. If the health care system rewards physicians for putting patients in the hospital (Germany), or punishes them for being innovative or working harder (Great Britain), then pneumatic retinopexy use will be limited. If the system of care is fully integrated so that the retinal surgeon can freely choose between office surgery, outpatient surgery, and hospitalization, then there will be greater use of pneumatic retinopexy. If there is a residual market economy with some remnant of supply, demand, and real pricing, then the procedure will be very popular. If the health care system is rigid, and local medical custom or payment scheme dictates that retinal detachments must be treated in hospitals, and if cost is irrelevant, then there will be limited use.

REFERENCES

1. Dominquez A. Cirugia precoz y ambulatoria del desprendimento de retina. Arch Soc Esp Oftalmol 1985; 48:47–54.
2. Hilton GF, Grizzard WS. Pneumatic retinopexy. A two-step outpatient operation without conjunctival incision. Ophthalmology 1986; 93:626–641.
3. Grizzard WS, Hilton GF, Hammer, ME, Taren D, Brinton DA. Pneumatic retinopexy failures. Cause, prevention, timing, and management. Ophthalmology 1995; 102;929–936.
4. Sebag J, Tang M. Pneumatic retinopexy using only air. Retina 1993; 13:270–271.
5. Chang TS, Pelzek CD, Nguyen RL, Purohit SS, Scott GR, Hay D. Inverted pneumatic retinopexy: a method of treating retinal detachments associated with inferior retinal breaks. Ophthalmology 2003; 110:589–594.
6. Cowley M, Conway BP, Campochiaro PA, Kaiser D, Gaskin H. Clinical risk factors for proliferative vitreoretinopathy. Arch Ophthalmol 1989; 107:1147–1151.
7. Grizzard WS, Hilton GF. Scleral buckling for retinal detachments complicated by periretinal proliferation. Arch Ophthalmol 1982; 100:419–422.
8. Tornambe PE, Hilton GF. The Retinal Detachment Study Group. Pneumatic retinopexy. A multicenter randomized controlled clinical trial comparing pneumatic retinopexy with scleral buckling. Ophthalmology 1989; 96:772–784.
9. Tornambe PE, Hilton GF, Brinton DA, et al. Pneumatic clinical trial comparing pneumatic retinopexy with scleral buckling. Ophthalmology 1991; 98:1115–1123.
10. Tornambe PE. Pneumatic retinopexy: the evolution of case selection and surgical technique. A twelve-year study of 302 eyes. Trans Am Ophthalmol Soc 1997; 95:551–578.
11. Mougharbel M, Koch FH, Boker T, Spitznas M. No cataract two years after pneumatic retinopexy. Ophthalmology 1994; 101:1191–1194.

THE LIBRARY
THE LEARNING AND DEVELOPMENT CENTRE
THE CALDERDALE ROYAL HOSPITAL
HALIFAX HX3 0PW

13 Fluid–air exchange/fluid–gas exchange

Kent W. Small

INSTRUMENTATION

- 20-cc syringe (for simple fluid gas exchange of vitreous hemorrhage)
- 50-cc syringe (for retinal detachments or macular holes)
- Arterial line tubing or IV line tubing
- 27-Gauge short needle
- 25-Gauge short needle
- Lid speculum (two for retinal detachments)
- Povidone iodine (Betadine) 10% swabs
- Topical povidone iodine 5% (if available)
- 2% Lidocaine without adrenaline (epinephrine)
- 4% Lidocaine (topical)
- Tuberculin syringe (2)
- Filter (2 μm)
- Cotton-tipped swabs (5)
- Eye pads (2)
- Moxifloxacin (Vigamox)
- Tobramycin and dexamethasone (Tobradex) ointment
- 4 × 4 sterile sponge

INDICATIONS AND CONTRAINDICATIONS

Indications

1. To clear the vitreous opacities. This is typically a recurrent vitreous hemorrhage in the setting of diabetic retinopathy. There are other potential settings such as clearing inflammatory debris after endophthalmitis.
2. To repair a retinal detachment without proliferative vitreoretinopathy (PVR).
3. To treat recurrent macular hole.

Contraindications

1. Absence of at least a relatively thorough posterior vitrectomy.
2. Lack of knowledge/assessment of the posterior anatomy. If the media are opaque, an ultrasound is needed to be certain there is no retinal detachment, tumor, etc.

INTRODUCTION

In-office fluid–air exchange is a simple procedure that can be used to treat a variety of conditions (Fig. 13.1). The major prerequisite for being able to do a fluid–gas exchange is that the eye must have had a previous vitrectomy. The procedure requires minimal formed vitreous to be present, otherwise a fluid–gas exchange would likely be ineffective and potentially cause serious complications.

I use fluid–gas exchange for indications for which I would also consider fluid washout. Instead of just flushing fluid (balanced salt solution [BSS]) through, gas or air can be flushed through without the fear of injecting an inappropriate or potentially contaminated fluid.

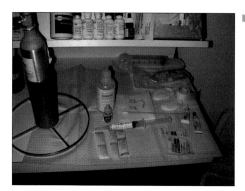

■ **FIGURE 13.1** Equipment setup for fluid–gas exchange for treating a retinal detachment.

I do not have Balanced Salt Solution Plus available in my office for phakic eyes and I do worry more about the sterility of a liquid that I am injecting into an eye than I do about a gas.

A B-scan ultrasound should always be performed within a couple of days of a fluid–gas exchange in order to allow the surgeon the most up-to-date and accurate information needed to avoid complications.

PREOPERATIVE CARE

While the use of preoperative antibiotics in this setting has not been proven to prevent endophthalmitis, I still prefer to place my patients on topical antibiotics. I like the newer generation topical antibiotics which have better ocular penetration such as moxifloxacin. I start the patient on moxifloxacin q.i.d. to begin 2 days prior to the fluid–gas exchange. If any evidence of blepharitis exists, I also begin the patient on lid hygiene measures.

THE TWO-NEEDLE APPROACH

Rationale

The two general approaches to performing an in-office fluid–gas exchange are the one-needle 'push–pull' approach or the two-needle continuous positive pressure approach. The one-needle approach is basically inserting a single needle in the eye and trying to inject gas, and then pulling the needle back to try to aspirate fluid. This has to be repeated several times to try to achieve a complete fluid–gas exchange. This results in a back and forth 'push and pull' of the syringe plunger and back and forth flow of air and gas through the needle. This single syringe method has the disadvantage of making the eye intermittently and perhaps abruptly hypotonous. I am actually more concerned with scleral infolding causing the retina, choroid or lens to move inward toward the tip of the needle and perhaps being injured by the needle. This is particularly true since this procedure is done without direct visualization of the needle. The two-needle approach allows the surgeon to always control the intraocular pressure (IOP) and the pressure will always be positive, thus avoiding hypotony/scleral infolding. Because of the to-and-fro movement of gas as well as fluid in the needle hub, the one-needle approach does not allow for as thorough a fluid–gas exchange and, in my opinion, has additional unnecessary risks.

The two-needle approach also allows for a single large bubble rather than 'fish eggs' which preclude adequate visualization and prevent any treatment of the underlying disease.

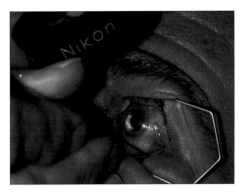

■ **FIGURE 13.2** In treating a retinal detachment, cryotherapy is performed first.

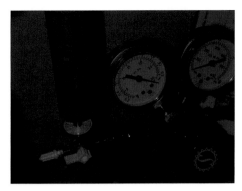

■ **FIGURE 13.3** After cryotherapy, 7 cc of 100% C_3F_8 gas is collected into the 50 cc syringe.

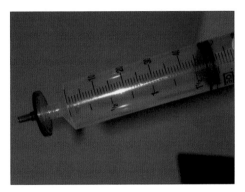

■ **FIGURE 13.4** The C_3F_8 gas is then diluted to 14% by pulling the plunger back to the 50 cc mark using filtered air.

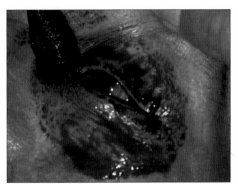

■ **FIGURE 13.5** The eye is prepared in a sterile fashion using povidone iodine.

Technique

Most of the following information will be on the two-needle approach (Figs 13.2–13.4). The initial preparation of the patient and the eye are identical to that for any intravitreal injection. First, proparacaine is instilled followed by a viscous tetracaine drop. The surgeon can either give a retrobulbar or peribulbar block with

13.1

2% lidocaine or administer subconjunctival 2% lidocaine nasally and temporally. The eye and periocular region are then prepared with povidone iodine swabs, being certain that some povidone iodine gets into the tear film and conjunctival surface (Fig. 13.5). Alternatively, topical povidone iodine 5% can be placed on the conjunctival surface. Next, a sterile lid speculum is inserted (Fig. 13.6).

The patient is then rolled into a lateral decubitus position and the surgeon sits down and adjusts the height of the stool and the patient (Fig. 13.7). It is important that the surgeon is comfortable in order to have maximal control and minimal extraneous movements.

Using a sterile tuberculin syringe to measure 3.8 mm posterior to the limbus, the 25-gauge (effluent) needle is inserted through the pars plana. The needle is left open and is not attached to anything. This needle is inserted into the dependent side of the eye (temporally for a standard diabetic vitreous hemorrhage). Then the 27-gauge (injecting) needle is inserted 3.8 mm posterior to the limbus using a sterile tuberculin syringe to measure

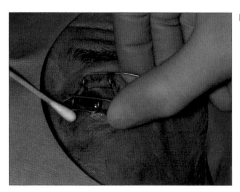

■ **FIGURE 13.6** A lid speculum is inserted.

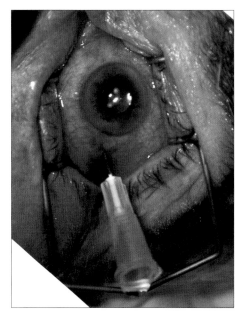

■ **FIGURE 13.7** This patient is placed in a left lateral decubitus position. Using a tuberculin syringe to measure 3.8 mm posterior to the limbus, the 25-gauge short needle, acting as the effluent needle, is inserted in the most dependent lateral position and left open.

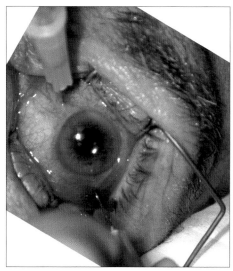

■ **FIGURE 13.8** The 27-gauge injecting needle is inserted 3.8 mm posterior to the limbus nasally in this patient. This is attached to a short tubing (arterial line tubing works nicely), which is attached to the 50 cc syringe of 14% C_3F_8 gas.

(Fig. 13.8). This is inserted through the least dependent side of the eye (nasally for a standard diabetic vitreous hemorrhage). This 27-gauge needle is attached to tubing, which is attached to a 20-cc syringe containing sterile filtered air.

Next, either the surgeon or the assistant slowly injects sterile filtered air by intermittently applying gentle pressure on the syringe plunger. Ideally I like to have an assistant perform this function so that I can gently ballott the eye to determine the approximate IOP. The surgeon needs to hold/steady the 27-gauge needle throughout the procedure. The 25-gauge effluent needle does not need to be stabilized. I like to use the 25-gauge needle for the effluent because it has a sufficient internal diameter to allow the fluid and blood to flow within a reasonable amount of time and yet it is self-sealing. As the air is injected and the bubble in the eye enlarges, it will eventually meet the tip of the 25-gauge needle. When this happens, there will be a sudden decrease in the resistance noted by the injecting person. In order to achieve maximal fluid–gas exchange, I then rotate the patient's head into more of a lateral decubitus position to ensure that the effluent needle is in as dependent a position as possible. This should cause the tip of the 25-gauge effluent needle to be submerged again, causing the injecting person to notice an increase in the resistance, and the surgeon needs to be aware of and monitor the elevation in IOP by palpation. As the bubble meets the tip of the 25-gauge effluent needle again, and air/bubbles begin to come out of the needle, it is backed slowly out of the eye. With each repositioning of the needle tip back into the fluid, the IOP will increase and fluid will once again come out of the needle tip. Repeat this maneuver of backing the needle out and injecting more gas till the 25-gauge needle is all the way out of the eye.

Once the 25-gauge effluent needle has been backed all the way out of the eye, it is then important to stop injecting to avoid excessive elevation of the IOP. Then adjust the IOP with the injecting needle/syringe, usually by aspirating a small amount of gas until the IOP feels normal. The 27-gauge injecting needle is then withdrawn. Next, indirect ophthalmoscopy is performed along with any needed cryotherapy or laser photocoagulation. Ideally there should be a single large bubble rather than 'fish eggs' to look through. Determine that there is no air or gas under the retina. If the fluid–gas exchange was performed for treating a retinal detachment, there will most likely still be fluid under the retina. Do not be alarmed by this—as long as the retinal hole is closed the subretinal fluid typically should reabsorb within a day or two. If you look into the posterior segment and find a 'fish eggs' formation of gas bubbles, I usually recommend just seeing the patient back the following day. Some have recommended 'thumping the eye' with the index finger. I have never found this necessary and it seems potentially risky as well as aesthetically unappealing.

FLUID–GAS EXCHANGE FOR VITREOUS HEMORRHAGES

When performing a fluid–gas exchange for a vitreous hemorrhage, the primary goal is to flush out the blood in order to clear the view for the patient and the surgeon. Often this is in the setting of diabetic retinopathy. Clearing the vitreous hemorrhage sooner, rather than waiting for spontaneous clearing, allows the surgeon to more aggressively and more appropriately treat the underlying cause, typically with laser photocoagulation or cryotherapy. Depending on the lens status, the surgeon may be able to place the treatment immediately after the fluid–gas exchange with laser photocoagulation or cryotherapy. Cryotherapy is particularly easy to apply after a fluid–gas exchange because the ice ball is usually more easily visualized by the surgeon than is laser photocoagulation. Additionally, laser photocoagulation is more difficult to apply because any remaining or residual blood easily blocks the laser. The combination of fluid–gas exchange and cryotherapy is especially useful in treating vitreous hemorrhages from central retinal vein occlusions. An intravitreal injection of bevacizumab (Avastin) is also helpful in treating rubeosis iridis from central retinal vein occlusion.

Because the goal is to merely clear the vitreous opacity and tamponade is not needed, I recommend using sterile air rather than a longer lasting gas mixture. Any fluid–gas exchange is not 100% complete. This usually leaves some residua of vitreous blood. If the surgeon really wanted a more complete exchange, then a washout should be performed preceding the gas exchange. This is relatively easy to accomplish by using 10 cc of sterile BSS. The surgeon can observe the red color of the effluent to determine when most of the vitreous hemorrhage has been cleared. Once the effluent appears clear, then a standard fluid–gas exchange can be performed. If a fluid washout is not performed, expect there to be a moderate amount of vitreous blood/haze for the first few days following the procedure. It is also important to warn the patient not to expect any significant improvement in vision for at least a week or two. The goal is basically to debulk the hemorrhage, not to clear it

100% immediately. If a significant amount of the blood is cleared, the remaining small amount should clear spontaneously. This is, of course, if the underlying cause is addressed with laser/cryotherapy or bevacizumab.

Because a tamponade is not the goal in this situation, positioning the patient during the procedure is not as critical an issue. Either way the patient needs to be in a lateral decubitus position with the temporal side of the treating eye being most dependent or down. Therefore, I position the needles in a way that I find most convenient/stable and secure. First, I insert the effluent 25-gauge needle temporally (dependent) with the patient in a lateral decubitus position; I then insert the nasal/influent (least dependent) 27-gauge needle.

FLUID–GAS EXCHANGE FOR RETINAL DETACHMENT

When there is adequate visualization of the retina, retinal detachment, and retinal tear, cryotherapy is performed first. After this is completed, the eye is re-prepped with povidone iodine and the fluid–gas exchange is performed. For this reason two specula are needed.

The positioning of the patient's head/eye during the fluid–gas exchange needs to be determined by the location of the detachment. It is advisable to have the effluent/dependent needle away from the area of the retinal detachment. The fear is that as the effluent needle is pulled slowly out of the eye, there will be a greater tendency of the subretinal fluid to shift toward the needle as well, possibly resulting in the needle tearing the retina or causing incarceration of the retina. For example, if the right eye has a temporal retinal detachment, the patient needs to be in a left lateral decubitus position. This has the unfortunate consequence of having the effluent flow over the patient's nose and perhaps drip into the fellow eye, which is rather disconcerting to the patient. To avoid this bit of unpleasantness, many paper or cloth towels need to be positioned to absorb the effluent.

There is, of course, the issue of the surgeon having a sufficient number of hands available to accomplish this procedure. Certainly the injecting needle, which is attached to tubing, which in turn is attached to the syringe, needs to be stabilized by the surgeon. It is possible to have an assistant do the actual injection of the gas while the surgeon stabilizes the needle. The surgeon then needs to intermittently palpate the sclera to ascertain the approximate IOP. It is important to remember that gas is compressible and fluid is not. The person doing the injection should inject a few cubic centimeters of gas and then wait for the surgeon to determine through palpation when to resume injecting. Once the effluent needle is in the intraocular gas bubble, then it is much safer to flush the gas through. If there is no assistant available, then the surgeon needs to stabilize the injecting needle with one hand and inject with the syringe with the other hand and let the effluent needle 'dangle'. The surgeon can approximate the IOP with palpation using the ring or little finger or with the movement of the needle.

Typically, the 25-gauge dependent effluent needle does not need to be stabilized as long as the patient is very still during the procedure. Allowing this needle to 'flap in the breeze', so to speak, is somewhat disconcerting to the surgeon. However, this seems to work well as long as the patient cooperates fully. The sclera seems to hold the needle in position adequately, preventing the needle tip from touching the lens or the retina. This is in part because there are no heavier devices attached to this needle such as tubing or syringe, etc. (It is important to note that it is the bare needle which is left hanging from the eye.) It is important not to allow the patient to move their eye excessively as this could cause the needle to be moved adversely against the lid.

FLUID–GAS EXCHANGE FOR RECURRENT MACULAR HOLE

The procedure for recurrent macular holes is essentially the same as that for a retinal detachment with a few exceptions. One exception is that there is no particular preference for the side—right or left—on which the patient needs to lie. Given that, I prefer the temporal side to be placed in the most dependent position/lateral decubitus. The other exception is that the sterile room air or gas is not used; instead 14% perfluoropropane (C_3F_8) is used.

POSTOPERATIVE CARE

While the postoperative use of antibiotics has not been proven effective in preventing endophthalmitis in this procedure, I prefer to continue the topical antibiotic for 4 days afterwards.

OUTCOMES

There is little published on fluid–gas exchange as an office procedure. A few publications of using fluid–gas exchange for macular holes have reported some success with this.[1-4] However, I tried this over 8 years ago without success and I abandoned the procedure for this particular indication. Perhaps I will reconsider it, although my success rate with the initial macular hole surgery is so high that the opportunity to try this procedure is infrequent now. My experience is that this can be a very effective procedure for treating retinal detachments as long as there is no PVR. It is also ideal with good outcomes in situations where a single small new retinal hole is found. For diabetic vitreous hemorrhages, the fluid–gas exchange sometimes has to be performed repetitively. Also, unless the underlying cause is treated, a recurrent hemorrhage may recur months or even years later.

Postoperative care involves topical antibiotics for a few days. If the fluid–gas procedure was performed for a retinal detachment, proper positioning instructions are mandatory for the patient. I don't feel that any patient can do proper face-down positioning. Therefore I prefer left or right side down (lateral decubitus) positioning which is much better tolerated by the patient. Additionally, lateral decubitus positioning with C_3F_8 should adequately tamponade the inferior retina.

COMPLICATIONS

1. Endophthalmitis
2. Elevated intraocular pressure
3. Migration of gas into the anterior chamber
4. Migration of gas under the retina
5. Hypotony

Certainly the most feared complication is endophthalmitis. While this is rare, I do like to monitor the patient closely after the procedure. For this I typically like to see the patient within 3–7 days postoperatively.

Elevated intraocular pressure rarely occurs when the gas used is air. If the gas used is a mixture of C_3F_8 or sulfur hexafluoride (SF_6) which should be an isovolumic, there can be an occasional intraocular pressure spike. This is more likely only if there is preexisting compromised outflow facility. In such suspected patients, I usually see the patient the next day.

Migration of gas into the anterior chamber (AC) is typically more of a nuisance than a complication by making adequate visualization of the posterior pole more difficult. Gas in the AC typically occurs because of some sort of disruption of the zonules or posterior capsule. Of course there is the issue that if gas migrated into the AC after the procedure is completed, then some of the gas is not 'doing its job' in the posterior pole. This, in my opinion, is usually not a serious issue and I recommend simply monitoring the situation. Concern about gas toxicity for the corneal endothelium I think is not clinically relevant.

Migration of gas under the retina is extremely rare. I have only seen this once when a fellow did a fluid–gas exchange on a giant retinal tear, which should never have been attempted in the first place. The other theoretical way that gas could get under the retina is if the gas-injecting needle is not placed sufficiently deep into the globe. I have seen gas going into the post lenticular hyaloidal space during a pneumatic retinopexy. In the setting of a total fluid–gas exchange, it is difficult to imagine that a larger volume of the gas could somehow be restricted to this space. Nevertheless, the gas can easily be aspirated through the same needle used to inject it with proper positioning of the patient.

Hypotony during the first postoperative day or two is not worrisome and should merely be monitored. As long as there is some intact conjunctiva, the needle sites should self-seal with little problem.

REFERENCES

1. Ohana E, Blumenkranz MS. Treatment of reopened macular hole after vitrectomy by laser and outpatient fluid–gas exchange. Ophthalmology 1998; 105:1398–1403.
2. Johnson RN, McDonald HR, Schatz H, Ai E. Outpatient postoperative fluid–gas exchange after early failed vitrectomy surgery for macular hole. Ophthalmology 1997; 104:2009–2013.
3. Stallman JB, Meyers SM. Repeated fluid–gas exchange for hypotony after vitreoretinal surgery for proliferative vitreoretinopathy. Am J Ophthalmol 1988; 106:147–153.
4. McDonald HR, Abrams GW, Irvine AR, Sipperley JO, Boyden BS, Fiore JV Jr, Zegarra H. The management of subretinal gas following attempted pneumatic retinal reattachment. Ophthalmology 1987; 94:319–326.
5. Landers MB 3rd, Robinson D, Olsen KR, Rinkoff J. Slit-lamp fluid–gas exchange and other office procedures following vitreoretinal surgery. Arch Ophthalmol 1985; 103:967–972.

14 Drainage of choroidal hemorrhage, detachment, or effusions

Maurice G. Syrquin, Bruce Taylor, Richard Winslow, Gregory Kozielec, and Marcus Allen

INSTRUMENTS AND DEVICES

- Cyclopentolate (Cyclogyl)
- Phenylephrine HCl (Sanofi-Synthelabo)
- Tobramycin and dexamethasone (Tobradex) (Alcon, Fort Worth, Texas)
- Marking pen
- Povidone iodine (Betadine) solution wash/prep
- Drape (Alcon, no. 8065117020)
- Stevens tenotomy scissors
- Jaffe lid speculum with rubber bands no. E0997
- Castroviejo 0.12 mm forceps no. E1796 Storz
- Blunt Westcott scissors no. E3320R
- Jameson muscle hook no. E0586
- Von Graphe muscle hook
- Gass eyelet muscle hook no. E4991
- 2-0 silk tie no. A185H
- Curved Schepens retractor no. E5008
- Keeler Fison indirect ophthalmoscope
- 20-diopter Volk lens
- 30-diopter Volk lens
- O'Connor scleral depressor/marker no. E5109
- Castroviejo 0.3 mm forceps no. E1797
- Mira TR4000 diathermy gray tip blunt T4
- No. 57 Beaver blade (Alcon no. 8065005701)
- Penetrating diathermy green conical tip T3 or indirect laser or 30-gauge needle no. S-24
- Barraquer cyclodialysis spatula no. E0484
- Balanced salt solution (BSS) 500 mL
- 1.5 mm infusion cannula
- Lewicky anterior chamber maintainer no. BD 585061, 20-gauge × 3.5 mm (self-retaining)
- For gravity flow, IV tubing with sterile extension (2)
- For gas forced infusion, VGFI tubing (Alcon no. 8065808002) connected to Accurus unit
- Castroviejo needle holder no. E3861, Storz
- 7-0 Vicryl no. J546
- Subconjunctival gentamicin 20 mg/0.5 mL, and dexamethasone (Decadron) 2 mg/0.5 mL
- Atropine
- Maxitrol (dexamethasone, neomycin, polymyxin B sulfate)
- Patch
- Fox shield

BOX 14.1 Etiology of choroidal detachment or hemorrhage

- Idiopathic
- Inflammatory
  - Intraocular surgery or trauma
- Hydrodynamic
  - Hypotony or wound leak

BOX 14.2 Classification of ciliochoroidal or uveal effusion

- Idiopathic
- Inflammatory
  - Intraocular surgery or trauma
  - Uveitis
  - Scleritis
  - Infected scleral buckle
  - Following photocoagulation and cryocoagulation
- Hydrodynamic
  - Dural arteriovenous fistula
  - Hypotony or wound leak
  - Nanophthalmos
  - Excessively thick sclera

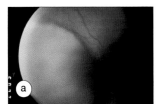 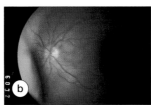 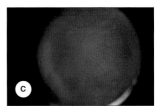

■ **FIGURE 14.1** (**a**) Serous choroidal detachment with orange/brown appearance. (**b**) Hemorrhagic choroidal detachment with darker appearance. (**c**) Shallow posterior hemorrhagic choroidal detachment.

INDICATIONS AND CONTRAINDICATIONS

Trauma

Blunt trauma following extracapsular, intracapsular, and clear cornea cataract surgery represents a large portion of choroidal detachments and hemorrhages. This trauma may result in wound dehiscence and prolapse of an intraocular lens, uvea, retina, and vitreous.[1]

Postoperative choroidal detachment

Choroidal detachment occurs in varying degrees of severity in approximately 24% of eyes following scleral buckling surgery for retinal detachments.[2] The majority of postoperative choroidal detachments are transudative (Fig. 14.1a); very few are hemorrhagic (Fig. 14.1b,c). Small choroidal detachments often pass unnoticed because they affect only the region of the pars plana ciliaris and the retinal periphery, and subside spontaneously.[3] Postoperative choroidal detachment appears as a solid, immobile orange-brown elevation of the fundus

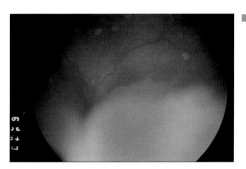

■ **FIGURE 14.2** Orange/brown coloration of choroidal detachment.

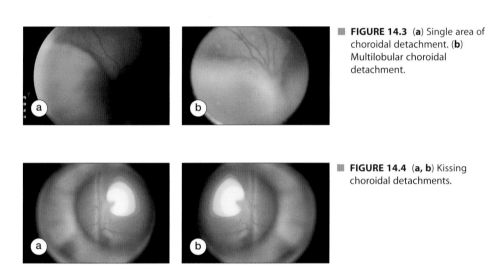

■ **FIGURE 14.3** (**a**) Single area of choroidal detachment. (**b**) Multilobular choroidal detachment.

■ **FIGURE 14.4** (**a, b**) Kissing choroidal detachments.

(Fig. 14.2). The detachment extends beyond the ora serrata, making the extreme fundus periphery visible without scleral depression. The choroidal elevation may be single or multilobular (Fig. 14.3). It may progress in an annular direction around the entire fundus periphery, or extend posteriorly to obscure the macula or optic disc.

Management of postoperative choroidal detachment

Most postoperative choroidal detachments subside spontaneously and require no treatment. When the choroidal elevation extends posterior to the equator and around the entire fundus periphery to result in a shallowing of the anterior chamber, 100 mg prednisone is given daily orally for 5–7 days. Drainage of subchoroidal fluid is indicated when the choroidal detachment involves the macula, or when temporal and nasal detachments extend posteriorly until they come in contact (Fig. 14.4).[4] These are termed 'kissing' choroidal detachments.[5]

Ciliochoroidal effusion (CCE)

Uveal effusion should not be considered a distinct disease entity. Actually the term refers to an abnormal intraocular accumulation of serous fluid due to a variety of conditions. In CCE, fluid leaks from the choriocapillaris into the choroid or subretinal space, or both. This results in choroidal and ciliary body detachment and a non-rhegmatogenous retinal detachment. Some causes of CCE have been identified but there are other cases in which no cause can be found.[6]

14.1

SURGICAL TECHNIQUE

Preoperative preparation

Clinical examinations with slit lamp biomicroscopy and indirect ophthalmoscopy are essential to determine the size and location of the choroidal clot size. If vitreous hemorrhage precludes a view, serial ultrasonography will be needed to assess the clot size, location, and retinal status.

Clot lysis usually occurs within 1–2 weeks after injury. Observation during this time will facilitate choroidal drainage and avoid exacerbating the choroidal hemorrhage.

A medical examination for preoperative clearance and informed consent should be obtained. The patient should be made nil per os (nothing by mouth/NPO) after midnight.

Procedure

A 360° conjunctival peritomy is performed. The intramuscular septum is dissected in all four quadrants using curved Stevens scissors. A 2-0 silk tie is slung on all four rectus muscles using a Von Graphe muscle hook. All four quadrants are inspected for signs of thinning staphylomata or any other ocular abnormalities. Indirect ophthalmoscopy with scleral depression using a Gass localizer is used to mark the area or quadrant of maximal choroidal effusion or hemorrhage (Fig. 14.5).

Drainage of subchoroidal fluid or hemorrhage in a phakic eye

A radial sclerotomy is made using a 57 Beaver blade in the previously marked point of maximal choroidal effusion or hemorrhage. The choroid is perforated with an S-24 needle or fine point diathermy. Once approximately 0.5 mL of fluid has been drained, Balanced Salt Solution Plus is injected into the pars plana 4 mm posterior to the limbus using a 30-gauge needle. This can be repeated until indirect ophthalmoscopy reveals the disappearance of the choroidal elevation.

Drainage of subchoroidal fluid or hemorrhage in an aphakic eye

Using the same radial sclerotomy and perforation technique in an aphakic or pseudophakic eye, the infusion is accomplished using a 1.5 mm anterior chamber infusion cannula or 25-gauge needle at the limbus connected to a BSS intraocular infusion bottle. In a vitrectomized eye, air can be used as well. Great care must be exercised to avoid high intraocular pressures which could cause incarcerations at the sclerotomy sites. Additional fluid may be released by carefully inserting an iris spatula tangentially into the sclerotomy in order to lyse any clots that may be impeding the drainage. After drainage, the sclerotomy should be left open for further drainage.

Drainage of ciliochoroidal (uveal) effusion

Simple drainage of subretinal fluid in conventional surgery for rhegmatogenous retinal detachment will not help this type of non-rhegmatogenous retinal detachment. Since the

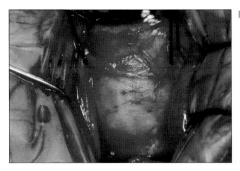

■ **FIGURE 14.5** Isolation of rectus muscles and exposure of quadrant for drainage of choroidal detachment.

CCE in nanophthalmos appears to be a consequence of the abnormally thick sclera, which obstructs vortex venous drainage, resection of sclera with decompression of the vortex veins is indicated.[6] However, there is controversy regarding vortex vein decompression, and partial-thickness scleral resection alone without vortex vein decompression can be successful. After identifying the vortex vein, an equatorial incision, 6–7 mm long, is made 5 mm anterior to the exit site of the vortex vein. Meridional incisions, 6 mm long, are then made on either side posteriorly. The incisions are carried down until a slate gray color, from pigment in the choroid, is seen and the sclera is dissected posteriorly so that the intrascleral portion of the vortex vein is exposed and unroofed or decompressed (Fig. 14.6). All four vortices are decompressed, and in each dissected scleral bed a sclerotomy is made to expose the choroid. The edges of the sclera at the sclerotomy site are treated with diathermy to cause shrinkage of the sclera and gaping of the sclerotomy to keep the sclerotomy open postoperatively. If significant choroidal detachment is present, fluid will escape from these sclerotomies. Subsequent hypotony is controlled by injection of BSS into the anterior chamber or through the pars plana.

Although subretinal fluid will gradually be absorbed after vortex vein decompression, it may be desirable to drain subretinal fluid to restore vision more rapidly if the detachment is extensive. The 'shifting fluid' phenomenon must be remembered when drainage of subretinal fluid is performed. The sclerotomy for drainage should be slightly posterior to the equator and positioned so that it is directed toward the center of gravity or floor of the operating room. Subretinal fluid in patients with CCE, including nanophthalmic effusion, is protein rich and heavy and will not run 'uphill'. After exposure of the choroid, it should be transilluminated and any choroidal vessels must be closed by diathermy to prevent hemorrhage. A 4-0 polyethylene suture is preplaced, mattress fashion, in the sclera for

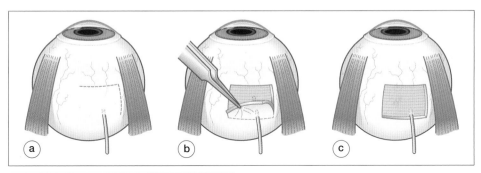

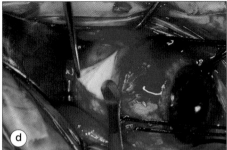

▓ **FIGURE 14.6** Technique for drainage of ciliochoroidal effusion and decompression of the vortex veins. (**a**) An incision is made circumferentially for approximately 6 mm in length. Then two incisions are made radially and posteriorly for approximately 6 mm in length. (**b**) A 57 blade is then used to dissect the partial thickness scleral flap so that the grayish/brownish color of the choroid is visible. (**c**) The partial thickness scleral tissue that has been dissected is then removed. (**d**) Intraoperative dissection of partial thickness sclera with 57 blade.

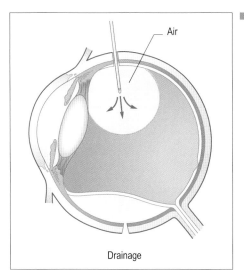

Air

Drainage

■ **FIGURE 14.7** Injection of air into the vitreous cavity through the pars plana to restore intraocular pressure after drainage of choroidal detachment.

subsequent closure of the drainage site. The drainage site should not involve vortex ampullae or the long posterior ciliary artery and nerve.

Just before penetration, the operating room table is tilted laterally and the patient's head rotated, so that the perforation site points toward the floor. A sharp, fine, perforating needle is then used to perforate the thickened choroid. Air or gas is injected at the most superior portion of the globe, through the pars plana, to restore normal intraocular pressure (Fig. 14.7).

Postoperatively the patient's head is positioned to keep the air (gas) in contact with the retina and away from the lens (phakic patients) to avoid inducing a cataract. Systemic steroids are generally used for 2–4 weeks to minimize postoperative inflammation.[7]

VIDEO

The video shows an example of a modified Brockhurst procedure in ciliochoroidal (uveal effusion) in a dwarf with nanophthalmos, extremely thick sclera, and a very hyperopic eye.

POSTOPERATIVE CARE

The patient is transported to the recovery room and discharged to home when discharge criteria are met. The patient is evaluated on postoperative day 1 and the shield is removed.

Postoperative medications and instructions

1. Cyclogel 1% (cyclopentolate) 1 gtt in the affected eye q.i.d.
2. Tobramycin and dexamethasone (Tobradex) 1 drop in the affected eye q.i.d.
3. Head of the bed at 45°.
4. No aspirin.
5. Signs and symptoms of infection and retinal detachment explained.
6. Follow-up in 1 week.

OUTCOMES

Outcomes are dependent on size, location, duration, and etiology of the choroidal detachment, hemorrhage or effusion and retinal status. Unfortunately these conditions may recur, particularly in patients with nanophthalmos requiring repeated procedures.

REFERENCES

1. Ryan SJ. Retina. Philadelphia: Saunders, 2008. Vol. 2, Section 6, Chapter 107:730.
2. Hawkins WR, Schepens CL. Choroidal detachment and retinal surgery: a clinical and experimental study. Am J Ophthalmol 1966; 62:812–819.
3. Schepens CL. Retinal detachment and allied diseases. Philadelphia: WB Saunders, 1983.
4. Freeman M, Tolentino F. Atlas of vitreoretinal surgery. Thieme: New York, 1989. Chapter 22:195.
5. Hilton GF, Wallyn RH. The removal of scleral buckles. Arch Ophthalmol 1978; 96:2061–2063.
6. Ryan SJ. Retina. Philadelphia: Saunders, 2008. Vol. 2, Section 6, Chapter 107:729.
7. Ryan SJ. Retina. Philadelphia: Saunders, 2008. Vol. 2, Section 6, Chapter 107:732–733.

15

Vitreous implants

Alex Bui, Sachin Mudvari, J. Michael Jumper, and Everett Ai

INDICATIONS AND CONTRAINDICATIONS

With the development of sustained-release intraocular drug implants, therapeutic concentrations can be achieved without the limitations of systemic, topical, or periocular administration. Vitreous implants allow long-term therapeutic drug levels while reducing the adverse effects from other modes of administration. There are currently two commercially available sustained-release implants: Vitrasert (dihydroxy propoxymethyl guanine 6 mg, Bausch & Lomb) indicated for the control of cytomegalovirus (CMV) retinitis and Retisert (fluocinolone acetonide 0.59 mg, Bausch & Lomb), designed to locally treat chronic, non-infectious uveitis affecting the posterior segment of the eye (Fig. 15.1). Intraocular steroids are contraindicated in viral diseases of the cornea and conjunctiva, including epithelial herpes simplex keratitis, vaccinia, and varicella, mycobacterial infections of the eye, fungal diseases of ocular structures, and in patients with a history of central serous retinopathy or advanced glaucoma.

Retisert

Intraocular inflammation results in blindness or visual impairment in 35% of uveitis patients and approximately 23% will undergo one or more surgical procedures due to complications.[1] Posterior uveitis can lead to vision loss by cataract formation, vascular occlusions, cystoid macular edema, epiretinal membranes, choroidal neovascular membranes, and optic disc atrophy. Corticosteroids are the mainstay for the treatment of intraocular inflammation but topical and systemic steroids have severe side effects with both short- and long-term use. In some cases of severe intraocular inflammation, immunosuppressive treatments are required in addition to steroids.[2] Major complications can occur with immunosuppressive agents such as severe infection, hypertension, liver dysfunction, and secondary malignancy.[3] Because of the adverse effects of systemic treatment of chronic posterior uveitis, a sustained-release steroid implant was developed. Retisert (fluocinolone acetonide 0.59 mg) is a sterile implant designed to release fluocinolone acetonide at a rate of 0.3 and 0.4 mcg/day over approximately 30 months.

In clinical trials, 227 patients with chronic (a 1-year or greater history) non-infectious uveitis affecting the posterior segment received a 0.59 mg Retisert implant.[4] The primary efficacy endpoint in both trials was the rate of recurrence in the posterior over the 34-week postimplantation period compared to the rate of recurrence in the 34-week period preimplantation. The rates of recurrence ranged from 7% to 14% for the 34-week period postimplantation as compared to 40% to 54% for the 34-week period preimplantation. There was also a decrease from baseline in systemic corticosteroid and/or immunosuppressive use over the follow-up period.

Vitrasert

Cytomegalovirus (CMV) is a species-specific DNA virus of the herpes group. Episodes of disease reactivation and progression can be expected in conditions characterized by impaired

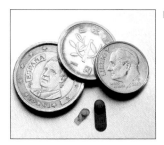

■ **FIGURE 15.1** Commercially available vitreous implants. Left: Retisert (fluocinolone acetonide 0.59 mg). Right: Vitrasert (dihydroxy propoxymethyl guanine 6 mg).

immunity, such as the acquired immunodeficiency syndrome (AIDS), transplant patients, and patients on chemotherapy.[5,6] In an immunocompromised host, CMV can disseminate hematogenously and cause a variety of systemic infections including encephalitis, pneumonitis, colitis, hepatitis, nephritis, and retinitis. CMV produces a necrotizing retinitis that enlarges by contiguous cell-to-cell spread. Clinically, retina infected with actively replicating virus becomes opaque and demonstrates the presence of multiple patches of granular appearing white dots which coalesce into a leading edge of infection with a variable amount of retinal hemorrhage. Infected regions of retinal tissue are gradually replaced over several weeks by atrophic tissue. CMV retinitis frequently demonstrates a radial or arcuate pattern of progression that may represent vascular or nerve fiber layer spread.

Prior to the development of highly active antiretroviral therapy (HAART), approximately 20% (range 12–46%) of AIDS patients in various studies developed CMV retinitis and required lifelong systemic medications.[7–9] Retinal detachments occurred in 38–50% of patients within a year of being diagnosed with CMV retinitis.[10,11] Compared with the rates reported in the pre-HAART era, there has been a 75% decline in the incidence of CMV retinitis since the introduction of HAART.[12,13] The use of HAART in AIDS patients appears to reduce the risk of retinal detachment by approximately 60%,[14] but among patients with CD4+ T-cell counts of < 50 cells/μL, the rates are more similar to those from the pre-HAART era.[15]

Ganciclovir (dihydroxy propoxymethyl guanine) is a virostatic agent that is a more potent inhibitor of CMV DNA polymerases than host cellular polymerases and has been the mainstay of CMV treatment since its clinical introduction in 1984. This drug is a purine analog and is similar in structure to acyclovir with the exception of an additional side-chain methoxyl group. Intracellular phosphorylation of ganciclovir to its active form in CMV-infected cells is 10 times higher than that inside uninfected cells. Uninfected bone marrow cells, however, are an exception and are more sensitive to ganciclovir than other host cells.[16] This accounts for the major toxicity of the drug—bone marrow suppression. Induction with intravenous ganciclovir is traditionally given b.i.d. at 5 mg/kg for 2–3 weeks, followed by maintenance of 5 mg/kg q.d. intravenously.

Foscarnet (trisodium phosphoformate) works as a reversible inhibitor of viral-specific DNA polymerases and HIV reverse transcriptase. Like ganciclovir, it is virostatic and a permanent maintenance dose is usually necessary. Unlike ganciclovir, however, myelosuppression is not a major concern with foscarnet. Alternatively, intravenous foscarnet can be used for active CMV at a dose of 60 mg/kg t.i.d. for 2–3 weeks for induction, and then 90–120 mg/kg for maintenance. The Study of Ocular Complications of AIDS Research (SOCA) Foscarnet–Ganciclovir CMV Retinitis Trial showed that foscarnet was associated with longer survival and a lower mortality rate than ganciclovir, but intravenous administration of the two drugs appeared equivalent in controlling CMV retinitis and preserving vision.[17] The difference in survival and mortality associated with foscarnet is thought to be due to two main factors. The drug has intrinsic activity against some retroviruses including HIV and it can be used concurrently with AZT (zidovudine) in AIDS patients, as opposed to ganciclovir, because the drug does not exacerbate bone marrow suppression. Since both drugs are virostatic, dormant CMV will typically relapse within 6 weeks if indefinite maintenance therapy is stopped in a patient without significant immune recovery.[18]

Long-term administration of intravenous ganciclovir is associated with myelosuppression and neutropenia in approximately a third of patients on initial or maintenance therapy.[19–21] Systemic foscarnet has been linked to seizures due to electrolyte imbalances and renal toxicity in approximately 15–30% of patients.[22–24] In an effort to reduce adverse effects in CMV retinitis patients treated with systemic ganciclovir, Henry and coworkers[25] used weekly to biweekly intravitreal ganciclovir injections of 200 mcg/0.1 mL. Repeat intravitreal injections enabled intraocular therapeutic levels without treatment-limiting side effects, but were associated with vitreous hemorrhage, endophthalmitis, cataract formation, and retinal detachment in up to 10% of patients with repeated injections.[26–29]

Spurred by the need for an alternative to either extended systemic or intravitreal ganciclovir, an intraocular device was developed for extended control of CMV retinitis.[30,31] The ganciclovir implant is a sustained-release intraocular drug delivery system used to treat CMV retinitis that provides a high and steady-state concentration of 1 mcg/h of ganciclovir in the vitreous cavity over a period of 7–8 months.[32] The implant is produced by coating a compressed 6 mg pellet of ganciclovir with ethylene vinyl acetate on all surfaces but the top surface and surrounded by a coat of polyvinyl chloride (Fig. 15.2). This device allows higher intraocular levels of ganciclovir than can be achieved with maintenance intravenous ganciclovir.[30,33,34]

The ganciclovir implant offers a number of advantages over systemic therapy, including the longest median time of control of retinitis reported to date, the elimination of the need for an indwelling catheter, and higher intraocular concentrations in patients with resistant CMV strains.[35,36] An advantage of systemic administration, however, is that patients treated with intravenous ganciclovir are less likely to have extraocular and fellow eye CMV infections.[8,37] Even with placement of an intraocular implant, it is important that the patient remains compliant with the antiretroviral protocol and maintenance CMV regimen to protect the fellow eye and overall health of the patient if immune recovery has not been meaningful.[38,39]

The Ganciclovir Implant Study Group showed that the median time to progression of retinitis was 221 days with the 1 mcg/h implant versus 71 days with ganciclovir administered intravenously. The risk of progression of retinitis was almost three times as great among patients treated with intravenous ganciclovir as among those treated with a ganciclovir implant.[36] Factors in the decision to place an implant include the patient's antiretroviral treatment history and potential for immunologic improvement, current CD4+ T-lymphocyte count, current plasma HIV RNA level, lifestyle preferences, and the location of CMV retinitis.

With the emergence of ganciclovir-resistant CMV, defined as a median inhibitory concentration (IC50) >6 μmol/L, an increased vitreous concentration is needed to suppress

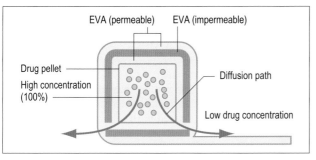

EVA (permeable)   EVA (impermeable)

Drug pellet
High concentration (100%)

Diffusion path

Low drug concentration

■ **FIGURE 15.2** Schematic of the ganciclovir intraocular delivery device. EVA, ethylene vinyl acetate; PVA, polyvinyl alcohol.

viral replication. Overall, approximately 3–8% of AIDS patients with systemic CMV and approximately 11–38% of patients previously treated with ganciclovir excrete CMV resistant to the drug.[40–42] Patients with ganciclovir resistance have been shown to respond to the sustained-release ganciclovir implant with an approximate 60% reduction in the risk of retinitis progression in these patients.[43–45]

INSTRUMENTATION

- Lid speculum
- Retrobulbar block with a 50:50 mixture of 2% lidocaine and 0.75% bupivacaine (Marcaine)
- Indirect ophthalmoscope
- 20-diopter lens
- Corneal shield
- Balanced salt solution (BSS)
- Angled tipped bipolar cautery
- 23-Gauge tapered endodiathermy
- 3-cc syringe with a 27-gauge needle
- 3-cc syringe with a 30-gauge needle
- 8-0 Nylon sutures
- Double-armed 8-0 Prolene (polypropylene) suture
- Curved needle drivers (2)
- Vannas scissors
- Blunt-tipped Westcott scissors
- 0.12 forceps
- Bishop–Harmon forceps
- Angled Macpherson forceps
- 6-0 Vicryl traction suture
- Calipers
- Marking pen
- 20-Gauge microvitreoretinal (MVR) blade
- No. 69 Beaver blade
- Weck-Cel sponges
- Dexamethasone 4 mg/0.5 mL subconjunctival injection
- Cefazolin 50–100 mg/1 mL subconjunctival injection

PREOPERATIVE PREPARATION

Induction and maintenance using intravenous ganciclovir or foscarnet is the mainstay of treatment of CMV retinitis. If recovery of immune function is not possible, indefinite treatment is needed, and an indwelling catheter and daily intravenous medication may be required. The costs and inherent risks of an indwelling catheter have been reduced by the development of an oral ganciclovir preparation. Valganciclovir is a monovalyl ester prodrug that, when administered orally, is rapidly hydrolyzed to the active compound ganciclovir. The absolute bioavailability of ganciclovir from valganciclovir is similar to that obtained with a dose of intravenous ganciclovir at 5 mg/kg of body weight.[46–49] Neutropenia, anemia, intravenous catheter-related adverse events, and sepsis were more common in those given intravenous ganciclovir for both induction and maintenance.

Cessation of anti-CMV therapy should only be considered in patients with a rise in the $CD4^+$ T-lymphocyte count of >50 cells/μL associated with suppression of the HIV plasma RNA levels to <200 copies/mL.[50–54] The location of the lesion and the status of the other eye should be considered before discontinuing therapy. It is recommended to restart maintenance therapy if the $CD4^+$ T-lymphocyte count decreases to 50–100 cells/μL, and continued ophthalmologic examinations are recommended in all patients with a history of CMV retinitis regardless of CD4⁺ T-lymphocyte count.

Special considerations may justify more aggressive interventions. When the retinitis threatens the optic nerve or macula, the patient has reduced vision in the fellow eye, or the patient has a declining CD4⁺ T-lymphocyte count despite HAART, aggressive treatment with an intraocular implant or intravitreal injections would be warranted as a bridge until immune recovery. However, if the lesion is peripheral, there is good vision in the fellow eye, and the patient is naive to HAART, treatment with intravenous therapy or oral valganciclovir may be preferred to spare the patient the morbidity of an intraocular procedure.[55]

Sanborn and coworkers defined parameters that helped guide their decision to proceed with intraocular ganciclovir implantation.[31] Progression was defined as an enlargement of the retinitis 750 μm beyond its margins or the appearance of a new lesion of at least 750 μm as seen on fundus photographs or fundus examination over a 2-week period. Non-progression was defined as a lack of progression of the retinitis with respect to retinal landmarks. Resolution was defined as non-progression and replacement of opacified retina with atrophic retinal pigmentation.

Holland et al. divided the retina into zones to describe the extent of involvement.[56] Zone 1 involvement (posterior and sight threatening) extended 3000 μm from the center of the fovea and 1500 μm from the disc. Zone 2 was anterior to zone 1 up to the equator and zone 3 was anterior to the equator (Fig. 15.3).

PROCEDURE

Following implantation of a vitreous implant, nearly all patients will experience an immediate and temporary decrease in visual acuity in the implanted eye which lasts for approximately 1–4 weeks postoperatively. This decrease in visual acuity is likely a result of the surgical procedure. When removing the implant from its packaging, care is taken not to grasp the device with toothed forceps or anywhere other than the securing strut as damage to the pellet may alter the diffusion rate of the drug. Care should be taken during implantation and explantation to avoid sheer forces on the implant that could disengage the drug reservoir from the suture tab. Aseptic technique should be

15.1

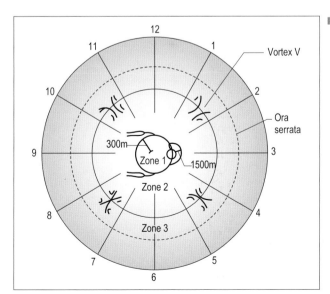

■ **FIGURE 15.3** Zones of retinal involvement in CMV retinitis.

maintained at all times prior to and during the surgical implantation procedure. No intra-ocular implant can be resterilized. The implant should be kept dry to prevent softening of the coating. A backup implant should be available as a precaution if the first one becomes unusable due to damage or loss of sterility.

The pupil is dilated with cyclopentolate (Cyclogyl) 2% and phenylephrine 2.5%. After administration of retrobulbar anesthesia consisting of 2% lidocaine and 0.75% bupivacaine 1:1 (volume:volume), the skin and conjunctiva are cleansed with 5% povidone iodine (Betadine). The eye is draped and a lid speculum is placed. The peripheral retina should be examined prior to surgery to identify any areas of peripheral traction, snowbanking, or retinal detachment, and these areas avoided as possible sites for implantation. A site should be chosen where the conjunctiva is healthy enough to cover the sutures used to close the wound and the sclera thick enough to prevent extrusion of the device.

Unlike the Retisert implant which comes with an anchoring strut ready for placement, the Vitrasert implant will need to be trimmed and a hole placed prior to insertion. The end of the implant is grasped firmly with a curved needle driver. The anchoring strut is trimmed with Westcott scissors so that the distance from the drug disk to the end of the anchoring strut is approximately 2.5 mm and leaving no sharp edges. Using the 27-gauge needle, create a puncture in the center of the strut no more than 0.5 mm from the end of the strut (Fig. 15.4). The implant is then prepared by passing a double-armed 8-0 poly-propylene suture on a TG-175 needle through the base of the anchoring strut. A single throw is made to prevent the implant tab from entering the sclera when the anchoring suture is tied. Browning reported a case of a posteriorly dislocated ganciclovir implant 6 years after original implantation.[57] Nylon may be a poorer choice for this purpose than polypropylene, which has less of a tendency to erode in an aqueous environment.

If the eye has had a previous vitrectomy, a 20- or 25-gauge pars plana infusion line can be placed in a separate quadrant to minimize globe collapse. A conjunctival peritomy is initiated with Bishop–Harmon forceps and blunt tipped Westcott scissors approximately 2 mm posterior to the temporal (or nasal) limbus and then radialized. The peritomy is extended inferiorly three clock hours to expose the inferotemporal quadrant. An angled tipped bipolar diathermy is used to achieve hemostasis of the surrounding sclera. Calipers and a marking pen are used to mark the sclera 4 mm posterior to the limbus, preferentially at the 7 o'clock position in the right eye or at 5 o'clock in the left eye. Proper placement of the implant in the pars plana is important as anterior positioning has been shown to lead to hyalinization and fibrosis of the ciliary body by histopathologic examination.[58] In

the event that a retinal detachment develops in a patient with CMV retinitis and silicone oil is used, inferior placement will allow the implant to rest within the inferior aqueous interface.

15.2
15.3

For the Vitrasert implant, a No. 69 Beaver blade is used to create a 5 mm scleral incision down to the choroid 4 mm from the limbus. In the case of the Retisert

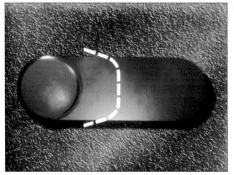

FIGURE 15.4 Vitrasert implant prior to preparation of the anchoring strut (right).

implant, a 3.5 mm scleral incision is made. The choroid is visualized and treated with a 23-gauge endodiathermy. A 20-gauge MVR blade is used to enter the pars plana and the incision is enlarged along its full length (Fig. 15.5a). With a vitrectomy cutter or a Weck-Cel with Westcott scissors, any vitreous prolapsed through the wound is excised. The lips of the incision are held open with two 0.12 forceps to confirm that a full thickness incision through the pars plana and underlying choroid has been made the full length of the

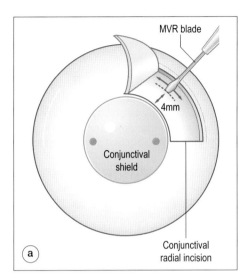

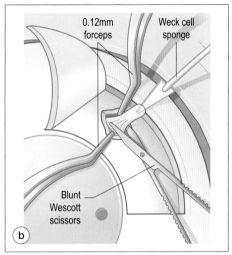

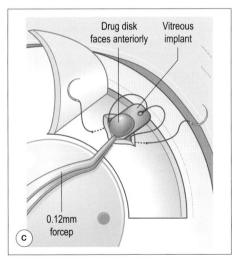

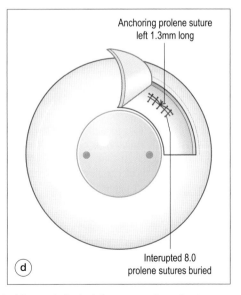

FIGURE 15.5 (a) Conjunctival peritomy and scleral incision made in the inferotemporal quadrant. (b) Inspection and preparation of the full thickness scleral incision prior to insertion of the vitreous implant. Prolapsed vitreous is removed using a Weck-Cel sponge and Westcott scissors or automated vitreous cutter. (c) Placement of the vitreous implant secured by the 8-0 prolene anchoring suture. (d) Closure of the scleral wound with interrupted 8-0 nylon sutures. The tails of the anchoring suture are flush against the sclera underneath the 8-0 nylon sutures.

incision (Fig. 15.5b). Any remaining choroidal tissue still intact should be cut so that inadvertent placement into the suprachoroidal space can be avoided.

The strut of the device is grasped with smooth-tipped forceps or needle driver and inserted into the eye with the drug pellet facing anteriorly. The double-armed 8-0 polypropylene suture is passed as an anchoring suture through either side of the scleral incision (Fig. 15.5c). The needle is passed full thickness through the anterior lip of the wound to the surface of the sclera. The second half of the polypropylene suture is passed in a similar fashion through the posterior lip of the wound. Extrusion of the implant may be avoided by trimming of the suture tab close to the anchoring suture, placing a single throw after threading the anchoring suture, and not tying it too tightly.[59] The anchoring suture is tied with moderate tension and the suture ends left 3 mm long. If the strut appears to be pulled into the wound when the anchoring suture is tightened, the suture should be loosened or adjacent 8-0 nylon sutures placed prior to tying the anchoring suture. Next, between three and five interrupted 8-0 nylon sutures are used to close the scleral incision with the ends of the anchoring suture secured flat against the sclera. The scleral sutures are rotated and buried with angled Macpherson forceps (Fig. 15.5d). The wound is inspected with a Weck-Cel sponge to assure proper closure without prolapsed vitreous or wound leak and that the strut of the implant is not exposed. BSS can be injected through the incision with a cannula or through the pars plana with a 30-gauge needle to restore intraocular pressure.

Indirect ophthalmoscopy verifies proper placement of the implant at the vitreous base. Gentle depression maybe performed to visualize the implant's location in the vitreous cavity (Fig. 15.6) The conjunctiva is closed with interrupted 6-0 plain gut sutures. Subconjunctival injections of cefazolin 100 mg/mL (Ancef, GlaxoSmithKline) and 4 mg/0.5 mL dexamethasone sodium phosphate are given so as to elevate the conjunctiva over the implant site. A sterile dressing is placed over the eye and the patient is seen the next day for follow-up.

REPLACING THE IMPLANT

Implant patients may require replacement of a device for continued treatment of their disease. The Retisert implant lasts for approximately 30 months. Replacement of a ganciclovir implant has been shown to be well tolerated and results in effective suppression of retinitis in a patient with previously controlled CMV.[60,61] The principal reason for progression of CMV retinitis after implantation is the device running out of drug.[35] An approximate 8-month effective duration of the implant corresponds well to the observed median times to progression in patients treated with intraocular ganciclovir devices of 221 days[36] and 226 days.[35] Reactivation of CMV due to depletion of the ganciclovir implant requires reimplantation. In implant patients without progression, the location of the retinitis and the overall health of the patient are important factors when deciding whether to wait for reactivation prior to reimplantation.

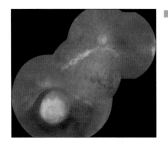

■ **FIGURE 15.6** A ganciclovir implant located at the vitreous base in a patient with CMV retinitis. (Courtesy of J. Michael Jumper, M.D.)

In CMV patients without appreciable immune reconstitution or vision-threatening lesions in zone 1 controlled by implantation, exchange of an implant based on the projected 8-month depletion of the device is reasonable. With patients experiencing immune recovery due to HAART and on concomitant oral maintenance valganciclovir, most patients have implants replaced when reactivation of retinitis occurs. Waiting for disease reactivation has some potential disadvantages. With each reactivation, there is increased loss of visual field, increased risk for visual loss (especially in the setting of zone 1 disease), and a higher risk of detachments with implant exchange in an eye with active retinitis.[60]

Implant replacement can be performed at the initial site, contiguous to the initial site, or in a separate site altogether as described by Morley et al.[61] The same-site technique (Fig. 15.7b) begins with an inferotemporal fornix-based conjunctival peritomy with careful dissection over the original incision. Any adherent episclera over the existing sutures is removed with Vannas scissors. The 8-0 nylon sutures closing the wound are cut with Vannas scissors and removed using 0.12 forceps. A stab incision is made with an MVR blade on either side of the 8-0 polypropylene anchoring suture and extended to the superior and inferior extent of the wound. Care must be taken not to cut the anchoring suture holding the device in place prematurely. With two 0.12 forceps, grasp either side of the wound and gently open the wound to visualize the strut. If the strut is not immediately visible, it is often found at the posterior lip of the incision. The end of the strut is grasped with 0.12 forceps and any fibrous sheath surrounding the implant is gently removed using the MVR blade. Once the implant is free of fibrous adhesions and the strut securely grasped, the anchoring suture is cut and the device brought just above the plane of the wound. Cut any vitreous adherent to the implant with Westcott scissors to minimize tractional forces. A vitreous cutter can remove any remaining prolapsed vitreous. Meticulous hemostasis of the sclera and of the wound with cautery and endodiathermy, respectively, can reduce the risk of subsequent vitreous hemorrhage from fibrovascular ingrowth or uveal tissue. Care is taken to avoid shrinkage of the wound due to excessive cautery that may make closure of the wound more difficult. The replacement implant is prepared and inserted in the manner described earlier. Additional nylon sutures may be necessary to prevent wound leak. Using the original site has the advantage of minimizing the size and number of circumferential incisions in the sclera. It is recommended to reuse the original incision for implantation only once to reduce the risk of complications from replacement surgery, as scleral thinning and scarring with subsequent surgery. Poor wound healing, wound leak, vitreous hemorrhage, increased risk of retinal detachment due to explantation, and separation of the drug pellet from the depleted implant are all potential disadvantages from same-site surgery and removal of an existing implant.[60–62]

Placing an implant contiguous with the first incision (Fig. 15.7c) involves a peritomy with careful preparation of the original site and the inferior sclera 4 mm from the 6 o'clock limbus. After hemostasis of the sclera, a 3-mm scleral wound contiguous to the original incision is extended parallel to the limbus with a MVR blade starting from the inferior edge of the original wound. The new wound incorporates approximately 2 mm of the previous wound and an additional 3 mm of previously undisturbed sclera. Choosing to extend the inferior aspect of the wound avoids damaging the long ciliary nerves and arteries at 3 and 9 o'clock. Remove any prolapsed vitreous with limited vitrectomy and inspect the wound with tooth forceps to assure that a full thickness incision has been made through the uvea and fibrous tissue. Since the wound incorporates some of the original incision, thorough hemostasis of the sclera and endodiathermy of the wound may decrease chances of postoperative vitreous hemorrhage from fibrovascular tissue growth at the original wound site. As with other implantation techniques, avoid excessive cautery to the wound. Secure the device as mentioned previously with 8-0 propylene and suture the wound with interrupted 8-0 nylon. Close the conjunctiva with 6-0 plain gut and administer subconjunctival antibiotics and steroid. Drawbacks to this approach include a large scleral incision

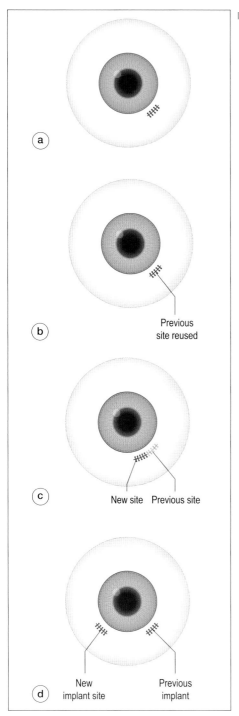

■ **FIGURE 15.7** Techniques of implant replacement as described by Morley et al.[67] (Adapted from Ophthalmology 1995;102(3):388–392.)

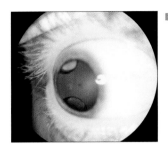

FIGURE 15.8 Use of a separate superotemporal site without explantation of the depleted inferior implant.

that compromises the integrity of the globe and the theoretical disruption of anterior segment circulation. A second implant in close proximity to the first may also dislodge or damage one or both implants if placed too close to one another.

In a separate-site technique for reimplantation (Fig. 15.7d), a conjunctival peritomy is performed in the inferonasal quadrant. Inferior placement of the implant is preferred as a second site since it allows positioning of the device in the aqueous phase in the event that silicone oil tamponade is required.[63–65] The device is otherwise prepared and placed the same as described with original inferotemporal placement. The advantage of this technique is the ease of insertion because there is no dissection and removal of the previous implant required (Fig. 15.8). Because there is less traction on the vitreous from dissection and removal of the depleted implant, a decreased risk for retinal detachment is likely.

POSTOPERATIVE CARE

The patient can be sent home with the eye patched and shielded till the next day visit. Vision, pressure, slit-lamp and dilated fundus examination should be performed at that time. Particular attention should be paid to the conjunctiva and sclera overlying the wound site, signs of hyphema or intraocular inflammation, lens appearance, vitreous hemorrhage, retinal detachment or breaks, and proper placement of the implant at the pars plana. The postoperative medication regimen is as follows:

1. Polytrim (trimethoprim sulfate and polymyxin B sulfate ophthalmic solution) 1 drop q.i.d. for 1 week.
2. Pred Forte 1% (prednisolone acetate) 1 drop q.i.d. tapered over 1 month.
3. Cyclogyl 2% (cyclopentolate) 1 drop b.i.d. for 1 week.
4. Vicodin (acetaminophen and hydrocodone) 1–2 tablets orally q 4 hours as needed for pain.

COMPLICATIONS

Vitreous implantation has been associated with surgical complications such as rhegmatogenous retinal detachment, severe vitreous hemorrhage, endophthalmitis, epiretinal membrane, cystoid macular edema, cataract, erosion of the implant through the sclera, hypotony, and temporary astigmatism.[35,36,39,66–68] Retinal detachment and vitreous hemorrhage are among the most common postoperative complications associated with implant placement, occurring in approximately 10% of patients.[35,36,69–71] The prevalence of endophthalmitis in eyes with ganciclovir implants is believed to be around 0.5%.[72,73] Previous studies have suggested that surgical complications of same-site implant replacement surgery—including detachment, vitreous hemorrhage, cataract, and hypotony—may be more common than with primary implant surgery.[55,61,70,73] The risk of complications may be reduced by choosing to insert an implant in a wholly different site rather than to do a same-site replacement procedure. The Retisert implant would theoretically have a higher rate of wound dehiscence, especially after exchanges using a same-site technique, given the inhibitory effect that corticosteroids have on wound healing.

The major adverse effects from Retisert implantation are IOP elevation and cataract formation. Patients must be monitored for elevated IOP. Some 60% of patients will require IOP-lowering medications to control IOP, with approximately 20% requiring filtering procedures to control IOP.[74] Within an average postimplantation period of approximately 2 years, some 90% of phakic eyes are expected to develop cataracts and require cataract surgery.[4]

REFERENCES

1. Rothova A, Suttorp-van Schulten MS, Frits Treffers W, Kijlstra A. Causes and frequency of blindness in patients with intraocular inflammatory disease. Br J Ophthalmol 1996; 80(4):332–336.

2. Menezo V, Lau C, Comer M, Lightman S. Clinical outcome of chronic immunosuppression in patients with non-infectious uveitis. Clin Experiment Ophthalmol 2005; 33(1):16–21.

3. Tamesis RR, Rodriguez A, Christen WG, et al. Systemic drug toxicity trends in immunosuppressive therapy of immune and inflammatory ocular disease. Ophthalmology 1996; 103(5):768–775.

4. Fluocinolone acetonide ophthalmic–Bausch & Lomb: fluocinolone acetonide Envision TD implant. Drugs R D 2005; 6(2):116–119.

5. McAuliffe PF, Hall MJ, Castro-Malaspina H, Heinemann MH. Use of the ganciclovir implant for treating cytomegalovirus retinitis secondary to immunosuppression after bone marrow transplantation. Am J Ophthalmol 1997; 123(5):702–703.

6. Derzko-Dzulynsky LA, Berger AR, Berinstein NL. Cytomegalovirus retinitis and low-grade non-Hodgkin's lymphoma: case report and review of the literature. Am J Hematol 1998; 57(3):228–232.

7. Jabs DA, Green WR, Fox R, et al. Ocular manifestations of acquired immune deficiency syndrome. Ophthalmology 1989; 96(7):1092–1099.

8. Gross JG, Bozzette SA, Mathews WC, et al. Longitudinal study of cytomegalovirus retinitis in acquired immune deficiency syndrome. Ophthalmology 1990; 97(5):681–686.

9. Holland GN, Pepose JS, Pettit TH, et al. Acquired immune deficiency syndrome. Ocular manifestations. Ophthalmology 1983; 90(8):859–873.

10. Jabs DA, Enger C, Haller J, de Bustros S. Retinal detachments in patients with cytomegalovirus retinitis. Arch Ophthalmol 1991; 109(6):794–799.

11. Rhegmatogenous retinal detachment in patients with cytomegalovirus retinitis: the Foscarnet–Ganciclovir Cytomegalovirus Retinitis Trial. The Studies of Ocular Complications of AIDS (SOCA) Research Group in collaboration with the AIDS Clinical Trials Group (ACTG). Am J Ophthalmol 1997; 124(1):61–70.

12. Palella FJ Jr, Delaney KM, Moorman AC, et al. Declining morbidity and mortality among patients with advanced human immunodeficiency virus infection. HIV Outpatient Study Investigators. N Engl J Med 1998; 338(13):853–860.

13. Jabs DA, Van Natta ML, Thorne JE, et al. Course of cytomegalovirus retinitis in the era of highly active antiretroviral therapy: 1. Retinitis progression. Ophthalmology 2004; 111(12):2224–2231.

14. Kempen JH, Jabs DA, Dunn JP, et al. Retinal detachment risk in cytomegalovirus retinitis related to the acquired immunodeficiency syndrome. Arch Ophthalmol 2001; 119(1):33–40.

15. Jabs DA, Van Natta ML, Thorne JE, et al. Course of cytomegalovirus retinitis in the era of highly active antiretroviral therapy: 2. Second eye involvement and retinal detachment. Ophthalmology 2004; 111(12):2232–2239.

16. Matthews T, Boehme R. Antiviral activity and mechanism of action of ganciclovir. Rev Infect Dis 1988; 10(Suppl 3):S490–S494.

17. Foscarnet–Ganciclovir Cytomegalovirus Retinitis Trial. 4. Visual outcomes. Studies of Ocular Complications of AIDS Research Group in collaboration with the AIDS Clinical Trials Group. Ophthalmology 1994; 101(7):1250–1261.

18. Teich SA, Cheung TW, Friedman AH. Systemic antiviral drugs used in ophthalmology. Surv Ophthalmol 1992; 37(1):19–53.

19. Holland GN, Sakamoto MJ, Hardy D, et al. Treatment of cytomegalovirus retinopathy in patients with acquired immunodeficiency

syndrome. Use of the experimental drug 9-[2-hydroxy-1-(hydroxymethyl)ethoxymethyl] guanine. Arch Ophthalmol 1986; 104(12):1794–1800.

20. Holland GN, Sidikaro Y, Kreiger AE, et al. Treatment of cytomegalovirus retinopathy with ganciclovir. Ophthalmology 1987; 94(7):815–823.

21. Spector SA, Weingeist T, Pollard RB, et al. A randomized, controlled study of intravenous ganciclovir therapy for cytomegalovirus peripheral retinitis in patients with AIDS. AIDS Clinical Trials Group and Cytomegalovirus Cooperative Study Group. J Infect Dis 1993; 168(3):557–563.

22. Palestine AG, Polis MA, De Smet MD, et al. A randomized, controlled trial of foscarnet in the treatment of cytomegalovirus retinitis in patients with AIDS. Ann Intern Med 1991; 115(9):665–673.

23. Lehoang P, Girard B, Robinet M, et al. Foscarnet in the treatment of cytomegalovirus retinitis in acquired immune deficiency syndrome. Ophthalmology 1989; 96(6):865–873; discussion 873–874.

24. Jacobson MA, O'Donnell JJ, Mills J. Foscarnet treatment of cytomegalovirus retinitis in patients with the acquired immunodeficiency syndrome. Antimicrob Agents Chemother 1989; 33(5):736–741.

25. Henry K, Cantrill H, Fletcher C, et al. Use of intravitreal ganciclovir (dihydroxy propoxymethyl guanine) for cytomegalovirus retinitis in a patient with AIDS. Am J Ophthalmol 1987; 103(1):17–23.

26. Cantrill HL, Henry K, Melroe NH, et al. Treatment of cytomegalovirus retinitis with intravitreal ganciclovir. Long-term results. Ophthalmology 1989; 96(3):367–374.

27. Ussery FM 3rd, Gibson SR, Conklin RH, et al. Intravitreal ganciclovir in the treatment of AIDS-associated cytomegalovirus retinitis. Ophthalmology 1988; 95(5):640–648.

28. Heinemann MH. Long-term intravitreal ganciclovir therapy for cytomegalovirus retinopathy. Arch Ophthalmol 1989; 107(12):1767–1772.

29. Cochereau-Massin I, Lehoang P, Lautier-Frau M, et al. Efficacy and tolerance of intravitreal ganciclovir in cytomegalovirus retinitis in acquired immune deficiency syndrome. Ophthalmology 1991; 98(9):1348–1353; discussion 1353–1355.

30. Smith TJ, Pearson PA, Blandford DL, et al. Intravitreal sustained-release ganciclovir. Arch Ophthalmol 1992; 110(2):255–258.

31. Sanborn GE, Anand R, Torti RE, et al. Sustained-release ganciclovir therapy for treatment of cytomegalovirus retinitis. Use of an intravitreal device. Arch Ophthalmol 1992; 110(2):188–195.

32. Chang M, Dunn JP. Ganciclovir implant in the treatment of cytomegalovirus retinitis. Expert Rev Med Devices 2005; 2(4):421–427.

33. Kuppermann BD, Quiceno JI, Flores-Aguilar M, et al. Intravitreal ganciclovir concentration after intravenous administration in AIDS patients with cytomegalovirus retinitis: implications for therapy. J Infect Dis 1993; 168(6):1506–1509.

34. Arevalo JF, Gonzalez C, Capparelli EV, et al. Intravitreous and plasma concentrations of ganciclovir and foscarnet after intravenous therapy in patients with AIDS and cytomegalovirus retinitis. J Infect Dis 1995; 172(4):951–956.

35. Martin DF, Parks DJ, Mellow SD, et al. Treatment of cytomegalovirus retinitis with an intraocular sustained-release ganciclovir implant. A randomized controlled clinical trial. Arch Ophthalmol 1994; 112(12):1531–1539.

36. Musch DC, Martin DF, Gordon JF, et al. Treatment of cytomegalovirus retinitis with a sustained-release ganciclovir implant. The Ganciclovir Implant Study Group. N Engl J Med 1997; 337(2):83–90.

37. Jabs DA, Enger C, Bartlett JG. Cytomegalovirus retinitis and acquired immunodeficiency syndrome. Arch Ophthalmol 1989; 107(1):75–80.

38. The ganciclovir implant plus oral ganciclovir versus parenteral cidofovir for the treatment of cytomegalovirus retinitis in patients with acquired immunodeficiency syndrome: The Ganciclovir Cidofovir Cytomegalovirus Retinitis Trial. Am J Ophthalmol 2001; 131(4):457–467.

39. Martin DF, Kuppermann BD, Wolitz RA, et al. Oral ganciclovir for patients with cytomegalovirus retinitis treated with a ganciclovir implant. Roche Ganciclovir Study Group. N Engl J Med 1999; 340(14):1063–1070.

40. Drew WL, Stempien MJ, Andrews J, et al. Cytomegalovirus (CMV) resistance in patients with CMV retinitis and AIDS treated with oral or intravenous ganciclovir. J Infect Dis 1999; 179(6):1352–1355.

41. Drew WL, Miner RC, Busch DF, et al. Prevalence of resistance in patients receiving ganciclovir for serious cytomegalovirus infection. J Infect Dis 1991; 163(4):716–719.

42. Jabs DA, Enger C, Dunn JP, Forman M. Cytomegalovirus retinitis and viral resistance: ganciclovir resistance. CMV Retinitis and Viral Resistance Study Group. J Infect Dis 1998; 177(3):770–773.

43. Jabs DA, Martin BK, Forman MS, et al. Cytomegalovirus resistance to ganciclovir and clinical outcomes of patients with cytomegalovirus retinitis. Am J Ophthalmol 2003; 135(1):26–34.

44. Hatton MP, Duker JS, Reichel E, et al. Treatment of relapsed cytomegalovirus retinitis with the sustained-release ganciclovir implant. Retina 1998; 18(1):50–55.

45. Kuo IC, Imai Y, Shum C, et al. Genotypic analysis of cytomegalovirus retinitis poorly responsive to intravenous ganciclovir but responsive to the ganciclovir implant. Am J Ophthalmol 2003; 135(1):20–25.

46. Jung D, Dorr A. Single-dose pharmacokinetics of valganciclovir in HIV- and CMV-seropositive subjects. J Clin Pharmacol 1999; 39(8):800–804.

47. Brown F, Banken L, Saywell K, Arum I. Pharmacokinetics of valganciclovir and ganciclovir following multiple oral dosages of valganciclovir in HIV- and CMV-seropositive volunteers. Clin Pharmacokinet 1999; 37(2):167–176.

48. Wiltshire H, Hirankarn S, Farrell C, et al. Pharmacokinetic profile of ganciclovir after its oral administration and from its prodrug, valganciclovir, in solid organ transplant recipients. Clin Pharmacokinet 2005; 44(5):495–507.

49. Martin DF, Sierra-Madero J, Walmsley S, et al. A controlled trial of valganciclovir as induction therapy for cytomegalovirus retinitis. N Engl J Med 2002; 346(15):1119–1126.

50. Macdonald JC, Torriani FJ, Morse LS, et al. Lack of reactivation of cytomegalovirus (CMV) retinitis after stopping CMV maintenance therapy in AIDS patients with sustained elevations in CD4 T cells in response to highly active antiretroviral therapy. J Infect Dis 1998; 177(5):1182–1187.

51. Tural C, Romeu J, Sirera G, et al. Long-lasting remission of cytomegalovirus retinitis without maintenance therapy in human immunodeficiency virus-infected patients. J Infect Dis 1998; 177(4):1080–1083.

52. Whitcup SM, Fortin E, Lindblad AS, et al. Discontinuation of anticytomegalovirus therapy in patients with HIV infection and cytomegalovirus retinitis. JAMA 1999; 282(17):1633–1637.

53. Vrabec TR, Baldassano VF, Whitcup SM. Discontinuation of maintenance therapy in patients with quiescent cytomegalovirus retinitis and elevated CD4⁺ counts. Ophthalmology 1998; 105(7):1259–1264.

54. Jabs DA, Bolton SG, Dunn JP, Palestine AG. Discontinuing anticytomegalovirus therapy in patients with immune reconstitution after combination antiretroviral therapy. Am J Ophthalmol 1998; 126(6):817–822.

55. Martin DF, Dunn JP, Davis JL, et al. Use of the ganciclovir implant for the treatment of cytomegalovirus retinitis in the era of potent antiretroviral therapy: recommendations of the International AIDS Society-USA panel. Am J Ophthalmol 1999; 127(3):329–339.

56. Holland GN, Buhles WC Jr, Mastre B, Kaplan HJ. A controlled retrospective study of ganciclovir treatment for cytomegalovirus retinopathy. Use of a standardized system for the assessment of disease outcome. UCLA CMV Retinopathy Study Group. Arch Ophthalmol 1989; 107(12):1759–1766.

57. Browning DJ. Dislocated ganciclovir implant from use of a nylon fixation suture. Retina 2003; 23(5):723–724.

58. Srivastava SK, Martin DF, Mellow SD, et al. Pathological findings in eyes with the ganciclovir implant. Ophthalmology 2005; 112(5):780–786.

59. Charles NC, Steiner GC. Ganciclovir intraocular implant. A clinicopathologic study. Ophthalmology 1996; 103(3):416–421.

60. Martin DF, Ferris FL, Parks DJ, et al. Ganciclovir implant exchange. Timing, surgical procedure, and complications. Arch Ophthalmol 1997; 115(11):1389–1394.

61. Morley MG, Duker JS, Ashton P, Robinson MR. Replacing ganciclovir implants. Ophthalmology 1995; 102(3):388–392.

62. Boyer DS, Posalski J. Potential complication associated with removal of ganciclovir implants. Am J Ophthalmol 1999; 127(3):349–350.

63. Perkins SL, Yang CH, Ashton PA, Jaffe GJ. Pharmacokinetics of the ganciclovir implant in the silicone-filled eye. Retina 2001; 21(1):10–14.

64. McGuire DE, McAulife P, Heinemann MH, Rahhal FM. Efficacy of the ganciclovir implant in the setting of silicone oil vitreous substitute. Retina 2000; 20(5):520–523.

65. Martidis A, Danis RP, Ciulla TA. Treating cytomegalovirus retinitis-related retinal detachment by combining silicone oil tamponade and ganciclovir implant. Ophthalmic Surg Lasers 2002; 33(2):135–139.

66. Lim JI, Wolitz RA, Dowling AH, et al. Visual and anatomic outcomes associated with posterior segment complications after ganciclovir implant procedures in patients with AIDS and cytomegalovirus retinitis. Am J Ophthalmol 1999; 127(3):288–293.

67. Virata SR, Kylstra JA. Delayed vitreous hemorrhage after placement of a ganciclovir implant for cytomegalovirus retinitis. Am J Ophthalmol 1997; 124(4):557–558.

68. Guembel HO, Krieglsteiner S, Rosenkranz C, et al. Complications after implantation of intraocular devices in patients with cytomegalovirus retinitis. Graefes Arch Clin Exp Ophthalmol 1999; 237(10):824–829.

69. Anand R, Nightingale SD, Fish RH, et al. Control of cytomegalovirus retinitis using sustained release of intraocular ganciclovir. Arch Ophthalmol 1993; 111(2):223–227.

70. Dunn JP, Van Natta M, Foster G, et al. Complications of ganciclovir implant surgery in patients with cytomegalovirus retinitis: the Ganciclovir Cidofovir Cytomegalovirus Retinitis Trial. Retina 2004; 24(1):41–50.

71. Marx JL, Kapusta MA, Patel SS, et al. Use of the ganciclovir implant in the treatment of recurrent cytomegalovirus retinitis. Arch Ophthalmol 1996; 114(7):815–820.

72. Shane TS, Martin DF. Endophthalmitis after ganciclovir implant in patients with AIDS and cytomegalovirus retinitis. Am J Ophthalmol 2003; 136(4):649–654.

73. Kappel PJ, Charonis AC, Holland GN, et al. Outcomes associated with ganciclovir implants in patients with AIDS-related cytomegalovirus retinitis. Ophthalmology 2006; 113(4):683 e1–8.

74. Jaffe GJ, McCallum RM, Branchaud B, et al. Long-term follow-up results of a pilot trial of a fluocinolone acetonide implant to treat posterior uveitis. Ophthalmology 2005; 112(7):1192–1198.

THE LIBRARY
THE LEARNING AND DEVELOPMENT CENTRE
THE CALDERDALE ROYAL HOSPITAL
HALIFAX HX3 0PW

16

Vitreous biopsy for endophthalmitis or cytology

Robert G. Josephberg

HISTORICAL PERSPECTIVE

In the years 1944 through 1966, 73% of patients with endophthalmitis ended up with hand-motion or less vision.[1] However, the results were dramatically improved in the 1970s and 1980s, after intravitreal antibiotics and pars plana vitrectomy were introduced.[2]

ENDOPHTHALMITIS VITRECTOMY STUDY (EVS)—1995[3]

The EVS included 420 patients, and was conducted to determine the necessity of immediate vitrectomy and the role of intravenous antibiotics in patient management after cataract surgery or secondary intraocular lens implants (IOLs) within 6 weeks of surgery (Figs 16.2 and 16.3). All operations were to be done within 6 hours of presentation to the retinal specialist. The view had to be sufficiently clear in the anterior segment to perform a vitrectomy or needle tap of the vitreous. This excluded many patients from the initial study, including those that were due to trauma or that had delayed onset, or that were associated with endogenous sources, glaucoma, filtering blebs, penetrating keratoplasty, or other causes.

Four treatment groups

Patients were assigned to one of four treatment groups. The first two groups underwent a three-port pars plana vitrectomy, with or without IV antibiotics. On average, up to 2 cc of vitreous fluid was removed. The second two groups underwent a vitreous tap (needle aspiration with a 25-gauge needle) or vitreous biopsy (0.1–0.3 cc) with an automated vitrector through a single sclerotomy in the operating room, again with or without IV antibiotics. All patients in the four treatment groups received systemic steroids.

EVS drug regimen

Intravitreal antibiotics consisted of vancomycin 1 mg/0.1 cc and amikacin 400 mcg/0.1 cc. Of note, no intravitreal steroids were used. Topical drops included vancomycin, amikacin, cycloplegics, and corticosteroids. Subconjunctival antibiotics consisted of vancomycin (25 mg), ceftazidime (100 mg), and dexamethasone (6 mg). Systemic medications were used for 5–10 days. They were prednisone (PO) 60 mg, amikacin (IV) 50 mg/kg every 12 hours, and ceftazidime (IV) 2 g every 8 hours. Oral ciprofloxacin was substituted for ceftazidime if the patient was allergic to penicillin.

Key points of EVS results

The average onset of signs and symptoms of endophthalmitis was 6 days after surgery. Of note, 25% were without pain and 14% had no hypopyon. Cultures were positive in only 69% of the cases. Of culture-positive cases, 94% were Gram positive, with the majority being *Staphylococcus* coagulase negative (70%), *Staphylococcus aureus* (10%), and *Streptococcus* species (11.5%). Only 6% were Gram-negative organisms. Of the Gram-positive cases, 84% achieved 20/100 vision or better, and 50% had better than 20/40 vision. It was evident that streptococci, *Staph. aureus* and Gram-negative organisms were more virulent and more difficult to sterilize in the vitreous cavity. In the EVS, less than 30% of these eyes with more virulent organisms achieved 20/100 or better, and 11% of all EVS patients

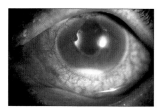

FIGURE 16.1 External ocular photograph of bacterial endophthalmitis.

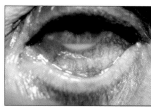

FIGURE 16.2 External photograph of secondary intraocular lens with hypopyon.

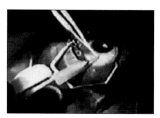

FIGURE 16.3 Primary cataract surgery with hypopyon 6 days postoperatively.

ended up with less than 5/200 vision. In all, 5% ended up with no light perception (NLP) vision. Patients presenting with LP vision and who had a vitrectomy had three times the chance of achieving 20/40 or better and 50% less incidence of NLP vision. Finally, it is important to note that 7% of all patients required reinjection of antibiotics because of worsening condition within 36–60 hours after the initial injection.

Generally, the eyes requiring reinjection had the worst outcomes because they harbored the more virulent organisms. In the EVS, a single injection of vancomycin and amikacin was insufficient to eradicate *Staph. epidermidis* (20%), *Staph. aureus* and streptococci (47%), and Gram-negative (75%) organisms upon retaps and recultures when the eye was clinically worsening at 36–60 hours. Infections also developed in 40.3% of patients (85 of 211) who had documented povidone iodine preoperatively and in 11.5% (10 of 87) who had documented intracameral antibiotics in the infusion bottle preoperatively. Retinal detachment rates were also noted to be lower in the vitrectomy arm versus the needle aspiration arm. Both anterior chamber and vitreous cultures should be obtained. In the EVS, 11% of anterior chamber cultures were positive when the vitreous was negative. Meticulous aseptic technique is the cornerstone of reducing the risk of infection. Povidone iodine preparation on the conjunctival surface is the only treatment that has been shown to reduce the risk of endophthalmitis. Although this is not completely proven, preoperative antibiotics also appear to lessen the risk.[4]

Conclusions of EVS

The intravenous antibiotics used at the time showed no additional benefit. Immediate vitrectomy (up to 6 hours) is of significant benefit to those who present with LP vision. However, when the vision is hand-motion or better, a vitreous needle aspiration (25-gauge) or an automated vitrector biopsy (up to 0.3 cc) done in the operating room proved to be as efficacious and was recommended.

INDICATIONS AND CONTRAINDICATIONS

Endophthalmitis, uveitis, and unknown vitreous opacities may be treated and diagnosed easily in the office, at the patient's bedside, or in the operating room, depending on the situation. Many of these cases have not been diagnosed or have not responded to medical or surgical treatments either locally or systemically. These patients may also manifest inflammatory signs in the vitreous that are a harbinger of a more serious disease that has yet to be diagnosed systemically. Obviously, for many reasons, the office is the most readily available site, and in acute endophthalmitis would be the quickest in terms of treatment which may be crucial to the outcome. Uveitis patients, while generally not an emergency, can also have a vitreous specimen easily obtained in the office.

Vitreous biopsies should preferably be done with a mechanical vitreous cutter because of the obvious inherent risks of trying to remove vitreous by needle aspiration alone, i.e.

retinal tears and obtaining minimal or no vitreous specimen at all. No-one wants a dry tap which happens all too frequently with needle aspirations.

Patients' medical conditions and other situations may dictate the place and timing of the surgery. If general anesthesia is needed, then the operating room would be the obvious appropriate arena. Children and adults that might be difficult to control or might be uncooperative would also be better served in an operating room setting. Vitreous biopsies using a one-port vitrectomy site are ideal for cases requiring a small vitreous aspirate (up to 1 cc) for fluid sampling and especially when the view into the eye is severely limited, i.e. corneal or lens clouding. These limited vitreous biopsies may be done in the office, operating room, or at the bedside with the appropriate instrumentation. If one wishes to do a full vitrectomy for therapeutic reasons, then a full vitrectomy using a three-port setup in the operating room would be appropriate. Many cases may easily be done in the operating room using one, two or three ports depending on the goals of the surgery.

INSTRUMENTS AND DEVICES

Vitreous biopsies may be done by various instruments that are now available. These include:

- the 23-gauge handheld portable sutureless vitrector made by Insight Instruments, the standard 20-gauge vitrectomy system, or
- the new 23- or 25-gauge sutureless vitrectomy system made by multiple manufacturers.

Plain needle aspiration (25- to 30-gauge), while always an option, is not recommended for vitreous aspiration. These needles may be useful to help further or to make the diagnosis through aqueous aspiration. Depending on the situation, clarity of the media, and the amount of vitreous to be removed, the above instruments may be tailored to meet the specific goals of the surgery.

Other necessary equipment includes:

- multiple 0.1–0.3 cc syringes,
- three-way stopcocks,
- blood culture bottles or culture media,
- microscope slides,
- lid speculum.

PREOPERATIVE REGIMEN

The preoperative regimen includes making sure that the appropriate tests and laboratory work that will be needed are in place. It is crucial to know what tests to order before you start and where to send the aqueous and vitreous specimens once they are obtained. Depending on whether the surgery will be performed in the office or operating room, different preparation regimens would be indicated. In the office no general sedation is warranted, whereas in the operating room sedation is routine. The patient must have the appropriate local or general anesthesia. In the operating room all levels and types of anesthesia are available while in the office or at the bedside you are limited to local anesthetics. I usually prefer a subconjunctival lidocaine (2%) injection in most cases but many times in acute endophthalmitis I give both a subconjunctival and a retrobulbar block because these patients are usually in severe pain. None of these cases is done under topical anesthesia. At this point I usually place a topical fluoroquinolone antibiotic drop into the eye.

After the above are administered, topical povidone iodine is applied to the periorbital region, eyelashes and conjunctiva. If corneal cultures are necessary for a corneal ulcer/infectious keratitis in a patient with endophthalmitis, then these precede the povidone iodine preparation. A lid speculum is then inserted into the eye and the sites of entry for the sclerotomies are chosen.

SURGICAL TECHNIQUE

Office-based vitrectomy with the sharp-tip cutter

16.1

1. Anesthesia, subconjunctival and/or retrobulbar, with 1% or 2% lidocaine.
2. Lid speculum.
3. Povidone iodine (Betadine) solution preparation of the conjunctiva, 5–6 drops (always use the 'solution' because other Betadine products contain detergent or alcohol).
4. Fill the cutter tip and tubing with balanced salt solution (BSS).
5. If simultaneous infusion is indicated, one may suture the infusion needle into place, and connect it to an elevated bottle of BSS.
6. Dry the injection site with a cotton-tipped applicator.
7. Introduce the sharp-tip cutter with a one-step stab incision 3.5 mm posterior to the limbus.
8. Observe the cutter tip with the slit lamp or indirect ophthalmoscope.
9. Activate the cutter, usually at the maximum rate of 300 cuts per minute, with the finger switch.
10. Instruct the technician to aspirate slowly with the syringe pointed toward the floor (allowing the inevitable air in the syringe to ascend upward and thereby facilitate the technician's observation of the precise volume of aspirated vitreous).
11. Aspirate up to approximately 1.0 mL for laboratory analysis (as in endophthalmitis or uveitis). Usually for endophthalmitis 0.3 cc is aspirated.
12. If simultaneous infusion was not utilized, maintain normal intraocular pressure with the surgeon's little finger, then restore normal intraocular pressure as the technician turns the stopcock and injects BSS. If indicated, leave sufficient volume to inject intraocular antibiotics and steroids.
13. Inspect the fundus with the indirect ophthalmoscope to rule out any possible complications and ensure patency of the central retinal artery.
14. Apply antibiotic ointment and other necessary drops or injections.
15. Utilize an eye pad.
16. Examine the patient on the first postoperative day.

Office-based vitrectomy with the blunt-tip cutter (recommended when operating near the retina or iris)

1. Proceed with items 1–6 in the prior section
2. Cauterize the conjunctiva at the incision site.
3. Stretch out the conjunctiva between two cotton-tipped applicators and firmly apply the transconjunctival cautery.
4. Stab incision with the 23-gauge microvitreoretinal (MVR) knife, then remove the knife.
5. Introduce the blunt-tip cutter into the eye.
6. Proceed with items 8–16 as listed.

Suspected endophthalmitis

The author's recommendation for investigation of suspected endophthalmitis is to perform an immediate tap of the anterior chamber and a full vitrectomy if light perception (LP) vision is seen upon initial presentation (Fig. 16.4). A vitrectomy biopsy should be performed if hand-motion or better vision is present (Fig. 16.5). This may be done either in the office or in the operating room barring no time delays. All specimens of both the anterior and posterior segments should be cultured on appropriate culture plates or media, such as blood agar, chocolate agar, fungal culture media, Sabaroud's media and thioglyco-late broth. Alternatively, specimens may be sent in appropriate blood culture bottles for

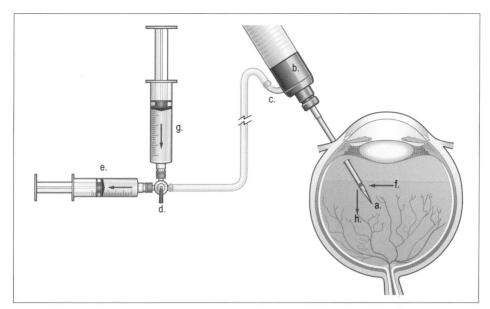

■ **FIGURE 16.4** A 27-gauge needle for aqueous aspiration. **A**, 23-Gauge needle/MVR blade tip of sutureless vitrector. **B**, Screw-on disposable vitrector probe to handheld motor handpiece. **C**, Aspirating cannula from vitrector probe for specimen. **D**, Three-way stopcock. **E**, 3 cc aspirating syringe of specimen. **F**, Vitreous flowing into vitrectomy port. **G**, 3 cc infusion syringe for drugs or saline. **H**, Infusion of drugs or saline from vitrectomy probe into vitreous.

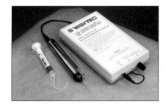

■ **FIGURE 16.5** Vitreous biopsy with handheld office sutureless vitrector.

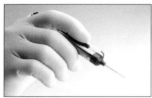

■ **FIGURE 16.6** Palm-size office vitrector with battery pack.

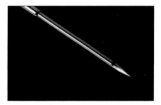

■ **FIGURE 16.7** Handheld motorized sutureless office vitrector.

growth. Gram stains are done on both the anterior and posterior fluids obtained. Often the Gram stain may be the only positive finding and may dictate the therapy.

Office vitrector

If the patient has hand-motion or better vision, I prefer to use a 23-gauge portable self-sealing office-based sutureless handheld automated battery-driven vitrector with an attached MVR blade made by Insight Instruments, Inc., Stuart, Florida. It is referred to as the Visitrec vitrectomy unit (Figs 16.6–16.8) and was developed by the author (RGJ). Note that the incision size is equivalent to the present 25-gauge systems which use a cannula and trocar system which make a 23-gauge opening in the sclera. The technique and equipment were presented by the author at the annual American Academy of Ophthalmology (AAO) meeting in 1996 and also at the Vitreous Society Annual Meeting

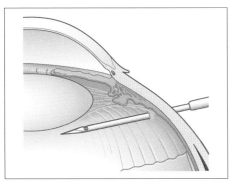

■ **FIGURE 16.8** A 23-gauge vitrectomy probe with attached MVR blade for transconjunctival office sutureless surgery. Note that the incision size is equivalent to the present 25-gauge systems which use a cannula and trocar system which make a 23-gauge opening in the sclera.

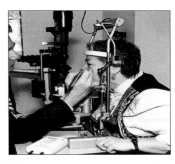

■ **FIGURE 16.9** Visitrec instrument inside the eye during pars plana vitreous biopsy. Self-sealing 23-gauge sutureless vitrector with MVR blade.

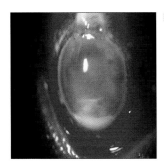

■ **FIGURE 16.10** Visitrec portable vitreous biopsy done at slit lamp.

in 1995. This self-sealing vitreous cutter was initially introduced as an abstract at the Association for Research in Vision and Ophthalmology (ARVO).[5,6]

Development of the Visitrec device

The Visitrec instrument (Fig. 16.9) was developed during the course of the EVS and became commercially available in 1994. It enables both rapid diagnosis and treatment which may begin in minutes in the office or emergency room setting. This machine optimizes the advantages of both the vitrectomy biopsy and the needle tap. Because of its unique design, the vitrectomy cutter with its attached MVR blade is inserted transconjunctivally through the sclera and pars plana. This device was the first commercially available sutureless vitrector. It has now been redesigned and renamed and is called the INTRECTOR made by Insight Instruments (Stuart, FLA). Both simultaneous infusion and aspiration are now capable through two separate channels in the 33-gauge sutureless needle tip based vitrectomy probe. It is designed to work in conjunction with the previous Visitrec units.

Candidates for office-based vitrectomy

Based upon the EVS and as reported by Mark Hammer (at AAO in 1998), 75% of EVS patients fall into the hand-motion or better vision category and could undergo this office-based vitrectomy procedure (Fig. 16.10).

Drug treatment regimen

The author's current drug treatment regimen includes intravitreal injections of vancomycin (2 mg/0.2 cc),[7,8] amikacin (250 mcg/0.1 cc)[9] or ceftazidime (2.25 mg/0.1 cc); dexamethasone (400 mcg/0.1 cc)[10] is also administered. A recent survey by retinal specialists has suggested that amikacin can cause macular toxicity.[9] In the EVS, one out of 420 patients possibly had amikacin toxicity at a dose of 400 mcg. Topically administered drops include vancomycin (25 mg/1 cc), and moxifloxacin or gatifloxacin (Tequin) along with cycloplegics and topical corticosteroids. Subconjunctival or periocular medications are optional. They could include vancomycin (25 mg/0.5 cc) or cefazolin (50 mg/0.5 cc) and dexamethasone (4 mg/1 cc). Systemic antibiotics are optional. Although not proven, systemic gatifloxacin (400 mg) may prove to be of benefit in future studies to help maintain the antibiotic level after the initial intravitreal injections. It has been shown in studies to have high intravitreal 'concentrations'.[11] At the present time, the mainstay of therapy and the gold standard of treatment are timely diagnosis and injection of initial intravitreal antibiotics.

Mixing of antibiotics and costs

All previous antibiotics mentioned are easily mixed in the office in under 5 min. The costs of the drugs are less than $20 and the portable vitrector probe costs about $80 per use. The total time to complete the procedure is less than 30 min. Routine repeated intravitreal antibiotics are given if the culture proves to be a virulent organism at 48–72 hours, and/or if the eye is getting worse. Endophthalmitis is an ocular emergency and should be treated no differently from septicemia. Both rapid diagnosis and treatment are essential. The EVS protocol is a valuable guideline.

Modern management shows 53% of patients have better than 20/40 vision after treatment. Assessment of visual acuity at onset dictates further management decisions. Make no mistake about it, the mainstay of treatment is immediate intravitreal antibiotics. Office vitrectomy or a needle tap allows for quicker treatments in hand-motion or better seeing eyes. Vitrectomy (three-port) at present is the treatment of choice for LP vision. It appears prudent that waiting 6 hours for an operating room to become available is not wise and more rapid treatment should theoretically lead to better outcomes.

Infectious endophthalmitis

Exogenous endophthalmitis is not the only condition that may be managed with a vitrectomy biopsy in the office setting. Endogenous infectious endophthalmitis, while the result of hematogenous spread, is usually seen in very debilitated and hospitalized patients. Bacterial sepsis is still the most likely cause, but other organisms such as fungi (*Candida*) are commonly found in many cases. Doing a vitreous biopsy with a mechanical portable vitrector at bedside is ideal rather than taking the patient to the operating room. We have used this technique many times in the intensive care unit at bedside where patients are on respirators or may be in a coma. Many of these patients have increased surgical risks and it is much more prudent for the physician to perform the vitreous biopsy at the patient's bedside. The procedure may be done with a local subconjunctival anesthetic and the vitrectomy biopsy completed in several minutes, without any fear of a dry tap or risk of vitreous traction with possible retinal tears, as may be seen with a needle tap. Gram stain and cultures can be performed immediately on the vitreous specimen for rapid identification of the organisms.

The overall frequency of posttraumatic infectious endophthalmitis is approximately 7%.[12] Because of the poor visual prognosis and the high association of *Bacillus cereus* in this setting, diagnostic suspicion calls for early intervention with a vitreous biopsy for culture and Gram stain. This early intervention, followed by the use of immediate antibiotics in rare cases, may be curative for this devastating pathogen. Both vancomycin and fluoroquinolones are very effective against this organism, which is found in endophthalmitis cases due to contamination by vegetation and those cases due to trauma in rural settings.

While the EVS only defined treatment guidelines for a specific subset of endophthalmitis patients, other types of exogenous or endogenous endophthalmitis cases are rampant. No prospective randomized study for many other types of infectious endophthalmitis cases which were not included in the EVS has ever been done. These cases include, but are not limited to, chronic postoperative (beyond 6 weeks), post trabeculectomy, post corneal transplant, endogenous, posttraumatic, and extensive corneal edema cases, precluding a good view even following routine cataract surgery. Cases of routine exogenous post cataract endophthalmitis were not included if the view was not clear enough to perform a vitrectomy. This precluded many of the worst cases from being entered into the EVS and was a selection study bias. Usually, the best prognostic cases start off with much clearer media. Most cases, however, while not considered EVS eligible, are still treated with standard treatment regimens. These include, for bacteria, intravitreal vancomycin 1 mg in 0.1 cc and ceftazidime 2.25 mg in 0.1 cc (or amikacin 0.4 mg in 0.1 cc). Dexamethasone 0.4 mg in 0.1 cc may or may not be given and was not studied in the EVS. If a fungal etiology is suspected, then dexamethasone may be withheld. If a fungal cause is suspected, then amphotericin 5 mcg in 0.1 cc, along with a systemic agent such as fluconazole, may be administered. The benefit of periocular, systemic, and/or topical antibiotics may be debated in various types of endophthalmitis. Most retinal specialists will administer and tailor their treatment of topical and/or systemic antibiotics depending on not only the causative organism but also the etiology. Any external cause such as infectious corneal ulcer or blebitis should be treated with both topical and periocular antibiotics.

If endogenous fungal endophthalmitis is suspected or proven, then intravitreal amphotericin may be used along with systemic fluconazole (Diflucan) as mentioned before. Since fluconazole penetrates into the vitreous cavity at very high levels, this or other similar antifungals may be given systemically for 2–4 weeks. Incipient fungal endophthalmitis with minimal vitreous involvement, in my experience, may be treated with systemic therapy alone, without intravitreal antifungals.

POSTOPERATIVE MANAGEMENT

After the surgery and depending on the type of case, most patients are comfortable and only need topical steroid/antibiotic combinations along with topical cycloplegics. If bacterial endophthalmitis is the cause of the problem, then frequent visits are usually necessary. Usually bacterial endophthalmitis cases are seen daily for the first 3 days so the treatment may be tailored to their clinical response. The initial treatment along with the subsequent culture reports and/or Gram stain results and the virulence of the organism are then considered. A repeat injection is then given with a single antibiotic at 48–72 hours if clinically indicated. Cases of unknown vitreous opacities and uveitis are seen the first day postoperatively and then 1 week later. As mentioned above, it is crucial to have the specimens sent to the appropriate laboratory with the tests requested. Contact your laboratory before you do the case if you have any questions about the case so that special stains or other testing methodology that are needed will be sent in an expeditious manner.

UVEITIS

While in most cases the etiology of intraocular inflammation is made by non-invasive techniques, identifying the cause in over 8% of cases of uveitis for suspected malignancy by systemic evaluation is inconclusive.[13]

INDICATIONS FOR DIAGNOSTIC VITREOUS BIOPSY

These indications fall into several categories, including those that are not only life threatening or sight threatening, but also chronic uveitis not responding to systemic antifungal therapies. For some of these unknown cases, or if we are suspicious of a malignancy or other atypical presentation, a vitreous biopsy may be quite useful. As discussed in previous sections, a vitreous biopsy specimen may be obtained with either a needle aspiration or a mechanical vitrectomy device. While a needle aspiration may be quick, it is not always easy. The risk of causing a retinal tear is rare.[14] By using a mechanical vitrector for a biopsy we are guaranteed to obtain enough vitreous for diagnostic testing without the well-known classic dry tap seen with a needle aspiration. This, as everyone is aware, can be a humbling and humiliating experience.

The entry point through the pars plana, in both phakic and pseudophakic patients, is 3.5 mm posterior to the temporal limbus. If a needle is used with its inherent risk, a 20- or 23-gauge needle should be used. Typically, only a very small amount of vitreous can be aspirated without cutting and this is usually in the syneretic (liquefied) portion that it is normally obtained with the needle aspiration technique. However, it is very difficult to almost impossible to aspirate the gel portion with a 23-gauge needle without causing traction.

When a limited diagnostic vitrectomy is required, an in-office mechanical sutureless transconjunctival vitrectomy at the slit lamp is an ideal option. This may also be done in the operating room setting. Both cost and setup time are minimal with few ancillary personnel needed. By increasing the amount of vitreous aspirate up to 1 cc, the potential is greater for higher diagnostic yield and other potential studies. While not only being diagnostic, it may also prove to be therapeutic by removing the visual incapacitating inflammatory cells and debris. As ocular hypotony may occur with a 1-cc vitreous aspirate, a three-way stopcock with either BSS or air may be sequentially used to reconstitute the eye. For a maximal, full and complete vitrectomy, the three-port pars plana vitrectomy done in the operating room is still the gold standard.

Remember that the removal of non-diluted vitreous for analysis is of the utmost importance and this must be done immediately. These cells may be labile and subject to death if not processed immediately.[15]

Steroids can be cytolytic to lymphoma cells and should not be used in suspected malignancy. The vitreous can be analyzed in various ways. These include cytology, pathology, immunophenotyping, flow cytometry, immunohistochemistry, antibody, cytokines, and molecular analysis using polymerase chain reaction (PCR). While Gram stains, Giemsa stains, and cultures are well accepted for fungal or bacteriological diagnosis, for suspected viral infections PCR analysis has been widely used. PCR analysis can be used for the diagnosis of herpes simplex virus (HSV), herpes zoster virus (HZV), cytomegalovirus (CMV), and toxoplasmosis. PCR is a technique involving amplification of nucleic acid sequences in DNA polymerase extension.[16] The list of organisms associated with PCR analysis includes most viruses, protozoa (toxoplasmosis) and many bacteria including *Streptococcus, Staphylococcus, Propionibacterium acnes, Mycobacteria, Pseudomonas, Bartonella* (Lyme disease), *Borrelia burgdorferi* (cat scratch disease), *Candida*, and intraocular malignancy.[17] Results can be obtained very quickly with 5 mL of an undiluted sample of aqueous or vitreous, with vitreous typically having a higher diagnostic yield. However, while PCR is extremely sensitive, it can produce both false-positive and false-negative results. An experienced laboratory needs to perform the test. Note that while a rapid diagnosis may be made, the procedure is both time-consuming and expensive.

In cases of suspected malignancy, trauma or autoimmune uveitis, cytology and immunocytochemistry may be very helpful.[18] By measuring CD4 helper cells and CD8 suppressor cells, flow cytometry, along with cytology and immunohistochemistry, may help with the diagnosis of malignancy, especially in cases of intraocular lymphoma.

The ratio of vitreous cytokines interleukin (IL)-10 to IL-6 is suggestive of lymphoma.[19] The classic but long forgotten and rarely used test for detecting organisms is the Goldman/Witmer antibody coefficient (AC).[20] It measures the ratio of vitreous to serum levels of antibody using the ELISA test. A coefficient greater than 3 is usually considered diagnostic. This test is most frequently used for *Toxocara canis* and *Toxoplasma gondii*. While there are many available diagnostic tests, the etiology remains elusive in many cases as documented in a series by Read and colleagues in 2002.[21] They demonstrated that cytology had only an 11% yield and PCR only a 39% yield in the cases they saw. The yield of diagnostic vitrectomy depends both on the likelihood of the pretest diagnosis and the appropriate screening and specimen handling. The surgeon must decide which studies are likely to yield a diagnosis and communicate this to the laboratory. Many local facilities are not equipped to handle PCR, immunohistochemistry and flow cytometry. Most hospitals outsource these tests. Coordination between the surgeon and laboratory is the key.

Case example 1

A 30-year-old male with a history of bilateral loss of vision presented with retinal lesions in the macula in both eyes. He had a history of HIV and was being treated in another facility unsuccessfully for *Candida*. An in-office automated vitreous biopsy was sent off for PCR and the results were positive for HZV. The diagnosis was consistent with progressive outer retinal necrosis (PORN).

Case example 2

A 6-year-old Caucasian female with congenital HIV presented with a history of totally blind right eye without any view secondary to an opacified cornea. Her only seeing left eye was thought to have a focal fungal, bacterial, or CMV infection in her macula. She was treated for several weeks for all of the above without regression. PCR vitreous analysis was done with a sutureless vitrector through a one-port site in the operating room. CMV resistant to the previous treatment was confirmed and the treatment drug was changed from ganciclovir to foscarnet. An immediate response was noted and she remained 20/20 in her only eye 10 years later.

Case example 3

A 34-year-old male with acute lymphoblastic leukemia in systemic remission developed bilateral retinal masses with vitreous opacities. Because he was in remission, it was thought to be infectious and not leukemic. A vitrectomy biopsy done at the slit lamp revealed the results by cytology in minutes. Leukemic cells were evident and immediate radiation was instituted in both eyes with a resolution of the masses and significant recovery of the vision within 2 weeks.

Case example 4

A 65-year-old male with sepsis had bilateral retinal masses. A vitrector biopsy done at the bedside revealed *Nocardia* before the systemic diagnosis was made and appropriate systemic antibiotics instituted.

CONCLUSION

In summary, diagnostic vitreous biopsy for endophthalmitis or cytology for uveitis or malignancy is an easily performed procedure with little risk. It may be done by needle aspiration, a three-port pars plana vitrectomy in the operating room or a portable office vitrector. With the proper analysis and appropriate testing and technique, an experienced laboratory may be very helpful in making a diagnosis in many cases.

Financial disclosure

Although the author previously had a financial interest in the Visitrec portable vitrector, he currently does not have any financial interest and his interest as been assumed by Insight Instruments, Inc., Stuart, Florida.

REFERENCES

1. Neveu M, Elliot AJ. Prophylaxis and treatment of endophthalmitis. Am J Ophthalmol 1959; 48:368–373.
2. Peyman GA, Vastine DW, Raichard M. Symposium. Postoperative endophthalmitis: experimental aspects and their clinical application. Ophthalmology 1978; 85:374–385.
3. Endophthalmitis Vitrectomy Study Group. Results of the Endophthalmitis Study. A randomized trial of immediate vitrectomy and of intravenous antibiotics for the treatment of postoperative bacterial endophthalmitis. Arch Ophthalmol 1995; 113:1479–1496.
4. Speaker MG, Menikoff JA. Prophylaxis of endophthalmitis with topical povidone iodine. Ophthalmology 1991; 98(12):1769–1775.
5. Singh S, Josephberg RJ, Zaidman GW. Office-based diagnostic pars plana vitrectomy. Invest Ophthalmol Vis Sci 1996; 37:402.
6. Hilton GF, Josephberg RG, Halperin LS. Office-based sutureless transconjunctival pars plana vitrectomy. Retina 2002; 22:725–732.
7. Pflugfelder SC, Hernandez E, Fliester SJ, et al. Intravitreal vancomycin, retinal toxicity clearance and interaction with gentamicin. Arch Ophthalmol 1987; 105:831–837.
8. Pavan PR, Oteizin E, Hughes B, et al. Exogenous endophthalmitis initially treated without systemic antibiotics. Ophthalmology 1994; 101:1289–1297.
9. Campochiaro PA, Lim JL. Aminoglycoside Toxicity Study Group. Arch Ophthalmol 1994; 112:48–53.
10. Schulman JA, Peyman GA. Intravitreal corticosteroids as an adjunct in the treatment of bacterial and fungal endophthalmitis. Retina 1992; 12:336–340.
11. Hariprasud SM, Mieler WF, Holy ER. Vitreous and aqueous penetration of orally administered gatifloxacin in humans. Arch Ophthalmol 2003; 121:345–350.
12. Brod RD, Flynn, HW Jr. Advances in the diagnosis and treatment of infectious endophthalmitis. Curr Opin Ophthalmol 1991; 2:306–314.
13. Rodriquez A, Calogne M, Pedroza Seres M, et al. Referral patterns of uveitis in a tertiary eye care center. Arch Ophthalmol 1996; 114:593–599.
14. Ausburger J. Invasive diagnostic technique for uveitis and simulating conditions. Trans Am Ophthalmol Soc 1990; 88:89–114.
15. Blumen Kranz MS, Ward T, Murphy S, et al. Applications and limitations of vitreoretinal biopsy techniques in intraocular large cell lymphoma. Retina 1992; 12:564–570.
16. Erlich HA, Gelfand D, Sninsky JJ. Recent advances in the polymerase chain reaction. Science 1991; 252:1643–1651.
17. Van Geldar RN. Applications of the polymerase chain reaction to diagnosis of ophthalmic disease. Surv Ophthalmol 2001; 46(3):248–258.
18. Davis JL, Solomon D, Nussenblatt RB, et al. Immunology to chemical staining of vitreous cells. Indications, techniques, and result. Ophthalmology 1992; 99:250–256.
19. Chan CC, Whitcup SM, Soluman D, Nussenblatt RB. Interleukin-10 in the vitreous of patients with primary intraocular lymphoma. Am J Ophthalmol 1995; 120:671–673.
20. Witmer R. Clinical implications of aqueous humor studies in uveitis. Am J Ophthalmol 1978; 86:39–44.
21. Read RW, Zamir E, Rad NA. Neoplastic masquerade syndromes. Surv Ophthalmology 2002; 47:81–124.

17

Treatment of advanced retinopathy of prematurity: peripheral retinal ablation

Antonio Capone Jr. and Anand Vinekar

INTRODUCTION

- The goal of retinopathy of prematurity (ROP) screening is to carefully monitor infants at risk for ROP and treat to prevent retinal detachment or scarring—all in the interest of optimization of visual outcome. Treatment involves laser ablation of avascular retina. As with any therapy in medicine, there are associated complications. This chapter presents an overview of the current approach to peripheral retinal ablation for ROP and treatment-associated complications.
- The ultimate goals of treatment of ROP are prevention of retinal detachment or scarring and optimization of visual outcome.
- Eyes with peripheral retinal ablation have superior anatomic and functional outcomes compared to eyes without ablation.
- Laser is the preferred method of peripheral retinal ablation for ROP.
- Anterior segment ischemia, though rare, is the most important complication of laser peripheral retinal ablation for ROP.

SURGICAL TECHNIQUE

Laser peripheral retinal ablation for ROP

ROP is a proliferative vascular disorder occurring in premature infants and is a leading cause of childhood blindness. The advancement of neonatology in recent decades has allowed babies with extremely low birth weights and young gestational ages to survive and potentially develop ROP. Peripheral retinal ablation has been effective in reducing the incidence of an unfavorable structural outcome and improving functional outcome in infants who develop ROP (since 1972), initially performed with cryotherapy.[1] In the Multicenter Trial of Cryotherapy for Retinopathy of Prematurity (CRYO-ROP) eyes of premature infants (birth weight less than 1251 g) with 'threshold ROP' were randomized to either cryotherapy or observation to establish whether peripheral retinal ablation could reduce the occurrence of an unfavorable visual outcome (20/200 or worse) or unfavorable structural outcome (retinal fold, retinal detachment, or retrolental fibroplasia).[2,3] At 10-year follow-up, eyes treated with cryotherapy were less likely to be legally blind (44% versus 62%), and were less likely to have an unfavorable structural outcome.[4]

Convenient portable units for indirect laser photocoagulation became available shortly after the publication of the CRYO-ROP study. Although the merit of cryopexy versus laser retinopexy for ROP has been hotly debated, laser is the current standard for treating ROP. Advantages of photocoagulation include ease of treatment, portability, and fewer systemic complications. Ng et al.[5] and Connolly et al.[6] recently reported long-term structural and functional outcomes using laser superior to those obtained with cryotherapy. Others have reported similar findings with shorter follow-up.[7–10]

The superiority of laser over cryopexy should come as no surprise. Laser has long been the standard of treatment in the management of other vasoproliferative retinopathies associated with diabetes, sickle cell disease, and retinal vascular occlusion. Laser photocoagulation is most effective for posterior (zone 1) disease: favorable anatomic results have been reported in 83% of eyes[11] versus only 25% of eyes with zone 1 disease treated with cryopexy.[12] Indications for using cryopexy instead of laser in the management of ROP include poor fundus visibility (vitreous hemorrhage or anterior segment problems), lack of availability of laser, and lack of treating physician familiarity with indirect laser retinopexy.

Equipment and anesthesia for laser surgery

17.1

It must be appreciated that some children will allow examination and treatment without anesthesia and others require it for accurate diagnosis and effective therapy. Sometimes it may be required that the procedure be carried out without anesthesia, if not tolerated by the child or family. The risks involved in anesthesia must be explained to the parents and formal written consent must be obtained. For an office examination alone, a lid speculum and scleral depression are often used, but with experience, the infant may be examined by using the doll's-eyes phenomenon and a 28-diopter lens with indirect ophthalmoscopy (Fig. 17.1). By turning the infant's head, the eyes will stay directed in the original field of gaze, bringing the peripheral retina into better view.

Laser photocoagulation may be performed using a number of different lasers.

The popular wavelengths in use are the: (1) 810-nm (infrared) diode laser; (2) 532-nm (visible) laser; and the (3) argon green (visible) laser. Unlike the argon, the other two are lighter and portable, can be plugged into a small wall socket, and even be easily transported to the neonatal intensive care unit, if so required (Fig. 17.2). The indirect ophthalmoscopic delivery system is used to deliver the laser (Fig. 17.3).

Pupillary dilation is achieved by using phenylephrine 2.5% and cyclopentolate 0.5% two to three times in both eyes after a gap of 15–20 min in between the drops. Sometimes due to the presence of tunica vasculosa lentis, posterior synechiae or very active disease, the pupil may dilate poorly. In such cases, care should be taken not to overuse the dilator drops as this may lead to systemic absorption and toxicity. Often the mechanical pressure caused by the scleral depressor during the laser procedure is able to dilate the pupil as the procedure is carried out.

An infant lid speculum is used to keep the eyelids open. This is useful especially in viewing and treating the superior and inferior retina. A pediatric scleral depressor or a

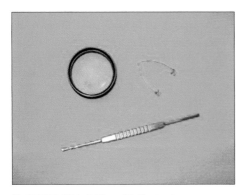

FIGURE 17.1 A 20- or 28-diopter lens, a pediatric speculum, and a pediatric scleral depressor are useful in both screening and treatment of ROP.

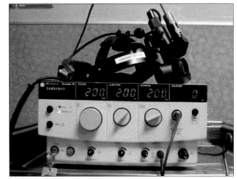

FIGURE 17.2 A portable laser console fitted with an indirect ophthalmoscopic delivery system is essential for laser treatment. Several laser wavelengths may be used. The 532 nm green wavelength laser console is seen in this picture.

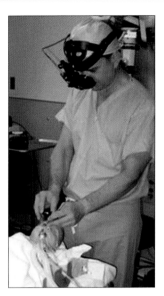

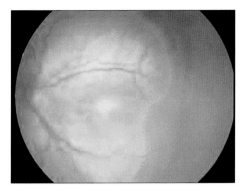

■ **FIGURE 17.4** In stage 3 ROP, there is extraretinal fibrovascular proliferation. The stage is characterized by the neovascularization that grows onto the vitreous at the ridge.

■ **FIGURE 17.3** The laser is delivered via the indirect ophthalmoscopy system. It may be performed under sedation or anesthesia with monitoring of systemic parameters.

modified lens loop is used to rotate and depress the globe to bring the desired quadrant of retina into view. An assistant keeps the cornea moist by periodically wetting it with balanced salt solution (BSS).

Timing of treatment—refining the definition of threshold disease

Threshold ROP in the CRYO-ROP study was defined as that severity of ROP for which a given eye had an equal chance (i.e. a 50/50 threshold) of spontaneous regression or progression to unfavorable outcome (defined atomically as the presence of a macular fold, retinal detachment involving zone 1, or obscuration of the posterior pole by cataract or retrolental fibrosis and later defined as Snellen equivalent of 20/200 or worse). Although initially based only on clinical estimation, threshold disease had become accepted as the point at which treatment should be administered. It was defined as stage 3 ROP in zone 1 or 2 occupying at least five contiguous clock hours or eight non-contiguous clock hours of retina[2] (Fig. 17.4). For eyes with zone 2 ROP, this estimation proved fairly precise; 62% of untreated eyes with threshold ROP went on to an untoward visual outcome. However, the estimation of a 50/50 threshold for eyes with zone 1 ROP was off the mark; untreated zone 1 eyes with threshold ROP had a 90% chance of untoward outcome.[3] Although the number of such eyes was small, the data suggested that the definition of threshold ROP used for zone 2 eyes may not be appropriate for zone 1 eyes.

Because zone 1 eyes almost always progress to threshold,[13] the question for such eyes and high-risk zone 2 eyes would appear not to be whether to treat, but when. Until recently, criteria for early treatment were lacking. This issue was investigated in the multicenter study of early treatment for retinopathy of prematurity (ETROP)[14] in which eyes with prethreshold ROP—also known as moderately severe ROP; any zone 1 ROP less than threshold; or zone 2 stage 2 with plus disease (dilation and tortuosity of posterior pole retinal vessels in at least two quadrants meeting or exceeding that of a standard photograph), or zone 2 stage 3 ROP without plus disease, or zone 2 stage 3 ROP with fewer than five contiguous or eight cumulative clock hours with plus disease—were randomized to early treatment once they attained 15% risk of unfavorable outcome or more. Comparison between untreated eyes, high-risk prethreshold eyes treated early, and high-risk eyes treated at threshold demonstrated that retinal ablative therapy is beneficial for: (1) any eye that has any stage of ROP in zone 1 with plus disease; (2) stage 3 ROP in zone 1 with or without plus disease; and (3) stage 2 or 3 ROP in zone 2 with plus disease.

Stage 1 ROP (Fig. 17.5) and stage 2 ROP without plus (Fig. 17.6) do not require laser treatment. In contrast, aggressive posterior ROP (Fig. 17.7) or posterior ROP, usually in zone 1 or posterior zone 2, may rapidly progress to detachment without passing through the classically described stages of the 'ridge' and 'extraretinal fibrovascular proliferation'. This type of ROP is characterized by flat neovascularization and retinal hemorrhages, and usually develops in very low birth weight babies. It requires earlier and aggressive treatment.

Indications for laser ablation—summary
The current guidelines for laser treatment are summarized in Table 17.1, adapted from the ETROP guidelines.[14]

TREATMENT PARAMETERS

Photocoagulation is delivered through a dilated pupil with a 20- or 28-diopter condensing lens. Initial laser settings vary depending on the laser wavelength and fundus pigmenta-

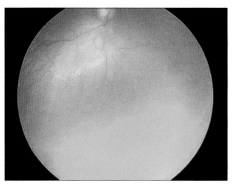

■ **FIGURE 17.5** Stage 1 ROP is seen as a tortuous, discontinuous grayish-white 'line of demarcation' between the vascularized (posterior) and avascular (peripheral) retina temporally.

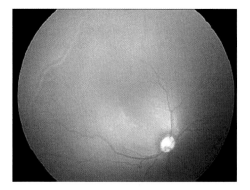

■ **FIGURE 17.6** Stage 2 ROP is characterized by the development of the 'ridge' which has obvious volume.

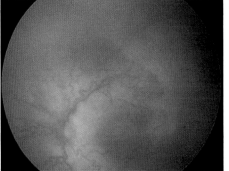

■ **FIGURE 17.7** Stage 3 aggressive posterior ROP (APROP) is characterized by flat neovascularization, rapidly progressing vascular changes, and intraretinal shunting without ridge tissue and hemorrhages.

TABLE 17.1 Guidelines for laser ablation[14]

Zone	Plus or no plus	Stage	Management
1	No plus	1	Follow
		2	Follow
		3	Treat
	Plus	1	Treat
		2	Treat
		3	Treat
2	No plus	1	Follow
		2	Follow
		3	Follow
	Plus	1	Follow
		2	Treat
		3	Treat

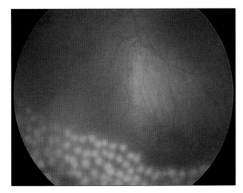

■ **FIGURE 17.8** The conventional treatment pattern is best described as nearly confluent with burns placed 0.5–1 burn widths apart.

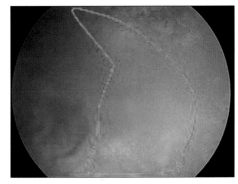

■ **FIGURE 17.9** Skip areas (green polygon) must be identified and subjected to supplement laser treatment.

tion. Settings of 200 mW for power and 100 mS for duration are used initially, and titrated until a laser burn with a gray or gray-white appearance is visible. The conventional treatment pattern is best described as nearly confluent, with burns placed 0.5–1 burn widths apart (Fig. 17.8). Treatment should extend from the ora serrata up to, but not including, the ridge for 360°. At the conclusion of the treatment session, the retina is inspected for 'skip areas' (Fig. 17.9) to ensure peripheral retinal ablation has been complete.

POSTOPERATIVE MANAGEMENT

Infants are placed on topical steroid drops four times daily for the week following laser. The eyes are reexamined within 1 week. Persistent plus disease or progressive fibrovascular proliferation may indicate inadequate treatment, in which case additional treatment is indicated.

COMPLICATIONS OF PERIPHERAL LASER RETINOPEXY FOR ROP

Similar to cryotherapy, transient conjunctival hyperemia can occur following laser peripheral retinal ablation.[15,16] This is due to the globe manipulation required when performing laser to ensure visualization and treatment of the entire avascular retina. Also, conjunctival hyperemia may be more pronounced with transscleral laser photoablation than with indirect ophthalmoscopic laser delivery.[16]

Corneal and iris defects are widely known potential complications of laser photoablation.[17–21] Irvine et al.[19] described small, white opacities estimated to be 10% excavations of the anterior cornea following indirect laser photoablation in adult patients. They postulated that these superficial corneal defects or burns may be secondary to laser energy absorbed by the edematous corneal epithelium or resulting from light scattering at the corneal surface. Corneal epithelial edema can occur and may be secondary to epithelial absorption of laser energy as well as epithelial exposure during treatment. Removal of the corneal epithelium helps maintain clarity during treatment.[18] Iris burns have been described and are probably due to inadvertent laser to the iris surface and absorption of energy by iris pigment. A subsequent mild iridocyclitis can occur, as can posterior synechiae.[19] Some advocate the use of transscleral laser delivery to prevent injury to the cornea and iris.[16] In addition, anterior chamber hyphema has been reported as a complication of laser photoablation.[9,22–24] These hyphemas most likely occur secondary to inadvertent lasering of the iris and iris vessels.

Angle-closure glaucoma is a known complication after laser photoablation, and has been described after panretinal photocoagulation for proliferative diabetic retinopathy.[25,26] After widespread photocoagulation, an exudative retinal and/or choroidal detachment can develop, causing forward rotation of the ciliary body with subsequent closure of the angle. Despite the numerous reports in the literature of using laser for treatment of ROP, only Lee et al. reported one patient who developed angle-closure glaucoma after laser treatment for ROP that required surgical iridectomies.[27]

Cataract formation has been reported as a complication of laser photoablation in elderly patients. Early reports theorized that the aged-lens changes, with possible pigmentation, make the lenses susceptible to laser energy absorption.[28,29] The clear lenses of preterm infants have also been shown to develop cataracts secondary to laser therapy; and these occurrences are well described.[10,17,22,23,30–37] One report indicated that cataracts occur in up to 6% of eyes treated for ROP.[37] Two types of cataract have been described, and both are believed to result from the thermal effects of laser. The first type appears as punctate or vacuolated focal opacities occurring at the capsular or subcapsular level. These focal opacities are believed to be visually insignificant and may spontaneously resolve over a period of 2–6 weeks.[34,35] Capone et al. suggest that the preterm infant lens is secondarily affected by laser by its proximity to the iris, iris pigment within broken iris synechiae to the anterior lens capsule, or the tunica vasculosa lentis, all of which may absorb energy and heat the lens.[11] In theory, there is reduced potential of thermal-induced cataract formation in infants with a prominent tunica vasculosa lentis with a diode laser (810 nm) than with an argon laser (514 nm) because the diode laser wavelength is less readily absorbed by blood vessels. The second type of cataract is visually significant and may appear immediately following laser or weeks after treatment.[30] The cataract appears as a dense opacity, sometimes total in nature, which obscures visualization of the fundus and requires cataract extraction. Although the etiology is of this type of cataract is unclear, Lambert et al. have proposed several explanations.[30] First, microperforations in the lens capsule may allow a phacoantigenic cause to the cataract formation. This explanation is supported by findings of Lambert et al. of posterior synechiae, iris atrophy, and pigment on the anterior lens capsule, suggesting an inflammatory component. A second explanation is that these forms of cataract represent anterior segment ischemia.

Ablation of the avascular retina, especially along the horizontal meridians at 3 and 9 o'clock, can theoretically damage or destroy the long posterior ciliary arteries and cause anterior segment ischemia. Despite limited discussion in the cryotherapy literature, there have been a number of reports of laser ablation leading to anterior segment ischemia.[17,30,38] Lambert et al. described a series of eight patients (10 eyes) who developed signs of anterior

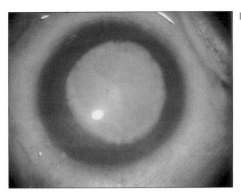

FIGURE 17.10 The right eye of a patient with zone 2 threshold retinopathy of prematurity treated 4 weeks earlier using a diode laser (1400 spots, 240 mW, 200 ms). There is a dense cataract with pigment on the anterior lens surface, posterior synechiae, a shallow anterior chamber with iridocorneal touch nasally, and mild corneal edema—all characteristic of anterior segment ischemia following laser.

segment ischemia including cataracts, corneal edema, iris atrophy, pupillary membranes, and shallow anterior chambers within 1–4 weeks after confluent treatment with argon or diode laser. Fifty percent of eyes developed retinal detachments before cataract surgery. On follow-up after cataract surgery, 9 of 10 eyes became phthisical.[30] Kaiser and Trese reported anterior segment ischemia occurring in 8 eyes of 5 patients following confluent treatment of cryotherapy or laser therapy[38] (Fig. 17.10). Finally, Fallaha et al.[17] reported on 2 of 87 eyes (2.3%) that underwent confluent laser photoablation for ROP and subsequently developed anterior segment ischemia. One possible modification of treatment application which may prevent this severe complication, as suggested by both Lambert et al. and Kaiser and Trese, is to lightly treat (with laser or cryotherapy) the horizontal meridians where the long posterior ciliary arteries are found.[17,30]

CONCLUSION

ROP management has changed over the last 20 years. Screening protocols and recommendations have helped refine intervention points for this potentially blinding condition. That most infants who are screened for ROP never develop threshold disease is indicative of the progress made in identifying and treating the disease. For those who do go on to develop ROP requiring therapy, however, effective therapies do exist. Although these therapies have inherent risks of complications, they are often successful in treating the disease.

REFERENCES

1. Yamashita Y. Studies on retinopathy of prematurity: III. Cryocautery for retinopathy of prematurity. Jpn J Ophthalmol 1972; 26:385–393.
2. Cryotherapy for Retinopathy of Prematurity Cooperative Group. Multicenter trial of cryotherapy for retinopathy of prematurity. Preliminary results. Arch Ophthalmol 1988; 106:471–479.
3. Cryotherapy for Retinopathy of Prematurity Cooperative Group. Multicenter trial of cryotherapy for retinopathy of prematurity: 3½-year outcome—structure and function. Arch Ophthalmol 1993; 111:339–344.
4. Multicenter Trial of Cryotherapy for Retinopathy of Prematurity: ophthalmological outcomes at 10 years. Arch Ophthalmol 2001; 119(8):1110–1118.
5. Ng EY, Connolly BP, McNamara JA, et al. A comparison of laser photocoagulation with cryotherapy for threshold retinopathy of prematurity at 10 years: Part 1. Visual function and structural outcome. Ophthalmology 2002; 109(5):928–934.
6. Connolly BP, Ng EY, McNamara JA, et al. A comparison of laser photocoagulation with cryotherapy for threshold retinopathy of prematurity at 10 years: Part 2. Refractive outcome. Ophthalmology 2002; 109(5):936–941.
7. Hunter DG, Repka MX. Diode laser photocoagulation for threshold retinopathy

of prematurity. A randomized study. Ophthalmology 1993; 100(2):238–244.

8. Robinson R, O'Keefe M. Cryotherapy for retinopathy of prematurity—a prospective study. Br J Ophthalmol 1992; 76(5):289–291.

9. Paysse EA, Lindsey JL, Coats DK, Contant CF Jr, Steinkuller PG. Therapeutic outcomes of cryotherapy versus transpupillary diode laser photocoagulation for threshold retinopathy of prematurity. J AAPOS 1999; 3(4):234–240.

10. McGregor ML, Wherley AJ, Fellows RR, Bremer DL, Rogers GL, Letson AD. A comparison of cryotherapy versus diode laser retinopexy in 100 consecutive infants treated for threshold retinopathy of prematurity. J AAPOS 1998; 2(6):360–364.

11. Capone A Jr, Diaz-Rohena R, Sternberg P Jr, et al. Diode laser photocoagulation for zone 1 threshold retinopathy of prematurity. Am J Ophthalmol 1993; 116:444–450.

12. Cryotherapy for Retinopathy of Prematurity Cooperative Group. Multicenter trial of cryotherapy for retinopathy of prematurity. Three-month outcome. Arch Ophthalmol 1990; 108:195–204.

13. Kivlin JD, Biglan AW, Gordon RA, et al. Cryotherapy for Retinopathy of Prematurity (CRYO–ROP) Cooperative Group. Early retinal vessel development and iris vessel dilatation as factors in retinopathy of prematurity. Arch Ophthalmol 1996; 114:150–154.

14. Early Treatment for Retinopathy of Prematurity Cooperative Group. Revised indications for the treatment of retinopathy of prematurity: results of the early treatment for retinopathy of prematurity randomized trial. Arch Ophthalmol 2003; 121:1684–1694.

15. McNamara JA, Tasman W, Vander JF, Brown GC. Diode laser photocoagulation for retinopathy of prematurity. Preliminary results. Arch Ophthalmol 1992; 110(12):1714–1716.

16. Seiberth V, Linderkamp O, Vardarli I. Transscleral vs transpupillary diode laser photocoagulation for the treatment of threshold retinopathy of prematurity. Arch Ophthalmol 1997; 115(10):1270–1275.

17. Fallaha N, Lynn MJ, Aaberg TM Jr, Lambert SR. Clinical outcome of confluent laser photoablation for retinopathy of prematurity. J AAPOS 2002; 6(2):81–85.

18. Landers MB 3rd, Toth CA, Semple HC, Morse LS. Treatment of retinopathy of prematurity with argon laser photocoagulation. Arch Ophthalmol 1992; 110(1):44–47.

19. Irvine WD, Smiddy WE, Nicholson DH. Corneal and iris burns with the laser indirect ophthalmoscope. Am J Ophthalmol 1990; 110(3):311–313.

20. Hunt L. Complications of indirect laser photocoagulation. Insight 1994; 19(4):24–25.

21. Lobes LA Jr, Bourgon P. Pupillary abnormalities induced by argon laser photocoagulation. Ophthalmology 1985; 92(2):234–23.

22. Seiberth V, Linderkamp O, Vardarli I, Knorz MC, Liesenhoff H. Diode laser photocoagulation for threshold retinopathy of prematurity in eyes with tunica vasculosa lentis. Am J Ophthalmol 1995; 119(6):748–751.

23. Simons BD, Wilson MC, Hertle RW, Schaefer DB. Bilateral hyphemas and cataracts after diode laser retinal photoablation for retinopathy of prematurity. J Pediatr Ophthalmol Strabismus 1998; 35(3):185–187.

24. Rundle P, McGinnity FG. Bilateral hyphaema following diode laser for retinopathy of prematurity. Br J Ophthalmol 1995; 79(11):1055–1056.

25. Prendiville PL, McDonnell PJ. Complications of laser surgery. Int Ophthalmol Clin 1992; 32(4):179–204.

26. Doft BH, Blankenship GW. Single versus multiple treatment sessions of argon laser panretinal photocoagulation for proliferative diabetic retinopathy. Ophthalmology 1982; 89(7):772–779.

27. Lee GA, Lee LR, Gole GA. Angle-closure glaucoma after laser treatment for retinopathy of prematurity. J AAPOS 1998; 2(6):383–384.

28. Lakhanpal V, Schocket SS, Richards RD, Nirankari VS. Photocoagulation-induced lens opacity. Arch Ophthalmol 1982; 100(7):1068–1070.

29. McCanna R, Chandra SR, Stevens TS, Myers FL, de Venecia G, Bresnick GH. Argon laser-induced cataract as a complication of retinal photocoagulation. Arch Ophthalmol 1982; 100(7):1071–1073.

30. Lambert SR, Capone A Jr, Cingle KA, Drack AV. Cataract and phthisis bulbi after laser photoablation for threshold retinopathy of prematurity. Am J Ophthalmol 2000; 129(5):585–591.

31. Christiansen SP, Bradford JD. Cataract following diode laser photoablation for retinopathy of prematurity. Arch Ophthalmol 1997; 115(2):275–276.

32. Pogrebniak AE, Bolling JP, Stewart MW. Argon laser-induced cataract in an infant with retinopathy of prematurity. Am J Ophthalmol 1994; 117(2):261–262.

33. Gold RS. Cataracts associated with treatment for retinopathy of prematurity. J Pediatr Ophthalmol Strabismus 1997; 34(2):123–124.

34. Capone A Jr, Drack AV. Transient lens changes after diode laser retinal photoablation for retinopathy of prematurity. Am J Ophthalmol 1994; 118(4):533–535.

35. Drack AV, Burke JP, Pulido JS, Keech RV. Transient punctate lenticular opacities as a complication of argon laser photoablation in an infant with retinopathy of prematurity. Am J Ophthalmol 1992; 113(5):583–584.

36. Campolattaro BN, Lueder GT. Cataract in infants treated with argon laser photocoagulation for threshold retinopathy of prematurity. Am J Ophthalmol 1995; 120(2):264–266.

37. Christiansen SP, Bradford JD. Cataract in infants treated with argon laser photocoagulation for threshold retinopathy of prematurity. Am J Ophthalmol 1995; 119(2):175–180.

38. Kaiser RS, Trese MT. Iris atrophy, cataracts, and hypotony following peripheral ablation for threshold retinopathy of prematurity. Arch Ophthalmol 2001; 119(4):615–617.

18 Scleral buckle surgery for retinal detachment associated with neonatal retinopathy of prematurity

Khaled A. Tawansy

Modern management in retinopathy of prematurity (ROP) includes timely screening of neonates at risk for retinal detachment and the recognition of aberrant vascular development and retinal ischemia. Early and appropriate ablation of the avascular retina in eyes at risk for progressive neovascular activity and retinal detachment has proven to be the most valuable intervention for preventing vision loss.[1] Despite significant efforts dedicated to widespread education and screening, including digital photographic screening for remote centers, ROP remains a major cause of childhood blindness in countries that are capable of sustaining premature infants (preemies).[2] The morphology of ROP varies between nations, likely relating to differences in maternal nutrition, neonatal management protocols (including monitoring of oxygen administration), and genetic variables. For example, most retinal detachments observed in Southern California occur in neonates under 28 weeks' gestation or 1000 g birth weight with posterior and highly active vascular disease; detachments observed in Southern India occur in babies between 28 and 34 weeks' gestation and between 1250 and 2500 g with zone 2 disease and a propensity for arteriovenous anastomosis without much vascular dilation and engorgement (plus) features.[3] Oxygen toxicity occurring from incubators with unregulated oxygen flow is at least one potential variable responsible for these differences.

VASCULOPATHY

In neonates with a critical level of retinopathy, as defined by the Cryotherapy for ROP and Early Treatment for ROP studies, appropriate timing of ablative therapy ensures the best likelihood of favorable outcome; approximately 85% go on to resolution of ischemia and neovascularization and long-term stable retinal anatomy.[4] Even in the approximately 15% that suffer retinal detachment, the prognosis is still excellent if thorough ablative laser has been performed and the vascular activity has resolved. Eyes with retinal detachment associated with dry fibrotic traction membranes have over 90% successful anatomic repair with lens-sparing vitrectomy (LSV), and most have the potential for excellent visual acuity.[5,6] The prognosis diminishes considerably when retinal detachment occurs in a vascularly active eye. This includes eyes that have missed the opportunity for ablative laser, as well as those where ablation is insufficient to reduce ischemic drive. Typically one finds a wide pink ridge with progressive circumferential contraction, a persistently active tunica vasculosa lentis (TVL) and hyaloidal artery, progressive subretinal lipid exudates, and engorgement of the retinal vessels with tortuosity in a child that has not yet reached the due date (Fig. 18.1).

Vitreous surgery in these active eyes is fraught with complications of hemorrhage, inadequate membrane removal and reproliferation. A retrospective analysis of eyes operated in Southern California showed that vascular activity is the highest predictor of surgical anatomic failure, with prognosis deteriorating from 90 to 15% or less depending on how many ischemic variables are present.[7] In these eyes the pediatric vitreous surgeon should proceed with caution, and might prefer to delay entering the eye until neovascularization

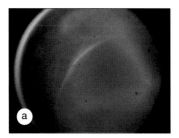 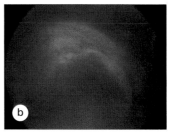

FIGURE 18.1 (**a, b**) Persistent neovascular activity involving a broad ridge with evolving tractional and exudative retinal detachment despite two prior sessions of ablative laser in two eyes. Because the macula is threatened, retinal reattachment surgery is warranted. Vitrectomy is not a good option because of the high risk of intraoperative hemorrhage and postoperative reproliferation. Scleral buckle with subretinal fluid drainage and cryotherapy of the ridge is a better option at this stage. It may relieve sufficient traction to prevent progressive detachment or stabilize the configuration until neovascularization quells and vitreous surgery becomes safer.

quells, even in the face of progressive macular detachment. Pharmacologic therapy with intravitreal angiostatic steroids and vascular endothelial growth factor inhibitors holds some promise in salvaging some of these severe cases, but prognosis for visual function remains grim. Two case series using intravitreal triamcinolone acetonide as an adjunct to surgery in vascularly active retinal detachments have shown a beneficial therapeutic effect.[8–10]

SURGICAL OPTIONS

Scleral buckle surgery is a viable option in these ischemic eyes with poor prognosis, possibly reversing posterior retinal detachment or delaying it until the environment for vitreous surgery becomes more favorable. In the subspecialty practice of ROP retinal surgery, this is the most common role for scleral buckle.

Successful repair of the ROP detachment depends on relief of the traction vectors, which tend to be:

1. circumferential along the ridge, contributing to vitreoschisis and peripheral retinal thinning,
2. from the ridge to the posterior pole, often in association with the hyaloid artery and membranes within Cloquet's canal and responsible for macular ectopia,
3. from the ridge to the anterior hyaloid face, including the ciliary body and the lens,
4. transvitreal from ridge to ridge, contributing to the volcano configuration of the retinal detachment.

The most effective relief of these intraocular traction vectors is achieved with lens-sparing vitreous surgery.[5,11] Systematic vitreous membrane dissection will reliably result in retinal relaxation. Because the neonatal retina under traction becomes stretched and redundant, it is common to find postoperative folds despite a well-executed and thorough dissection.

A well-placed scleral buckle can relieve a significant component of the anteroposterior and circumferential traction.[12–14] In experienced hands, retinal reattachment rates of approximately 70% can be achieved.[12–14] In some cases, buckling can be combined with vitreous surgery. This is most often performed when the ridge is very anterior and its attachment to the anterior hyaloid cannot be relieved because of possible damage to the crystalline lens. Scleral buckle in this situation may allow an eye to remain phakic, which is important not only in preventing amblyopia in these highly susceptible eyes but also for avoiding the high risk of cyclitic membrane formation associated with early lensectomy.

Lens dissection is especially difficult in eyes with active TVL, and inadequate lens dissection is second only to persistent vascular activity as a cause of reproliferation and anatomic failure.[7]

PARADIGMS

In vitreoretinal surgery for ROP, it is important that for each eye the choice and order of surgical intervention be considered carefully and individualized. The traditional paradigm of first buckle, then vitrectomy when buckle fails is often not appropriate. Buckle is one of several tools available in the armamentarium of the retinal surgeon that should be applied in select cases when it is the best option after that eye's retinal morphology and specific features have been studied. In this regard, we find it very helpful to study panoramic images of the retina before surgery to determine configuration, degree of vascular activity, and location or extent of traction vectors.

A retinal surgeon should consider offering scleral buckle for an eye with stage 4 or open stage 5 retinal detachment when it is the most appropriate intervention for that eye. Because most peripheral ROP detachments show progression over time, observation of these detachments is not recommended. If the eye has been well ablated and the detachment is generally dry and associated with fibrous traction that is predominantly posterior to the equator, lens-sparing vitrectomy is the most appropriate intervention with anatomic and visual success rates above 90%.[5,6,15] Because of the anatomic constraints of the neonatal eye, typically one-sixth of the adult volume, and the potential for irreversible complications, vitreous surgery in ROP should be reserved for centers with considerable experience in this area. Scleral buckle surgery should be considered in eyes with vascularly active ROP, especially when occurring before the due date, as well as those with a rhegmatogenous component, those with residual or recurrent detachment after appropriate and thorough vitrectomy, and those where dissection adjacent to the ridge is avoided because of its location close to the lens.

INDICATIONS

As discussed above, heavy retinal vascular activity is a good reason to avoid intraocular surgery in the eye with acute ROP. This is the number one indication for scleral buckle in our patients. We have a grading points system that incorporates five variables with scores assigned from 0 to 2 for each[7]:
1. The presence of an active tunica vasculosa lentis
2. The presence of hemorrhage in the vitreous or on the retina more than two disc diameters in size
3. The amount of extraretinal or intraretinal neovascularization
4. The extent of plus disease (posterior pole vessel dilation and tortuosity)
5. The width and extent of the shunt or ridge.

A total of 10 points can be assigned to the vascular activity score. In a series of 310 vitrectomies for active ROP performed by three surgeons over a 10-year period, there appeared to be a linear relationship between the vascular activity score and the anatomic success rate, ranging from 90% for scores of 1–2, to 15% for scores of 8–10.

Two additional situations have been particularly appropriate for scleral buckle in ROP. The first is an eye that has had appropriate vitreous surgery but failed to reattach or reattached and then went on to detach again. If the primary vitrectomy has been performed with the above principles involved, then one must decide whether detachment has recurred or persisted because of new membrane formation or because of membranes that could not safely be removed. In the latter situation we have found that scleral buckle is preferable to vitrectomy, with a slightly higher anatomic success rate (70 vs. 59%), lower rate of lensectomy (0 vs. 88%), and lower rate of retinal breaks and phthisis.[13]

The final indication is eyes with ROP and a rhegmatogenous component. Retinal breaks occur in neonatal ROP under five circumstances, in order of decreasing frequency:[16]

1. Complication of vitrectomy surgery, either as a dialysis created at the entry or inadvertent break caused by an instrument
2. Complication of external drainage of subretinal fluid during scleral buckle
3. Complication of ablative laser into retina that is shallowly detached
4. After ridge contracts in response to heavy confluent laser, typically a giant tear at the margin between treated and untreated retina
5. Spontaneously as a result of membrane contraction not associated with recent ablative therapy, typically a smaller break created in thin retina associated with heavy membranes.

Although retinal breaks in ROP almost always require vitrectomy and tamponade with gas or oil, placement of a buckle to support the vitreous base and retinal break can make the difference between success and failure.

INSTRUMENTATION

One major advantage of buckle surgery is the simplicity of instrumentation relative to intraocular surgery. The following is a list of preferred items

Non-disposable items
- Wire lid speculum
- Westcott blunt and sharp scissors
- Stevens tenotomy scissors
- 0.3 or 0.5 toothed forceps
- Bishop toothed forceps
- Locking straight fine-tipped needle holders (2)
- Schepens retractor, preferably pediatric size
- Scleral depressor and marker
- Handle for Beaver blade
- Gass muscle hooks
- Heavy smooth utility forceps (2)
- Indirect ophthalmoscope
- 20- or 28-diopter condensing lens, sterile
- Indirect laser and/or cryotherapy unit
- Diathermy unit
- Loops or operating microscope per surgeon preference

Disposables items
- Sterile drapes, towels, and plastic bags
- Sterile gowns and gloves
- Silicone band (240 or 41 Myra or equivalent)
- Balanced salt solution
- Povidone iodine (Betadine) paint
- Antibiotics and steroids for subconjunctival injection
  - Cefazolin 50 mg/mL (0.5 mL)
  - Dexamethasone 4 mg/mL (0.5 mL)
- 2-0 silk ties to pass around muscles
- 5-0 nylon suture on S-24 needle for intrascleral passes
- 4-0 polyglactin (Vicryl) for clove hitch
- 8-0 polyglactin to close Tenon's capsule and conjunctiva
- 6-0 polyglactin to close sclerotomy drain
- No. 57 Beaver blade or equivalent

- Cotton-tipped applicators
- 27-Gauge needle and small syringe for paracentesis
- Postoperative topical medications
- Atropine 1% solution
- Antibiotic ointment with or without steroid
- Acetazolamide for intravenous injection
- Sterile gauze eye patch and plastic 1-inch tape
- Ice packs for postoperative application

PREOPERATIVE PREPARATION

A thorough preoperative evaluation by the patient's neonatologist or pediatrician is important to ensure that systemic health is optimized prior to surgery. Routine preoperative
laboratory tests should be reviewed within a few days of surgery, including complete blood
and platelet count, prothrombin and partial thrombin time, and basic metabolic panel.
General anesthesia is used with endotracheal intubation or a laryngeal mask airway. An
anesthesiologist comfortable with the care of premature neonates is much preferred. The
day prior to surgery, the eyelids and lashes are cleansed with gentle soap. A detailed
informed consent is obtained from the parents or legal guardian. A careful explanation of
the surgical objectives and potential complications is performed, with ample opportunity
for the family to ask questions. The consent is documented in the chart and witnessed by
the nursing staff.

One hour before surgery, the pupils are dilated with a combination of cyclopentolate
1%, phenylephrine 2.5%, tropicamide 1%, and flurbiprofen 0.03%. A careful study of the
retinal configuration is done during an examination under anesthesia, and the findings
are documented with fundus drawings and/or retinal photography. This will help the
surgeon plan the approach.

SURGICAL TECHNIQUE

Once a decision has been made to apply a scleral buckle, some consideration of technique
is warranted. Most literature has described encircling the neonatal eye with a band, typically placed at the equator, then division of the encircling element 3–6 months later to
allow growth of the eye and avoid migration or extrusion. Although this is a reasonable
approach, I will herein describe a practical technique where the band is placed at the ridge
and tied with a dissolving suture, allowing growth of the eye without division of the buckle.
This technique has evolved from personal experience with 300 cases over 10 years.

A 360° conjunctival peritomy is created at the limbus. The connective tissue is then
bluntly dissected from the sclera in each quadrant using curved Stevens scissors, and the
underlying sclera is carefully examined, looking for areas of scleral ectasia or staphyloma.
One should also visualize and avoid injury to the vortex veins. If the sclera is adequate,
then the 2-0 silk sutures are passed around the rectus muscle insertions using a Gass
hook (Fig. 18.2). Care is taken to avoid looping the obliques or splitting any of the rectus
muscles. The heavy neonatal Tenon's fascia and intermuscular connective tissue is dissected away from the muscle insertions with sharp scissors to prevent its entrapment by
the encircling exoplant.

A thin band (Myra 240 or 41 style exoplant) is then passed under the rectus muscles.
The free ends are placed in the quadrant with least vitreous traction. The band is placed at
the height of the neovascular ridge. This position is identified with indirect ophthalmoscopy
and marked after gentle scleral indentation. The horizontal mattress nylon sutures are
placed intrascleral, ideally at 50% depth and parallel to the limbus (Fig. 18.3). This maneuver requires careful attention as the neonatal sclera is significantly thinner than in adults
and an inadvertent perforation could have devastating consequences. Typically one or two

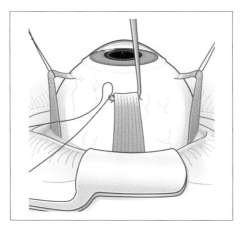

■ **FIGURE 18.2** Silk suture passed around superior rectus muscle with a Gass hook while the sutures through the medial and lateral rectus are retracted; the hook is kept anterior to avoid catching the superior oblique tendon.

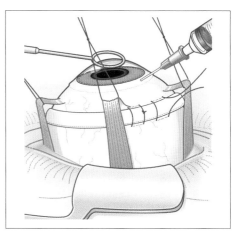

■ **FIGURE 18.3** Horizontal mattress 5-0 nylon sutures placed in the superotemporal quadrant around the Myra 41 band which has been positioned to support the neovascular ridge. One suture has been temporarily tied with a slip knot. In order to make room for additional imbrication created by the second suture, an anterior chamber paracentesis is performed with a 27-gauge needle Luer-locked to an empty syringe. The needle is positioned in the mid anterior chamber overlying the iris to help avoid injury to the lens, and the pressure is being assessed with a cotton tip applicator. The free ends of the band are overlapped in the superonasal quadrant.

sutures are placed in each quadrant, spaced 1–2 mm wider than the buckle to give adequate imbrication at the ROP ridge. Only the quadrants with active traction need to be buckled. Segmental elements are often used in eyes with isolated traction, most often temporally. Problems with migration are not often seen if the element is well secured.

We usually tie the nylon mattress sutures temporarily with a slip knot in the quadrants with greatest traction, and then examine the retina with indirect ophthalmoscopy. Once it has been verified that the band has the desired height and location, the knots can be made permanent and sutures are trimmed. If the intraocular pressure (IOP) has risen from the tightening of the sutures, then anterior chamber paracentesis is performed. A 27-gauge sharp needle Luer-locked to a small syringe with the plunger removed is passed through the limbus and over the iris, taking care to avoid injury to the lens (Fig. 18.3). Anterior chamber fluid is allowed to passively egress until the IOP normalizes or the chamber becomes too shallow. If the latter occurs while the IOP is still high, one must wait for the chamber to reform or consider alternative means of lowering the pressure such as systemic carbonic anhydrase inhibitors or osmotic diuretics or vitreous tap. At all times one must be mindful of the IOP as the newborn is highly susceptible to ischemic optic nerve injury.

Important intraoperative decisions are whether to drain subretinal fluid or ablate the retina with cryotherapy or laser. Drainage of subretinal fluid can be helpful in reducing volume to allow for adequate height of the buckle when the horizontal mattress sutures are tightened. After relief of traction with a buckle, it may take weeks for the retinal pigment epithelium to remove all the subretinal fluid. If the fluid is of sufficient volume, involving one or more quadrants with a height of ≥2 mm, then drainage may significantly hasten recovery. The decision to drain is based on clinical judgment and the experience of the surgeon, as this is the step that can most often result in complications. While sub-retinal hemorrhage and retinal incarcerations are significant problems, they can usually be managed without disastrous consequences. Perforation of the retina can be particularly devastating to the eye with acute ROP as discussed below.

To avoid incarceration, the quadrant with the most fluid is selected for drainage, and the eye is palpated to ensure that the pressure is not elevated. Fluid is drained slowly through a small choroidal perforation. A scleral dissection is made with a 57 Beaver blade posterior to the buckle. To avoid hemorrhage, the incision is made close to the horizontal rectus muscles, avoiding the vortex veins. Transillumination of the globe through the pupil can further outline the scleral emissary vessels and guide the surgeon to a safe site. Per-pendicular to the limbus, a careful dissection of scleral fibers is performed with the curved part of the blade that is held on a slight angle (Fig. 18.4). Once the choroid is reached, a 2-mm knuckle is allowed to protrude. The margins of the sclerotomy and the exposed choroid are lightly treated with diathermy. A 6-0 Vicryl purse-string suture is placed around the sclerotomy to allow rapid closure if the eye becomes too soft. The choroid is perforated with a needle passed tangentially, just grasping the outer fibers and pulling outwards.

Fluid is allowed to egress slowly until the eye becomes hypotonous, then the sclerotomy is closed with the preplaced Vicryl. At this point any loose mattress sutures can be tight-ened; if the eye remains soft then fluid or air is injected through a pars plicata paracentesis to restore volume. The sclerotomy can then be reopened as necessary if there is residual

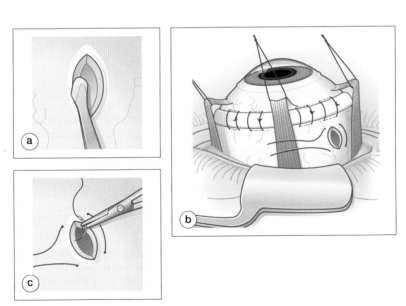

FIGURE 18.4 Drainage sclerotomy placed in the superotemporal quadrant posterior to the encircling band and close to the lateral rectus muscle, avoiding the vortex vessels. The encircling band is in position and the nylon mattress sutures have been loosely tied in slip knots. (**a**) A 57 Beaver blade is held at an angle and used to dissect scleral fibers until a knuckle of choroids is exposed. The margins of the scleral cutdown and the choroidal bed are treated with diathermy. (**b**) A 6-0 polyglactin suture is placed as a purse-string around the dissection to allow rapid closure of the drain. (**c**) An S-24 needle is passed tangentially, catching the outer choroidal tissue and perforating it without risking perforation of the retina. The subretinal fluid is allowed to drain passively. Once the eye has become soft, the drain can be closed temporarily with the purse-string and the horizontal sutures around the buckle can be tightened further, giving additional support.

subretinal fluid, but always when the pressure is normal (below 20 mmHg). If drainage does not occur after perforation of the choroid, a new site is chosen for scleral dissection and no deep needle passes are made. After successful drainage, the site is closed permanently to prevent growth of fibrovascular tissue in this area. The eye is left soft (5–10 mmHg) enough to allow additional tightening of the horizontal mattress sutures and overlap of the band if needed.

Once subretinal fluid is drained, there may be an opportunity to safely ablate previously detached areas of avascular retina with cryotherapy or laser. This is a particularly important step when retinal detachment occurs in an ischemic eye, in order to prepare for the possibility of subsequent vitrectomy and reduce the vasoproliferative response. Either ablative technique is acceptable; however, if the view is adequate, laser is preferred. Cryotherapy is usually associated with an increase in subretinal exudation in the first postoperative week, which may result in macular detachment and a worse visual prognosis.

In eyes with significant circumferential traction, it is desirable to encircle the eye and tie the free ends of the band together to give height and support. If a Myra 270 (Watske) sleeve is used, then division of the band will be necessary later. A preferred alternative is to use a clove hitch of 4-0 polyglactin suture, which will hydrolyze and dissolve over the subsequent 3 months. This will give the desired level of support for the month or two when it is most needed, then relax as the eye grows. Since adopting this approach we have not noted issues with migration or strangulation. On follow-up examinations as long as 9 years, restriction of growth has not been observed and division of the band has not been required. The clove hitch is made by creating two loops with the suture then overlapping them with the trailing loop in front. The loops are placed around the overlapping ends of the band which have been drawn to give a snug fit around the eye. The free ends of the polyglactin suture are pulled to lock the clove hitch, and a standard knot is placed over it (Fig. 18.5).

Once the buckle has been secured in a satisfactory position and the issues of drainage, peripheral ablation, and encirclement are resolved, the eye can be closed. The band is trimmed and inspected in all quadrants, ensuring that Tenon's fascia has not been entrapped by the band or the placed sutures. This can be a source of postoperative restriction in motility. The pressure is left low–normal and the optic nerve is visualized to ensure good perfusion. The silk sutures are removed and a double layer closure of Tenon's fascia and conjunctiva is performed with interrupted 8-0 polyglactin. Subconjunctival injections of dexamethasone and cefazolin or alternative antibiotic are given, and the eye is patched over atropine and antibiotic ointment. One dose of acetazolamide 5 mg/kg is given intravenously at the end of the case.

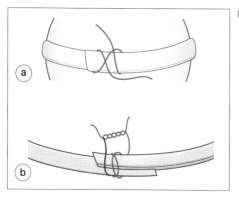

■ FIGURE 18.5 (a, b) Polyglactin 4-0 suture tied as a clove hitch around the free ends of the encircling band, which have been overlapped in the superonasal quadrant and drawn to give a snug fit of the band around the eye.

POSTOPERATIVE CARE

To minimize orbital congestion, we recommend positioning the child with the head elevated 30–40°, and application of ice packs over the eye patch as tolerated. The patch is removed 24 hours after surgery and topical prednisolone acetate and a broad-spectrum antibiotic are administered four times per day. The eye is examined 24 hours after surgery and monitored closely for pressure fluctuations or other potential postoperative complications such as angle closure. The latter is usually associated with a buckle that is too high and that induces anterior rotation of the lens–iris diaphragm. Treatment includes frequent topical steroids and cycloplegics in combination with topical and systemic aqueous suppressants. If the pressure cannot be controlled, then the buckle should be divided or removed.

Within a few days of surgery, the postoperative orbital congestion and chemosis should resolve, allowing detailed examination of the fundus. Ideally there should be a smooth indent of the buckle against the neovascular ridge with resolution of the traction and subretinal fluid (Fig. 18.6). If a significant amount of cryotherapy had been used for ablation of the avascular retina or ridge, there may be an initial increase in exudative detachment in the first postoperative week before resolution later.

COMPLICATIONS

Complications of scleral buckling such as hemorrhage or retinal incarceration often relate to drainage or deep passage of the intrascleral sutures. Certainly it is best to avoid these potential problems by giving close attention to those critical steps and optimizing visualization through the use of good lighting and loops or a microscope as needed.

If retinal incarceration occurs, one must decide whether it is significant enough to warrant further intervention that can be risky. Many small incarcerations will smoothen out spontaneously with time. A radial sponge or silicone wedge (Myra 135) can be extended from the encircling band to give additional height to the involved retina and help relax the associated folds. One may be able to relieve incarceration by vitrectomy and gentle aspiration of the involved retina with a soft-tipped cannula or anterior displacement of subretinal fluid with perfluorocarbon liquid, but these maneuvers are associated with a high risk of retinal perforation. They are only considered when the incarceration creates a fold through the macula.

Hemorrhage can occur into the vitreous cavity or subretinal space. Many critically ill preemies have thrombocytopenia or liver dysfunction, and a careful preoperative assessment and correction of deficiencies is warranted to minimize potential bleeding. When it

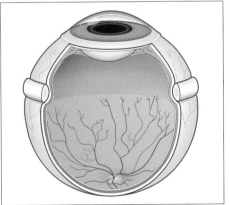

■ **FIGURE 18.6** Postoperative appearance with support of the neovascular ridge and associated circumferential traction with a high encircling band. There is persistent plus disease and activity at the ridge but the subretinal fluid has resolved.

does occur, one must examine the retina carefully to rule out perforation. Most mild vitreous hemorrhage can be observed and may clear without complications. If the vitreous hemorrhage is more significant, then one must weigh the potential risks and benefits of simultaneous vitrectomy.

Most subretinal hemorrhage can also be observed for spontaneous clearing unless a thick hemorrhagic macular detachment occurs. In this situation it is sometimes possible to mobilize the blood anteriorly by vitrectomy, detachment of the hyaloid, and injection of a heavy perfluorocarbon liquid. Laser can then be used to barricade the blood and prevent its posterior migration.

An additional potential problem is choroidal effusion. This usually relates to a buckle that is placed to high or too tight. This is less often a problem in babies than in adults and can generally be prevented by maintaining proper distance between the intrascleral passes, avoiding excess tightening of the overlapped free ends, and avoiding prolonged periods of hypotony. Postoperative choroidal effusion will almost always improve with time but this can take several weeks, and may be hastened by a short course of systemic steroids.

Retinal breaks are a more significant complication and are to be avoided as a first priority as they are difficult to manage successfully. Eyes with neonatal ROP detachments that develop a break rarely have a good visual outcome. In approximately 50% of cases, retinal reattachment with a stable anatomic outcome can be achieved.[14] This may help growth of the eye and prevent phthisis. The operative approach involves placement of an anterior Myra 240 encircling band to support the vitreous base and relieve residual traction. A vitrectomy is then performed with aggressive detachment and removal of the posterior hyaloid. Intraocular triamcinolone or fluorescein may be used to stain the vitreous for more complete removal. The vitreous is dissected from the optic disc to at least the anterior edge of the break. All accessible membranes are removed. A gentle fluid–air exchange is then performed with drainage of subretinal fluid through the break.

If one is able to drain all the fluid and flatten the break, then laser photocoagulation may be applied at its margins followed by silicone oil tamponade. In most cases, however, residual traction will cause air to accumulate in the subretinal space. Under these conditions it is best to return to fluid, then perform a wedge-shaped relaxing retinotomy sized four to six clock hours. This is extended from the break anteriorly towards the ora serrata. The fluid–air exchange is then repeated, with or without the assistance of perfluorocarbon heavy liquid, and laser retinopexy is applied to the margins of the retinotomy. Critical to this technique is the complete removal of hyaloid posterior to the retinotomy, otherwise the retina will contract into a central mass and become inoperable. At that point, further maneuvers will only cause injury and should be avoided. Silicone oil 5000 centistokes is used as the vitreous substitute of choice in these cases, both because of its long-term tamponading effect and also to help reduce progression to phthisis.

Practical and theoretical concerns

There are some practical and theoretical concerns regarding the buckling of neonatal eyes with ROP. Buckles do nothing to relieve posterior traction vectors that can disorganize the macula. They tend to be avoided in retinal vascular diseases because of the potential to worsen ischemia. Anterior segment ischemia is a well-recognized potential complication of laser ablation of the avascular retina. The risk is minimized by keeping the laser power to the minimum necessary to achieve a light white or yellow burn (generally 200–350 mW, always below 500); it is equally important to avoid excessive scleral depression, limit the number of laser spots administered per session (generally 1500 or less per eye), and avoid heavy treatment at 3 and 9 o'clock where the long posterior ciliary neurovascular bundle travels. In highly ischemic eyes with severe ROP, heavy laser ablation may be necessary and appropriate to gain adequate control of the disease. These eyes are more susceptible to ischemia which can manifest later. We have on occasion observed anterior segment ischemia develop after scleral buckling of eyes that had previous heavy laser. Eyes with buckles that develop hypotony, cyclitic membrane, cataract, or corneal edema should be considered for possible removal of the buckle to improve circulation.

Additional considerations include induced myopia and astigmatism caused by a high buckle. The myopia will be minimized when the scleral foreshortening by the horizontal mattress sutures is the primary source of buckle height, rather than the encirclement. Postoperative pain and edema are slightly greater in buckle surgery than in vitrectomy but in general they are minimal and well tolerated by most neonates. Postoperative strabismus occurs most commonly as a result of entrapped Tenon's fascia and intermuscular connective tissue. It can be minimized with a thorough dissection prior to passing the band. Glaucoma occurs in ROP by a variety of mechanisms and can be exacerbated by scleral buckle surgery.

ADDITIONAL CONSIDERATIONS

Smoldering ROP

In most eyes with ROP retinal detachments that have responded to laser ablation, lens-sparing vitrectomy alone is the most appropriate intervention and has excellent success in experienced hands. If the ridge and associated traction are adjacent to the crystalline lens, and especially if the traction has caused a fold to extend onto the lens, then entering the eye at the iris root could cause retinal tears, and scleral buckle is a better option. This type of detachment is a subtype of ROP that has been labeled smoldering ROP. This phenotype is being observed with increasing frequency in very small preemies, typically 23–26 weeks' gestation, with delayed retinal vascular maturation but minimal vascular activity.[17,18] Many of these preemies have coexisting central nervous system disease and they may suffer an early insult to the pleuripotent mesenchymal tissue at the optic nerve that is preprogrammed for vasculogenesis.[17,18] These eyes develop late macular dragging and retinal detachment, typically after 45 weeks' gestation. They involve zone 3 and anterior zone 2 with minimal plus disease or neovascularization at the ridge (Fig. 18.7). They respond very nicely to an encircling band that supports the vitreous base.

Combined scleral buckle and vitrectomy

There are some few cases, between 5 and 10% in our series, in which pars plana vitrectomy is planned with scleral buckle. In these eyes there is some posterior traction, typically membranes associated with a persistent hyaloidal artery that can only be removed with vitrectomy, but some of the anterior peripheral traction requires scleral buckle.

In these combined cases, there is more room for maneuvering during vitrectomy if it is performed before the buckle. Typically the encircling band and horizontal mattress sutures are placed but not tightened. A two-port vitrectomy is performed with sclerotomies placed 180° apart. An irrigating light pipe is utilized to avoid potential trauma to the lens or ridge that can be created by a separate infusion cannula. Once the vitreous dissection is completed, a fluid–air exchange is performed and the sclerotomies are closed. The buckle can then be tightened to an appropriate height.

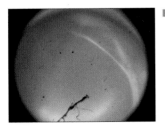

■ **FIGURE 18.7** Delayed retinal vascular maturation with fibrotic tractional detachment occurring at 51 weeks post conception in an eye with minimal plus disease (smoldering ROP). Because of the typically anterior location of the ridge adjacent to the crystalline lens, scleral buckle is an ideal procedure for this detachment.

ROP detachments in older children and adults

While this chapter focuses on retinal detachments occurring in neonates with acute ROP, it is well recognized that ROP is a lifelong problem with a high potential for rhegmatogenous detachments to occur later in life. These tend be retinal defects in ischemic or ablated retina anterior to the equator, including atrophic holes, flap tears, and giant tears. It is advantageous to treat these holes and flap tears with a broad scleral buckle, such as a Myra 276, 286, or 287 tire. The defects can be readily closed while avoiding the potential problems of vitrectomy in these eyes, including difficult and incomplete hyaloidal removal and a propensity for secondary proliferative vitreoretinopathy.

CONCLUSIONS

Scleral buckle procedures are appropriate for a select group of ROP retinal detachments. These include eyes with:

- open configuration,
- high neovascular activity,
- anterior disease that involves lens (which can be spared),
- predominately circumferential traction,
- failed primary LSV or late re-detachment,
- late onset of traction,
- rhegmatogenous component.

Scleral buckle is a valuable tool for the pediatric retinal surgeon and when used appropriately can help to rescue eyes with an otherwise poor prognosis. It is no longer the primary procedure for the majority of routine dry ROP retinal detachments, as this has been supplanted by lens-sparing vitrectomy. In current practice scleral buckle has specific indications. When a thoughtful treatment strategy is tailored specifically for each eye, taking account the location of the ridge, the degree of neovascular activity, as well as the distribution of the traction vectors, scleral buckle can be a gratifying procedure for the patient and surgeon, increasing the breadth of cases that can be successfully repaired.

REFERENCES

1. Repka MX, Tung B, Good WV, et al. Outcome of eyes developing retinal detachment during the Early Treatment for Retinopathy of Prematurity (ETROP) study. Arch Ophthalmol 2006; 124(1):24–30.
2. Good WV, Hardy RJ, Dobson V, et al. The incidence and course of retinopathy of prematurity: findings from the Early Treatment for Retinopathy of Prematurity study. Pediatrics 2005; 116(1):15–23.
3. Pons ME, Shah P, Lee H, Narendran V, Tawansy KA. Comparison of threshold ROP in Southern India and Southern California. Invest Ophthalmol Vis Sci 2005; 46:e4103.
4. Good WV, Early Treatment for Retinopathy of Prematurity Cooperative Group. Final results of the Early Treatment for Retinopathy of Prematurity (ETROP) randomized trial. Trans Am Ophthalmol Soc 2004; 102:233–248.
5. Capone A Jr, Trese MT. Lens-sparing vitreous surgery for tractional stage 4A retinopathy of prematurity retinal detachments. Ophthalmology 2001; 108(11):2068–2070.
6. Prenner JL, Capone A Jr, Trese MT. Visual outcomes after lens-sparing vitrectomy for stage 4A retinopathy of prematurity. Ophthalmology 2004; 111(12):2271–2273.
7. Tawansy KA, Lee H. Predictors of anatomic failure in surgery for advanced neonatal ROP retinal detachments. Invest Ophthalmol Vis Sci 2004; 45:e3535.
8. Tawansy KA, Lakhanpal RR, de Juan E Jr. Intraocular triamcinolone in the management of zone 1 retinopathy of prematurity refractory to laser ablation of the avascular retina. Invest Ophthalmol Vis Sci 2003; 44:e600.
9. Tawansy KA, Lakhanpal RR, de Juan E Jr. Intra-vitreal triamcinolone for severe ROP refractory to laser ablation: one year results. Invest Ophthalmol Vis Sci 2005; 46:e3493.
10. Lakhanpal RR, Fortun JA, Chan-Kai B, Holz ER. Lensectomy and vitrectomy with and without intravitreal triamcinolone acetonide for vascularly active stage 5

retinal detachments in retinopathy of prematurity. Retina 2006; 26(7):736–740.

11. Trese MT. Two-hand dissection technique during closed vitrectomy for retinopathy of prematurity. Am J Ophthalmol 1986; 101(2):251–252.

12. Tawansy KA, Samuel M. Retinopathy of prematurity: practical surgical management in the new millennium. Clinical report and clinicians corner. Techniques Ophthalmol 2004; 2(2):60–65.

13. Samuel M, Tawansy KA. The modern role of scleral buckle in ROP retinal detachment. American Society of Retinal Specialists Annual Meeting, San Diego, August 2004.

14. Hinz BJ, de Juan E Jr, Repka MX. Scleral buckle surgery for active stage 4A retinopathy of prematurity. Ophthalmology 1998; 105(10):1827–1830.

15. Capone A Jr, Trese MT. Take good care of my baby: evolving standards of care for retinopathy of prematurity. Ophthalmology 2002; 109(5):831–833.

16. Samuel MA, Tawansy KA, Oppenheimer N, Russell MK, de Carvalho RAP, Kupperman BA. Rhegmatogenous retinal detachment in neonatal ROP. Invest Ophthalmol Vis Sci 2005; 46:e4104.

17. Lam HD, Tawansy KA, Samuel MA, Lee H. Delayed retinal vascular maturation and late onset macular dragging and retinal detachment in neonates with retinopathy of prematurity. Invest Ophthalmol Vis Sci 2004; 45:e4027.

18. Tawansy KA, Lee H, de Juan E Jr. Smoldering retinopathy of prematurity. Vail Vitrectomy Meeting, Vail, Colorado, March 2004.

Vitrectomy surgery for retinopathy of prematurity

Michael T. Trese

INSTRUMENTS

For most surgeries a 20-gauge system is preferable. The flexibility of the 25-gauge system makes accessing certain surgical spaces difficult and, therefore, not usable in challenging surgeries. Both a wide-field viewing system and a posterior pole lens are needed.

Vitrectomy with lensectomy

If the lens cannot be preserved during surgery due to a closed surgical space then an anterior approach must be taken and the lens removed. This can be done with a two- or three-port procedure.

Two-port lensectomy vitrectomy requires the vitrector and a manual infusion (we use a 23-gauge butterfly needle stabilized with a hemostat, irrigating with lactated Ringers solution). When the lens is removed, the butterfly irrigation is replaced with an irrigating light pipe. A three-port system uses a 90° anterior infusion cannula, secured at the limbus with a 7-0 Vicryl suture. The vitrector is used for the lensectomy, with high vacuum and a low cutting rate. In the three-port procedure, the anterior infusion is used throughout the surgery and either a light pipe or lighted pick can be used for illumination. Additional instruments include membrane peeler cutter (MPC) scissors, irrigating spatula, and intraocular forceps. It is important to have available an endolaser probe, viscoelastic, and silicone oil.

Lens-sparing vitrectomy

The first step in performing lens sparing vitreous surgery is identifying the ports of entry. There must exist a space between the lens and the detached retina to allow for entry of the instruments. If the ciliary processes can be visualized and a space for entry identified, a lens-sparing procedure can be accomplished. In the premature infant the pars plana is not yet developed, requiring sclerotomies that are more anterior than in standard vitreous surgery. The sclerotomies are made approximately 1 mm posterior to the limbus at the 9 and 3 o'clock positions with a 19- or 20-gauge microvitreoretinal (MVR) blade.

A two-port surgery is used for lens-sparing vitrectomy. An infusing light pipe (either with or without a pick) is used for illumination and intraocular pressure maintenance. A vitrector, MPC scissors, irrigating spatula, and intraocular scissors are generally required.

SURGICAL TECHNIQUE

Preoperative considerations

Eyes with retinopathy of prematurity (ROP) which progresses to retinal detachment following peripheral laser ablation may be exudative, tractional, or a combination of the two. Primarily exudative retinal detachment does not require surgical intervention. Tractional retinal detachments are due to organized primary vitreous contracting and pulling anteriorly on the underlying retina. Most stage 4a (Fig. 19.1) and even stage 4b (Fig. 19.2) eyes can be addressed with a lens-sparing technique. Most stage 5 eyes will require a lensectomy for adequate surgical exposure. A subset of stage 5 (Fig. 19.3) eyes will have a surgical

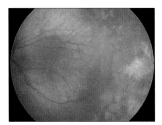

■ **FIGURE 19.1** Stage 4a ROP. The peripheral retina is detached but the fovea remains dry.

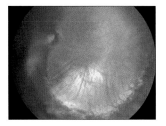

■ **FIGURE 19.2** Stage 4b ROP. The peripheral retina is detached and there is fluid under the fovea.

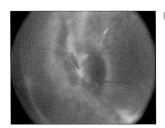

■ **FIGURE 19.3** Stage 5 ROP. The entire retina is detached. Overlying organized vitreous and fibrotic tissues create multiple tissue planes.

space that allows for a lens-sparing procedure. Despite adequate laser ablation, some eyes will demonstrate persistent plus disease. Although surgical intervention at the earliest sign of detachment is ideal, the presence of continued vascular activity is a contraindication for surgery. Although the detached retina may progress during this time, an improved surgical result will be attained.

Surgical approach

A conjunctival peritomy is made with sharp dissection, exposing 9 and 3 o'clock (this can be two T-incisions or 180° superiorly) for a two-port approach. The conjunctiva must be opened 360° if an anterior infusion cannula (three-port system) will be used (an option for pressure maintenance if the lens is to be taken). The primary goal of surgery is to transect the vectors exerting traction on the retina. Several planes of contractile tissues form and progressively detach the retina. These tissues develop between the: (1) ridge and the eye wall; (2) ridge and the ciliary processes; (3) ridge to the posterior lens capsule (4) ridge to ridge (5) posterior pole to ridge and (6) posterior pole to posterior lens capsule. All of these tissue planes will exist in an eye with a tractional retinal detachment due to retinopathy of prematurity. The dominant tractional forces, however, will determine the various configurations of retinal detachment that may be encountered. The end-goal of the surgery is to relax the tractional forces sufficiently to allow the posterior retina to fall towards the eye wall and assume a more natural configuration. With time (weeks to years), the underlying retinal pigment epithelium will resorb the subretinal fluid and/or blood and reattach the retina. The peripheral retina is addressed in regards to relieving tractional forces that may disallow the posterior retina to reattach. However, the final anatomy of the peripheral retina itself is less important as the retina is often redundant in the ROP eye.

Vitrectomy with lensectomy

Lensectomy is required when the surgical space is closed and the detached retina meets or closely approaches the posterior lens and/or ciliary processes. Because of the anterior position of the retina in these cases, the entrance into the eye must be through the iris root to ensure that a sharp incision of the retina does not occur. After the sclerotomies are made, if a permanent anterior infusion is not being used, the irrigating butterfly cannula is introduced into the substance of the lens through the nasal port. The vitrector, via the temporal port, is used to remove the lens with high vacuum and a low cutting rate. After removing the lens the capsule is removed in its entirety. At this point the iris must also be trimmed back to prevent postoperative scarring to underlying tissues. Bleeding from the iris is generally self-limited. If bleeding continues, intraocular diathermy with a 23-gauge tip can be performed. Attention is then turned to relieving the tractional elements of the vitreous. The goals at this point are the same as those for lens-sparing vitrectomy and will be addressed in the following section.

Lens-sparing vitrectomy

19.1

After identifying that an open surgical space is present, two sclerotomies are made entering the pars plicata, approximately 1 mm posterior to the limbus. First ensure that the instruments are easily viewed and not caught in any organized vitreous. The primary vitreous is predominant and creates sheets of organized vitreous. The primary vasculature is also in varying states of regression and creates scaffolding that accounts for the many vectors of traction. These extend from the posterior pole to the posterior lens (stalk tissue), branch from the stalk to the peripheral retina, from the ridge tissue to the eye wall, from the ridge to the ciliary processes and posterior lens, and also form a ridge to ridge sheet. These must be dissected to allow for relaxation of the retina. This can be achieved using the vitrector and MPC scissors. It is often difficult to identify the planes between organized vitreous and retina, as the retina is often thin and dysplastic. The irrigating spatula is helpful in this regard. Aggressive removal of vitreous and fibrous tissue is not necessary for successful surgery, but rather dissection and radicalization of tractional tissues. The posterior hyaloid cannot be separated from the retina in an infant, and this should not be attempted without the aid of enzymatic cleavage (plasmin) of the hyaloid–retinal interface. A posterior retinal break is a devastating event in this surgery and can occur easily due to the thin, poorly developed peripheral retina. The final anatomic retina will not assume a normal configuration but is not necessary for a visually functional retina. Upon completion of the surgical dissection, a fluid–air exchange is performed. This helps to avoid wound incarceration while suturing the incisions as well as pneumatically reapproximating the retina to the underlying pigment epithelium.

Postoperatively the infant is placed in a face-down position overnight, maximizing the pneumatic effect. The air bubble will aid in displacing the subretinal fluid away from the posterior pole while allowing the retina to assume a concave figure. It may also aid in further dissecting any remaining tractional vectors anteriorly. The subretinal fluid resorption can take weeks to years depending on the predominant constituents. Serous fluid will resorb quickly, while subretinal cholesterol crystals may remain for years.

OUTCOME

Results can be divided into anatomic success and functional success. Anatomic success consists of partial or total retinal reattachment. The posterior pole is the most important region to attain reattachment, as the retinal redundancy renders the attachment of the peripheral retina less important so long as the tractional components have been addressed. The rate of attachment for stage 4 ROP is greater than 85% with a single surgery.[1-3] Vitrectomy also has a higher success rate when compared to scleral buckling.[4] Vitrectomy in stage 4a ROP is also successful at interrupting progression to stage 4b or stage 5 retinal detachment.[3] Factors associated with surgical failure are retinal tears and vitreous hemorrhage.[5]

Final functional success, as ascertained by visual acuity, is harder to verify. Natural history data show that stage 4b and stage 5 eyes without intervention go on to no light

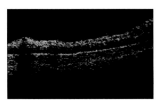

FIGURE 19.4 OCT demonstrating poor foveal development in a stage 4 eye 6 months after vitrectomy.

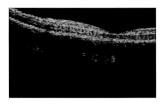

FIGURE 19.5 OCT demonstrating good foveal development in a stage 4 eye 6 months after vitrectomy.

perception.[6] Visual acuity after vitrectomy for stage 4a ROP eyes is very good, with an average vision of 20/58.[3,7] Even stage 5 eyes have improved visual acuity following surgical intervention.[8] Foveal structure, however, is generally atypical to some extent. The degree of foveal development, as determined by a foveal depression on optical coherence tomography (OCT) (Figs 19.4 and 19.5) and the presence of a foveal avascular zone (FAZ) on a fluorescein angiogram, appears to correlate highly with final visual function.

Patients with ROP are at an increased risk of rhegmatogenous retinal detachment (RRD).[9,10] Regressed ROP eyes typically have multiple breaks occurring at the equator or more posteriorly.[11] Previously vitrectomized eyes that develop an RRD have a high success rate for reattachment with subsequent surgery and maintain good vision.[9-11]

REFERENCES

1. Lakhanpal RR, Sun RL, Albini TA, Holz ER. Anatomic success rate after 3-port lens-sparing vitrectomy in stage 4A or 4B retinopathy of prematurity. Ophthalmology 2005; 112(9):1569–1573.
2. Hubbard GB 3rd, Cherwick DH, Burian G. Lens-sparing vitrectomy for stage 4 retinopathy of prematurity. Ophthalmology 2004; 111(12):2274–2277.
3. Capone A Jr, Trese MT. Lens-sparing vitreous surgery for tractional stage 4A retinopathy of prematurity retinal detachments. Ophthalmology 2001; 108(11):2068–2070.
4. Hartnett ME, Maguluri S, Thompson HW, McColm JR. Comparison of retinal outcomes after scleral buckle or lens-sparing vitrectomy for stage 4 retinopathy of prematurity. Retina 2004; 24(5):753–757.
5. Kono T, Oshima K, Fuchino Y. Surgical results and visual outcomes of vitreous surgery for advanced stages of retinopathy of prematurity. Jpn J Ophthalmol 2000; 44(6):661–667.
6. Pendegast SD, Trese MT. Bilateral visual improvement following lens-sparing vitrectomy for threshold 4B ROP [letter]. Retina 1996.
7. Prenner JL, Capone A Jr, Trese MT. Visual outcomes after lens-sparing vitrectomy for stage 4A retinopathy of prematurity. Ophthalmology 2004; 111(12):2271–2273.
8. Hartnett ME, Rodier DW, McColm JR, Thompson HW. Long-term vision results measured with Teller Acuity Cards and a new Light Perception/Projection Scale after management of late stages of retinopathy of prematurity. Arch Ophthalmol 2003; 121(7):991–996.
9. Tufail A, Singh AJ, Haynes RJ, Dodd CR, McLeod D, Charteris DG. Late onset vitreoretinal complications of regressed retinopathy of prematurity. Br J Ophthalmol 2004; 88(2):243–246.
10. Terasaki H, Hirose T. Late-onset retinal detachment associated with regressed retinopathy of prematurity. Jpn J Ophthalmol 2003; 47(5):492–497.
11. Kaiser RS, Trese MT, Williams GA, Cox MS Jr. Adult retinopathy of prematurity: outcomes of rhegmatogenous retinal detachments and retinal tears. Ophthalmology 2001; 108(9):1647–1653.

20 Surgery for intraocular tumors

Bertil Damato and Carl Groenewald

There are many different intraocular tumors, most of which can be treated by a variety of methods, each modality having countless technical variations.[1] The aim of this chapter, therefore, is to describe the surgical techniques used by the authors in the treatment of uveal melanoma, other tumors and methods being referred to only briefly.

PREOPERATIVE MANAGEMENT

Ocular assessment

In addition to standard examination of both eyes, specific ophthalmic procedures, such as echography, are required to define the nature, size and extent of the tumor, both to select the most appropriate treatment and to be able to assess the likely outcome.

Systemic investigation

The purposes of preoperative systemic examination are to:(1) identify any conditions that might require special care during general anesthesia; (2) locate the primary tumor if the ocular lesion is a metastasis; and (3) detect any systemic metastases if the patient has a uveal melanoma. Opinion is divided as to whether liver imaging should be performed in all patients with uveal melanoma or just those with an increased risk (e.g. tumor diameter exceeding 16 mm), the latter approach preferred by the authors. With regard to ocular metastases, it is debatable as to whether systemic examinations should be performed in the first instance or, as we prefer, once the differential diagnosis has been narrowed by ocular tumor biopsy.

Counseling

As with treatment for any condition, proper counseling is essential if the patient is to be satisfied with the surgical result. In particular, patients with an ocular tumor are distressed by their fear of cancer, concerns about losing the eye, and apprehension about visual handicap.

It is difficult for patients to understand and remember all they are told at the initial consultation with the ocular oncologist, especially if they are distressed. The author (BD) manages this problem in several ways, such as giving each new patient an audiocassette tape recording of the actual discussion that has taken place.

As with other treatments, it is important to manage the patient's expectations, especially if there is a chance of visual deterioration or loss of the eye. In ocular oncology, special measures need to be taken to address any psychological difficulties experienced by patients and their relatives.

SURGICAL PROCEDURES

Tumor biopsy
Instruments and devices

- Wire speculum
- 25-Gauge vitrectomy system
- Gallipot

- Pathology specimen container with the pathologist's preferred fixative
- Cytogenetics container, with transport medium

Indications and contraindications

Tumor biopsy is indicated to establish a diagnosis if clinical examinations are inconclusive. It is not conventional to perform biopsy primarily for the purpose of grading the malignancy of a uveal melanoma. Cytogenetic studies have recently been shown to have high prognostic value, however, so that we now perform prognostic biopsy wherever possible.[2] Others have also started performing prognostic biopsy.[2]

Surgical technique

The ports are inserted in the usual fashion, while pulling the conjunctiva towards the limbus (Fig. 20.1). The vitreous cutter is passed through the retina into the tumor, using the standard cutting rate and suction to aspirate tissue. Vitrectomy is not required. The cutter is repeatedly withdrawn from the tumor to aspirate a small amount of vitreous, thereby preventing blockage. The vitreous cutter is removed from the eye and the specimen back-flushed into a gallipot, which is examined under the operating microscope to ensure that tumor fragments are visible. This sample is poured into a bottle containing a small amount of fixative (e.g. 10% neutral buffered formalin) and sent to the pathology laboratory in the usual fashion. The procedure can be repeated if a second specimen is required for cytogenetic studies. At the end of the procedure, the ports are removed, and cotton buds are used to apply pressure to the sclerotomies and to stroke the conjunctiva back into position. Retinal diathermy and gas tamponade are not required.

When combined with insertion of tantalum markers or a radioactive plaque, the biopsy must be performed last, with the ports placed in undisturbed conjunctiva. This allows the plaque or marker insertion to be completed without hindrance from any vitreous hemorrhage or hypotony. We prefer to perform prognostic biopsy of uveal melanoma on the last day of proton beam radiotherapy so that any vitreous hemorrhage does not interfere with treatment.

Outcome

A preliminary study of 14 patients reported uneventful surgery in all patients (Fig. 20.2).[3] A positive diagnosis was achieved in 13, albeit at the second attempt in one patient. The

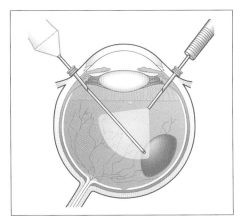

FIGURE 20.1 Technique of 25-gauge biopsy. The procedure is performed without vitrectomy, retinopexy, or tamponade. The scleral ports (blue) reduce any risk of tumor seeding to entry sites.

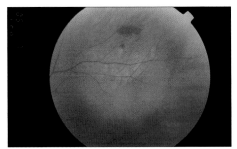

FIGURE 20.2 Amelanotic choroidal tumor, measuring 9.8 × 8.9 × 2.7 mm, located superotemporally in the left eye of a 68-year-old man. Residual hemorrhages are present from a 15-G biopsy performed 2 weeks before. The tumor proved to be a melanoma and the patient received proton beam radiotherapy. Six months later the vision was 20/30.

most frequent complication was vitreous hemorrhage, which tended to be mild and to resolve spontaneously, except perhaps with small, juxtapapillary tumors, when there was a greater chance of damaging a major choroidal vessel. Since the publication, over 40 such procedures have been performed at our center, with only one patient developing rhegmatogenous retinal detachment. The 25-gauge vitreous cutter has also been used to biopsy iris tumors.[4]

Brachytherapy
Instruments and devices
- Extraocular tray consisting of
  - Barraquer speculum
  - Conjunctival spring scissors
  - Moorfields forceps (2 pairs)
  - St Martins forceps
  - Pointed scissors
  - 90° fiberoptic transilluminator
  - Marker pen
  - Barraquer needle holder
  - Bulldog clamps (4)
  - Watson retractor
  - Calipers
- Plaque template and radioactive plaque
- Sutures
  - 2 × 6-0 Polysorb
  - 2 × 4-0 Ethibond
  - 1 × 5-0 half-circle Vicryl
  - 1 × 5-0 half-circle Ethibond

Indications and contraindications
The indications for ruthenium plaque radiotherapy are small and medium-sized melanomas, small uveal metastases, selected iris melanomas, selected vascular uveal and retinal tumors, and adjunctive therapy after local resection.

Surgical technique
After draping the patient, binocular indirect ophthalmoscopy is performed to confirm that the correct eye is being operated upon and to check the tumor location. A 180° conjunctival peritomy is made (Fig. 20.3). If a rectus muscle passes over the tumor, it is disinserted. Before the muscle is cut, the distance between the knots of the preplaced sutures and the cornea is recorded. Two traction sutures are placed in the sclera, about 90° apart and over pars plana, in case the sclera is inadvertently perforated. The oblique muscle is also disinserted if it is likely to get in the way of the plaque.

The tumor margins are localized by transillumination using a 21-gauge illuminator with its tip pre-bent by 90°. The tip of the transilluminator is passed under the edge of the conjunctival opening and around the globe so that it lies directly opposite the tumor. Alternatively, transpupillary transillumination can be performed. The tumor margins are marked on the sclera with a pen.

First a transparent, plastic template (i.e. 'dummy plaque') is sutured in place, with the knots fastened by releasable bows, and when its correct position is confirmed it is replaced with the radioactive plaque, using the same sutures. A 15-mm plaque is used for tumors up to 10 mm in diameter, with a 20-mm plaque being selected if the tumor diameter is 11–16 mm and a 25-mm plaque if the tumor diameter is greater than this. If the tumor is peripheral, the plaque is positioned so that it is centered on the tumor with a safety margin of at least 2 mm in all directions. If the tumor extends post-equatorially, then the plaque is positioned eccentrically, with its posterior edge overlapping the posterior tumor

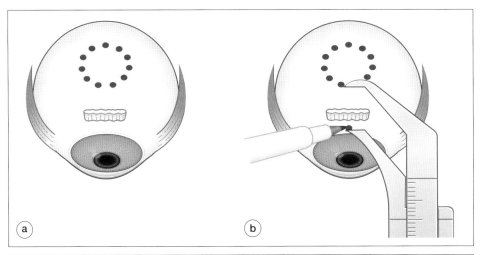

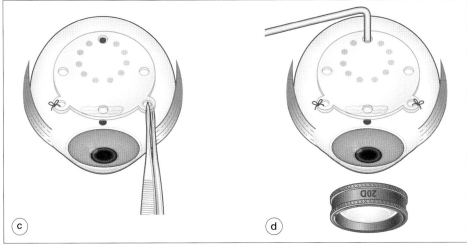

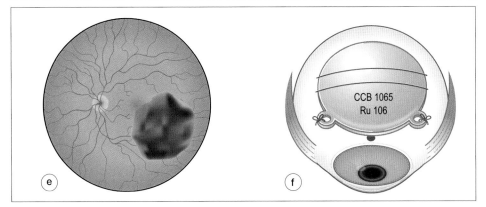

■ **FIGURE 20.3** Technique of plaque insertion. (**a**) Conjunctival peritomy, muscle disinsertion and demarcation of tumor margins on sclera (with transilluminations). (**b**) Marking point for positioning anterior plaque edge. (**c**) Positioning transparent plaque template, indenting sclera with tips of forceps to mark points for scleral suture. (**d**) Performing transscleral transillumination with right-angled fiberoptic light source. (**e**) Ophthalmoscopic view of transillumination at edge of tumor ('sunset sign'). (**f**) Insertion of radioactive plaque, with mattress suture to ensure firm apposition against eye.

margin by about 1 mm if the tumor is further than 4 DD (disc diameters) from the optic disc or fovea. If the tumor extends closer to the optic disc or fovea than 4 DD, the plaque is positioned with its posterior edge aligned with the posterior tumor margin. This is achieved by referring to the preoperative echographic tumor measurements, then subtracting the longitudinal tumor diameter from the plaque diameter and marking the sclera this distance in front of the anterior tumor margin (e.g. if the longitudinal tumor diameter is 9 mm and is treated with a 15-mm plaque, the sclera is marked 6 mm anterior to the anterior tumor edge). The dummy plaque is placed on the sclera and is held by one lug with Moorfields forceps (these forceps have pointed tips so that they create a pair of marker dimples in the sclera). The forceps are held with the tips equidistant from the limbus, so that each scleral suture is placed transversely when it is passed from one dimple to the next. Once the first lug is sutured in place (with a bow), the anterior edge of the plaque is aligned with the ink-mark on the sclera, holding the plaque with the second lug, again using pointed forceps to mark the entry and exit points of the scleral suture.

The position of the plaque is checked by performing binocular indirect ophthalmoscopy with transillumination, passing the tip of the right-angled transilluminator through each of the four perforations in the dummy plaque. If the intention is to align the posterior plaque edge with the posterior tumor margin, then on ophthalmoscopy the posterior tumor margin should be silhouetted against the glow from the transilluminator (i.e. 'sunset sign'). If the plaque is not in the correct position, the scleral sutures are adjusted and the process is repeated.

Once the dummy plaque is positioned correctly, a mattress suture is placed over the plaque, but left untied. The bows at the lugs are released, and the template replaced by the radioactive plaque. Care is taken to hold the plaque only by its lugs and not to touch the undersurface of the plaque, which is very delicate. The lug sutures are tightly fastened. The mattress suture is also tightened as much as possible and tied, ensuring that the plaque is securely fixed and firmly applied against the wall of the eye.

Any disinserted oblique muscle is replaced into its correct anatomic position by suturing it to the mattress suture or to the sclera with a sling. The rectus muscle is also repositioned by suturing it to its stump. If this is not possible, because the plaque lies over the muscle stump, the muscle is attached to the sclera with a sling, ensuring that the knot-to-limbus distance is the same as before (see above). The conjunctiva is closed in the usual fashion.

Dosimetry is calculated by a radiation physicist, using the Astrahan program or other software.[5] The plaque is removed once the desired dose of radiation has been administered, which in our hospital is a minimum of 300 Gy to the sclera and a minimum of 85 Gy to the tumor apex. The reasons for the minimum scleral dose are: (1) to provide an adequate radiation safety margin where the tumor is not overlapped by the plaque; and (2) to produce an area of visible choroidal atrophy, which facilitates postoperative surveillance. Many tumors receive apex radiation doses well in excess of 85 Gy so that the chances of central tumor recurrence are reduced. Such high doses are safe with ruthenium brachytherapy because of the limited range of beta irradiation, especially if the plaque is far from optic disc and fovea (i.e. eccentrically if necessary). When removing the plaque, care is taken to reposition any rectus muscles so that the knot-to-limbus distance is the same as before disinsertion. Any detached oblique muscle is left disinserted as it will be held in place by adhesions.

Some technical variations include: (1) using a different isotope, such as iodine-125, palladium-102, or strontium-90; (2) not using a template, or using one consisting of a metal ring; (3) never decentering the plaque and always administering a safety margin of at least 1 mm; (4) checking plaque position by echography or using a template fitted with transilluminators or using a transilluminator fitted with a diathermy (for scleral marking); and (5) using different dosimetry, administering an apex dose of 85 Gy irrespective of the scleral dose. Notched and crescentic plaques are available for juxtapapillary and ciliary

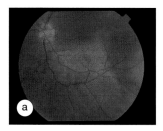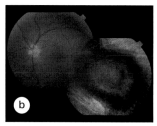

■ FIGURE 20.4 Left fundus of a 54-year-old man treated with ruthenium plaque brachytherapy.
(**a**) Preoperative photograph showing inferotemporal choroidal melanoma, measuring 11.4 × 8.3 ×
2.8 mm. (**b**) Fundus appearance 15 months after treatment, showing choroidal atrophy extending
almost to the posterior tumor margin. The tumor thickness had diminished to 0.9 mm. The visual
acuity 27 months after treatment was 20/30, as at initial presentation.

body tumors, respectively. The author (BD) prefers to treat such tumors with proton beam
radiotherapy.

Outcome

An analysis of 458 patients treated with ruthenium plaque radiotherapy indicates a 97%
actuarial rate of local tumor control at 7 years, the main risk factor for local recurrence being
largest tumor diameter (Fig. 20.4).[6] The actuarial rate of conservation of vision of 20/40 or
better was 55% at 9 years, risk factors for visual loss being posterior tumor extension, temporal location, increased tumor thickness, and older age.[7] Visual loss was also more likely
in diabetic patients and if the tumor had perforated retina. Even when optic disc and fovea
receive negligible doses of radiation visual loss can occur as a result of exudation from the
irradiated tumor and this can be treated by administering transpupillary thermotherapy to
the residual tumor or by intravitreal injection of triamcinolone. The role of bevacizumab
(Avastin) is being investigated.

Good results have been reported following treatment of unresectable iris melanomas
with customized iodine-125 plaques.[8]

Proton beam radiotherapy
Instruments and devices
- Extraocular tray (as for brachytherapy)
- 4 × 2.5 mm tantalum markers
- Thorpe caliper
- Sutures
  - 2 × 6-0 Polysorb
  - 2 × 5-0 Mersilene
  - 1 × 4-0 Ethibond
  - 1 × 7-0 Vicryl

Indications and contraindications

Some authors use proton beam radiotherapy as the only form of conservational therapy
for uveal melanoma. The authors' indications for proton beam radiotherapy include:
(1) choroidal melanomas that cannot easily be treated with plaque because of large size or
proximity to optic disc; and (2) iris melanomas, as a means of avoiding a surgical iris defect
and photophobia.

Surgical technique for insertion of tantalum markers

The tumor margins are identified as for brachytherapy. At least three tantalum markers
are sutured to the sclera adjacent to or near the tumor margins (Fig. 20.5). With anterior

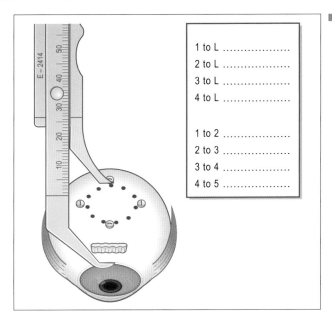

■ **FIGURE 20.5** Insertion of tantalum markers. Drawing showing location of markers and measurements.

1 to L	....
2 to L	....
3 to L	....
4 to L	....
1 to 2	....
2 to 3	....
3 to 4	....
4 to 5	....

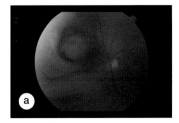
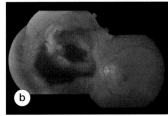

■ **FIGURE 20.6** Left fundus of a 68-year-old woman with superonasal choroidal melanoma in the left eye. (**a**) Pretreatment photograph showing a collar-stud tumor measuring 10.5 × 9.3 mm in its basal dimensions, with a thickness of 5.6 mm. The visual acuity was 20/30. (**b**) Fundus appearance 45 months after treatment. The tumor appeared atrophic and on echography the tumor thickness was 1.6 mm. Despite mild radiation-induced abnormalities around the optic disc, the visual acuity remained 20/30.

tumors, markers are inserted at least 4 mm from limbus and more than 2.5 mm from tumor margin, to avoid extrusion through conjunctiva. Using calipers, measurements are taken of distances between: (1) each marker and tumor margin; (2) all markers; (3) each marker and limbus; and (4) limbus diameter. The conjunctiva is closed in the usual manner.

Further details regarding proton beam radiotherapy are described elsewhere.[9]

Outcome

The author (BD) has reported his experience with 349 choroidal melanomas treated with proton beam radiotherapy when other conservational methods were considered inappropriate (Fig. 20.6).[10] The 5-year actuarial rates were 3.5% for local tumor recurrence, 9.4% for enucleation, 79.1% for conservation of vision of counting fingers or better, 61.1% for conservation of vision of 20/200 or better, and 44.8% for conservation of vision of 20/40 or better. Proton beam radiotherapy caused external eye and eyelid complications that do not occur with brachytherapy and the author's impression is that it caused more exudative complications than ruthenium brachytherapy. With small tumors, exudation was treatable

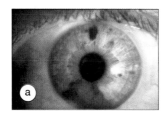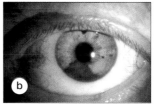

■ FIGURE 20.7 Proton beam radiotherapy of iris melanoma. (**a**) Left anterior segment of a 51-year-old woman with a 4.2 × 3.2 × 2.0 mm tumor involving the inferonasal iris. (**b**) Ocular appearance 57 months after radiotherapy and 8 months after phacoemulsification. Almost 9 years after radiotherapy the visual acuity was 20/20 and the tumor thickness was 0.8 mm.

with transpupillary thermotherapy and intravitreal steroids, but larger tumors required surgical excision, either by endoresection or transsclerally (see below).

Proton beam radiotherapy of iris melanoma tends to cause little morbidity, at least in the first few years after treatment (Fig. 20.7).[11] The main complications are: (1) cataract; (2) glaucoma from drainage obstruction by tumor or melanomacrophages in eyes that previously used to be treated by enucleation; (3) ocular discomfort in some patients, worse in bright light; and (4) local tumor recurrence if the extent of diffuse melanoma is underestimated. Proton beam radiotherapy has made it possible to conserve eyes with extensive iris melanomas, which previously were unsalvageable.

Transscleral local resection
Instruments and devices
- Extraocular tray
- Marker pen
- 90° transilluminator
- Feather blade
- Desmarres scarifier
- Microvitreoretinal (MVR) blade
- O'Malley corneal lens
- Vitrectomy set
- Corneoscleral scissors
- 2 × notched and 2 × toothed Colibri forceps
- Notched microforceps (straight)
- Brunswick syringe
- 20-ml syringe
- Air filter
- Castroviejo needle holder
- Barraquer needle holder
- Sutures
  - 4 × 4-0 silk
  - 2 × 6-0 Polysorb
  - 2 × 4-0 Ethibond
  - 3 × 8-0 Ethilon
- Containers for pathology and cytogenetic specimens

Indications and contraindications
The indications for transscleral local resection are: (1) choroidal melanomas considered too bulky for radiotherapy; (2) small ciliary body tumors, such as melanoma, if histology is required; (3) exudative retinal detachment and/or neovascular glaucoma caused by

residual tumor after radiotherapy;[12] and (4) benign tumors such as leiomyoma and neurilemmoma.

Local resection of uveal melanoma is contraindicated by: (1) basal tumor diameter greater than 16 mm; (2) involvement of more than three clock hours of angle or ciliary body; (3) diffuse tumor margins; and (4) bulky, posterior, extraocular extension.

Surgical technique

The conjunctiva is opened and the tumor localized as for brachytherapy. A lamellar scleral flap is prepared using a Desmarres scarifier (Fig. 20.8). The flap is as thick as possible and is hinged posteriorly for tumors extending posterior to the ora serrata and at the limbus if the tumor is small and anterior. The flap is polyhedral to facilitate wound apposition during closure; with posterior tumors the flap is wider

20.1
20.2

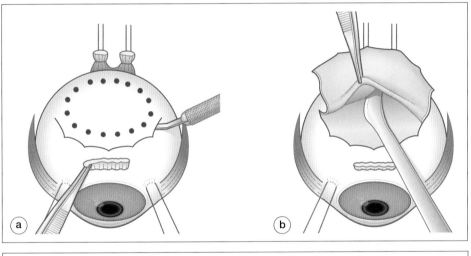

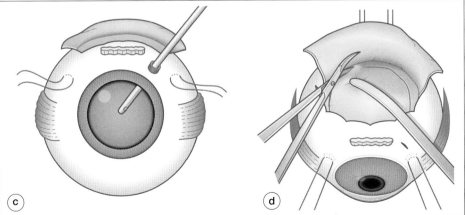

■ **FIGURE 20.8** Choroidectomy technique. (**a**) Making superficial scleral incisions to create a polyhedral scleral flap, wider posteriorly. (**b**) Lamellar scleral dissection, making flap as thick as possible. (**c**) Limited vitrectomy, performed without infusion, using a contact lens and illumination from the operating microscope. (**d**) Deep scleral incisions, creating a stepped wound edge. (**e**) Ripping choroids with notched microforceps. (**f**) Tumor resection, using deep scleral lamella as a handle. (**g**) Suturing scleral flap, avoiding subretinal hematoma by indenting eye and exerting gentle traction on globe. (**h**) Adjunctive brachytherapy with 25 mm ruthenium plaque.

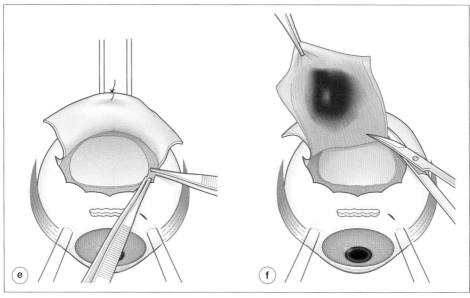

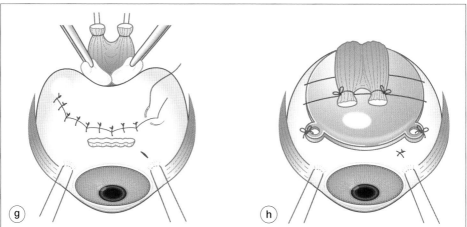

■ **FIGURE 20.8** Cont'd

posteriorly to facilitate access to the tumor. Before being divided, any vortex veins in the region of the flap are cauterized, both behind the globe and within the sclera. The globe is decompressed by limited pars plana vitrectomy, using a corneal contact lens and light from the operating microscope to visualize the posterior segment, and ocular indentation instead of infusion.

Deep scleral incisions are made by pinching the sclera with forceps and shaving the sclera with a blade. The deep sclera is divided with scissors around the tumor, first laterally, then posteriorly, and finally anteriorly. The deep scleral opening is smaller than the external scleral opening so as to create a 1–2 mm step in the scleral wound edge to facilitate closure.

Hemorrhage is minimized by lowering the systolic blood pressure to approximately 45 mmHg, with cerebral monitoring.[13]

If the tumor involves choroid, the uvea is opened posterior to the ora serrata. This is done by gently grasping the choroid with two pairs of notched microforceps and pulling them apart to rip the uveal tissue until a small opening is created. The uveal dissection is then continued with blunt-tipped spring scissors. The uvea is first divided along the anterior tumor margin. If such surgery extends anterior to the ora serrata the ciliary epithelium is first separated from the uvea by blunt dissection, using the flat surface of the scissors. Using the anterior edge of the deep scleral lamella as a handle, the tumor is gently lifted out of the eye while dissecting the uvea first along each lateral tumor margin and finally posteriorly. If the tumor is adherent to retina, the two tissues are separated by blunt dissection, if possible. If the tumor has actually invaded retina, then if it has previously been irradiated it is top-sliced with a Bard Parker scalpel and its apex left in situ. With non-irradiated tumors, such a procedure is associated with an increased risk of tumor dissemination in the eye so that it may be preferable to excise the infiltrated retina along with the tumor and perform appropriate vitreoretinal surgery at the end of the local resection.

With ciliary body tumors, the general principles are the same, except that it is not usually possible to conserve ciliary epithelium. Vitreous prolapse through the scleral window may require limited vitrectomy, preferably through a separate sclerotomy so as to conserve an intact vitreous face.

Once the tumor excision is complete, the scleral flap is sutured with interrupted 8-0 nylon sutures. Near the limbus it may be preferable to use absorbable sutures, unless adjunctive radiotherapy is planned. To prevent subretinal hematoma developing during scleral closure, it is important to indent the eye immediately posterior to the flap until the retina is bulging slightly through the scleral window. As soon as suturing of the scleral flap is complete, the eye is reformed with balanced salt solution, injected into the eye with a syringe.

Any retinal tear requires immediate vitreoretinal surgery, which consists of total vitrectomy, removal of subretinal blood, flattening of the retina with heavy liquid, retinopexy, and tamponade with silicone or heavy silicone, which is removed after about 12 weeks.

If adjunctive brachytherapy is administered, the plaque is inserted at the end of the local resection. The author's preferred method is to use a 25-mm ruthenium applicator. Such adjunctive brachytherapy is delayed by a month if cyclectomy is performed to prevent cyclodialysis and ocular hypotony. If tumor excision is apparently complete, there may be scope for waiting until histological and cytogenetic results are available before deciding whether this treatment is necessary.

The eye is closed as for brachytherapy. For the first postoperative day, the patient is postured so that any hemorrhage from the uveal coloboma margins gravitates away from the fovea.

Outcome

Between 1984 and 2004 the author performed 344 transscleral resections for uveal melanomas involving choroid and the results for patients resident in Britain have recently been reported (Fig. 20.9).[14] The 8-year actuarial rates of ocular conservation ranged from 81% to 57% depending on the number of risk factors present, which were: basal tumor diameter exceeding 15 mm; tumor height more than 8 mm; and tumor extension to within 3 mm of optic disc or fovea. In the absence of risk factors, 43% of eyes with vision of 20/40 or better retained such good vision. Retinal detachment tended to occur in the immediate postoperative period and was more common with thick tumors (i.e. more than 8 mm).[15] Local tumor recurrence rates were higher if the tumor diameter exceeded 15 mm, if the posterior margin extended close to optic disc or fovea, or if the tumor contained epithelioid cells.[16] Adjunctive brachytherapy was introduced relatively late so that further follow-up is needed.

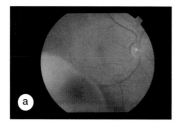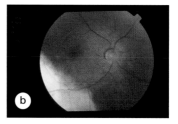

FIGURE 20.9 Right fundus of a 67-year-old man. (**a**) Preoperative photograph showing an inferotemporal choroidal melanoma, measuring 15.6 × 11.6 × 7.6 mm. The visual acuity was 6/5 with the affected eye but only 6/60 with the left eye. Postoperatively, the patient developed a subfoveal hematoma, which was removed without delay. (**b**) Fundus appearance 9 months postoperatively, when the visual acuity was 20/30.

Transretinal endoresection
Instruments and devices
- Vitrectomy set
- Containers for pathology and cytogenetic specimens

Indications and contraindications
Primary endoresection of melanoma is highly controversial because of concerns about tumor seeding to other parts of the eye and systematically. Such fears are based on intuitive assumptions about metastatic disease (Damato, B, BJO. In press). This operation is therefore indicated only in exceptional cases, if it offers the only hope for conserving useful vision, and if the patient accepts the unorthodox nature of the surgery. Secondary endoresection is useful as a treatment for exudation from bulky, posterior residual tumor after previous radiotherapy (i.e. 'toxic tumor syndrome').

Surgical technique
Total pars plana vitrectomy is performed (Fig. 20.10). The systemic blood pressure is lowered and the ocular infusion pressure increased, so as to reduce hemorrhage. The vitreous cutter is passed through the retina into the apex of the tumor, which is removed piecemeal. First, a crater in the tumor is formed into which any hemorrhage pools. Next, the walls of the crater and the tumor margins are removed, taking care not to damage the adjacent retina, which is held away from the vitreous cutter with a second instrument. Endodiathermy is applied to the scleral bed and the margins of the surgical coloboma to destroy any residual tumor and reduce postoperative hemorrhage. Fluid–air exchange is performed to flatten the retina so that two rows of laser burns can be placed all around the margins of the uveal coloboma to achieve retinopexy. The eye is filled with silicone, which is removed after about 12 weeks. Postoperatively, the patient is postured to enhance tamponade and to encourage any hemorrhage to gravitate away from the fovea.

Outcome
The author (BD) has reported results obtained with his first 52 endoresections, of which 11 were secondary (Fig. 20.11).[17] The main complication was rhegmatogenous retinal detachment, which has become less common with improved methods for detecting and treating entry-site retinal tears. Tumor dissemination around the eye was rare and occurred only in a patient who was lost to follow-up and whose marginal tumor recurrence was not immediately detected and treated.[18] Extraocular recurrence was also rare, and occurred in a patient whose intrascleral tumor was inadequately treated.[19]

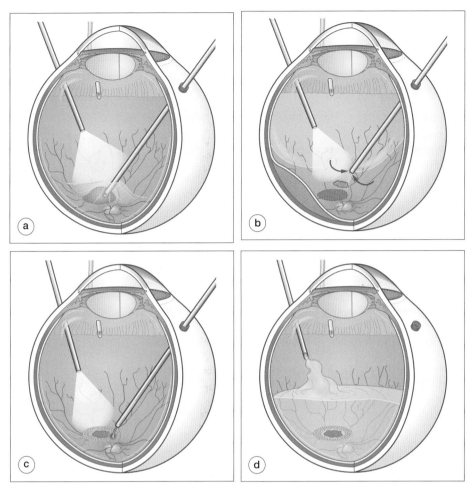

■ **FIGURE 20.10** Endoresection technique. (**a**) Tumor excision, through retinotomy. (**b**) Fluid–air exchange, to flatten retina. (**c**) Endolaser photocoagulation/retinopexy. (**d**) Air–silicone exchange.

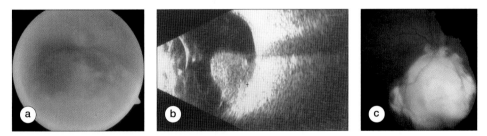

■ **FIGURE 20.11** Right fundus of a 65-year-old man treated by endoresection. (**a**) Preoperative photograph, showing an inferonasal, collar-stud melanoma. (**b**) Ultrasound scan showed the tumor to measure 10.4 × 9.6 × 9.6 mm and to extend close to optic disc. (**c**) Fundus appearance 45 months after treatment, when the visual acuity with pseudophakic correction was 20/40.

POSTOPERATIVE MANAGEMENT

Long-term ocular surveillance is required after conservational treatment of uveal melanoma, because local tumor recurrence can occur many years after treatment. As there is no consensus as to whether systemic screening for metastasis is valuable, it should be recommended to all patients or only those with a poor prognosis (i.e. tumors with monosomy 3), the latter being our practice. The first author (BD) and associates have developed a neural network for producing personalized survival curves for individual patients.[20] Radiation-induced complications tend to increase with time and their treatment forms an important part of patient management.

CONCLUSIONS

The surgical treatment of intraocular tumors is evolving rapidly, mostly because of impressive technological advances that are taking place. With uveal melanomas, progress is also being driven by changing attitudes regarding the impact (or, more precisely, the apparent lack of impact) of treatment on survival.[21] There is a growing suspicion, for example, that medium-sized and large melanomas with any metastatic potential have already disseminated to other parts of the body by the time the patient initially presents, in which case any ocular treatment is perhaps only palliative. It is not known whether, after metastatic spread has commenced, life is prolonged by treating the ocular tumor, thereby reducing metastatic burden.

Increasingly, patients with ocular tumors are being treated by ophthalmologists with special expertise in ocular oncology, who have a range of therapeutic modalities at their disposal, and who are supported by a multidisciplinary team so as to maximize all opportunities for enhancing patient well-being.

REFERENCES

1. Singh AD, Damato BE, Pe'er J, Murphree AL, Perry JD. Clinical ophthalmic oncology. Edinburgh: Saunders, 2006.
2. Damato B, Duke C, Coupland CE, et al. Cytogenetics of uveal melanoma: a 7-year clinical experience. Ophthalmology 2007; 114:1925–1931.
3. Sen J, Groenewald C, Hiscott PS, Smith PA, Damato BE. Transretinal choroidal tumor biopsy with a 25-gauge vitrector. Ophthalmology 2006; 113:1028–1031.
4. Finger PT, Latkany P, Kurli M, Iacob C. The Finger iridectomy technique: small incision biopsy of anterior segment tumours. Br J Ophthalmol 2005; 89:946–949.
5. Astrahan MA. Improved treatment planning for COMS eye plaques. Int J Radiat Oncol Biol Phys 2005; 61:1227–1242.
6. Damato B, Patel I, Campbell IR, Mayles HM, Errington RD. Local tumor control after (106)Ru brachytherapy of choroidal melanoma. Int J Radiat Oncol Biol Phys 2005; 63:385–391.
7. Damato B, Patel I, Campbell IR, Mayles HM, Errington RD. Visual acuity after Ruthenium(106) brachytherapy of choroidal melanomas. Int J Radiat Oncol Biol Phys 2005; 63:392–400.
8. Shields CL, Naseripour M, Shields JA, Freire J, Cater J. Custom-designed plaque radiotherapy for nonresectable iris melanoma in 38 patients: tumor control and ocular complications. Am J Ophthalmol 2003; 135:648–656.
9. Gragoudas ES, Marie LA. Uveal melanoma: proton beam irradiation. Ophthalmol Clin North Am 2005; 18:111–118, ix.
10. Damato B, Kacperek A, Chopra M, Campbell IR, Errington RD. Proton beam radiotherapy of choroidal melanoma: the Liverpool–Clatterbridge experience. Int J Radiat Oncol Biol Phys 2005; 62:1405–1411.
11. Damato B, Kacperek A, Chopra M, Sheen MA, Campbell IR, Errington RD. Proton beam radiotherapy of iris melanoma. Int J Radiat Oncol Biol Phys 2005; 63:109–115.

12. Damato BE, Foulds WS. In: Ryan SJ et al., eds. Retina, 4th edn. Philadelphia: Mosby; 2006:769–778.

13. Damato B, Jones AG. Uveal melanoma: resection techniques. Ophthalmol Clin North Am 2005; 18:119–128, ix.

14. Damato B. The role of eyewall resection in uveal melanoma management. Int Ophthalmol Clin 2006; 46:81–93.

15. Damato B, Groenewald CP, McGalliard JN, Wong D. Rhegmatogenous retinal detachment after transscleral local resection of choroidal melanoma. Ophthalmology 2002; 109:2137–2143.

16. Damato BE, Paul J, Foulds WS. Risk factors for residual and recurrent uveal melanoma after trans-scleral local resection. Br J Ophthalmol 1996; 80:102–108.

17. Damato B, Groenewald C, McGalliard J, Wong D. Endoresection of choroidal melanoma. Br J Ophthalmol 1998; 82:213–218.

18. Hadden PW, Hiscott PS, Damato BE. Histopathology of eyes enucleated after endoresection of choroidal melanoma. Ophthalmology 2004; 111:154–160.

19. Damato B, Wong D, Green FD, Mackenzie JM. Intrascleral recurrence of uveal melanoma after transretinal 'endoresection'. Br J Ophthalmol 2001; 85:114–115.

20. Damato B, Eleuteri A, Fisher AC, Coupland SE, Taktak AF. Artificial neural networks estimating survival probability after treatment of choroidal melanoma. Ophthalmology. 2008. In press.

21. Damato B. Treatment of primary intraocular melanoma. Expert Rev Anticancer Ther 2006; 6:493–506.

THE LIBRARY
THE LEARNING AND DEVELOPMENT CENTRE
THE CALDERDALE ROYAL HOSPITAL
HALIFAX HX3 0PW

21 Vitrectomy technology and techniques

Steve Charles

Techniques and technology have evolved hand-in-hand since the inception of vitreous surgery over three decades ago.[1-4] A better understanding of the physics and engineering principles underlying vitreous surgery should result in convergence on best practice techniques and technology because all surgeons work with the same set of diseases, pathoanatomy, and engineering/physics principles. Physicians and surgeons worldwide recognize that there are far more similarities than differences in the diseases and biologic principles involved in the patients they treat. Wide variation in surgical practice for a given surgical scenario is an indication of incomplete understanding of the principles involved and/or inadequate dissemination of information.

WOUND CONSTRUCTION AND SUTURELESS SURGERY

Rapid transition from large incision, full-function probes to three-port, 20-gauge surgery[5] took place three decades ago. We are now almost 5 years into a transition to transconjunctival, sutureless 23- and 25-gauge surgery.

Three-port surgery is far superior to full-function single incision techniques because the wounds are much smaller and the infusion is separate from cutting/aspiration and other functions, increasing surgical flexibility and reducing turbulence. Unlike phacoemulsification, continuous infusion is essential to vitrectomy and is made possible by a separate infusion port.

Sutureless surgery was made possible because of 23- and 25-gauge tools which require sclerotomies that are significantly smaller than the 20-gauge tools, as well as new wound construction techniques. Conjunctival displacement prior to insertion of the trocar/cannula allows the conjunctiva to be repositioned at the end of the procedure so that it covers the sclerotomies. Although straight-in 25-gauge incisions rarely leak, especially if fluid–air exchange is used at the end of the case, the author now recommends making a scleral tunnel for 25-gauge sutureless surgery to reduce even further the risk of wound leaks. This method of wound construction has also been referred to as angulated or oblique wound construction and is obligatory for the significantly larger 23-gauge wounds. The 23- and 25-gauge wounds are made by starting with the trocar tangential to the sclera, limbus parallel, and inserting the trocar until the cannula is in contact with the sclera and then changing the angle and inserting straight in. The cannulas should be removed in a tangential manner similar to the initial phase of insertion while applying light pressure over the scleral tunnel similar to the way pressure is applied as a needle is withdrawn from a vein.

Patients have much less discomfort and faster visual recovery with 25-gauge surgery than with 20-gauge, and the conjunctiva and episcleral tissues are not damaged which is an advantage in the context of glaucoma filtering procedures. While 23-gauge surgery is superior to 20-gauge surgery with respect to patient comfort, there is greater conjunctival damage than with 25-gauge because the wounds are larger and conjunctival damage occurs with various devices used to stabilize the eye to counteract greater translational and torsional forces during trocar/cannula insertion. Although some surgeons believe that vitreous should be left in the sutureless 23- and 25-gauge wounds to reduce wound leaks, the author believes that this results in more wound-related retinal breaks and can result in vitreous wicks. Some surgeons believe that 23- and 25-gauge wounds have a greater risk of post-operative endophthalmitis; however, it is the author's contention that vitreous wicks and the unwise elimination of the use of subconjunctival antibiotics are responsible for the apparent increased risk.

FLUIDICS AND CUTTING

21.1
21.2
21.3

Fluidics cannot be discussed without an understanding of the effect of the cutting rate on fluidic resistance at the port. There has been an evolution of cutter actuation over the past three decades which has resulted in a significant increase in cutting rates. Although it has been stated that 'fast cutting' results in 'better cutting', there is no evidence that collagen fibers are cut 'better' with higher cutting rates. Faster cutting rate (cuts per minute, cpm) does not mean higher cutter velocity (mm per sec); cutter velocity is determined in pneumatic systems mostly by actuation pressure (pounds per square inch, psi), spring rate (with current axial cutters), and friction between the inner and outer needle. The InnoVit utilizes dual actuation of a transverse piston without spring return rather than single actuation of a diaphragm with spring return as used in pneumatic axial cutters. Cutter velocity is determined with current electric cutters by the rotational velocity of the electric motor. Moreover, there is minimal, if any, evidence that achievable higher cutter velocities result in inertial cutting. The best examples of inertial cutting are weed eaters and phacoemulsification. Vitreous collagen fibers and epiretinal membranes are primarily severed by shearing, one square edge moving past another square edge. Scissors and vitreous cutters use shear while knives use sharpness to create high force (stress) per unit area.

It has also been stated that fast cutting results in greater cutting efficiency; efficiency is defined as vitreous volume removed per unit volume of infusion fluid. Fast cutting (high cutting rate) does not affect the amount of vitreous removed per unit volume of infusion fluid; efficiency is technique driven. It is essential to always keep the cutter port engaged in vitreous and always advance while suction is applied—never pull back. This approach minimizes vitreoretinal traction as well as improving efficiency. Previous generations of vitreous cutters and aspiration systems required 'standoff' vitrectomy technique—keep the probe away from the vitreous and use high vacuum to pull vitreous into the port. This is a dangerous and unnecessary technique and should be avoided.

There two advantages of high cutting rates: (1) port-based flow limiting; and (2) minimizing vitreoretinal traction due to travel of uncut vitreous collagen fibers through the port. Port-based flow limiting, a term coined by the author, increases fluidic stability and reduces fluid surge after sudden elastic deformation of epiretinal membrane (or similar dense material) through the port. The metric for fluidic stability is 'pulse flow', a term also coined by the author, which is defined as the fluid volume passing through the port during an open–close cycle. Port-based flow limiting decreases pulse flow, thereby decreasing movement of detached retina and pulsatile vitreoretinal traction on attached retina, and reducing the frequency of iatrogenic retinal breaks. Port-based flow limiting is produced by higher cutting rates, smaller lumens, and lower duty cycle. High cutting rates result in higher fluidic resistance at the port because the inner needle obstructs flow through the port each time it closes. Duty cycle is defined as the percentage of port-open to port-closed time. When the cutter rapidly closes and rapidly reopens there is less fluidic resistance than when the port dwells in the closed position. Although some have stated that a 50% duty cycle is ideal, this is not the case in a clinical setting because of the wide variety of material properties encountered: air, perfluorooctane (PFO), balanced salt solution (BSS), vitreous, dense hemorrhage, dense epiretinal membrane, silicone oil, and sclerotic lens nucleus (in order of increasing resistance to mechanical deformation and fluid flow). For this reason pneumatic cutters with an inherent variable duty cycle are preferred over electric cutters with a fixed 50% duty cycle. Fluidic resistance is proportional to the fourth power of the lumen diameter; 25-gauge cutters have higher port-based flow limiting than 23-gauge cutters and much more than 20-gauge at the same cutting rates. 25-Gauge cutters at 1500 cpm produce the same pulse flow as 23-gauge cutters at 2500 cpm, and both produce less pulsatile vitreoretinal traction and less fluid surge after sudden elastic deformation of dense tissue through the port than 20-gauge cutters at the same cutting rate.

Pneumatic cutters are much lighter and more compact than electric cutters because pneumatic actuation has an approximate 10 times advantage in force : mass and force : volume ratios. Lighter tools produce less fatigue, less tremor, and enhance dexterity (Weber–Fechner law).

Best practice is to always use the highest cutting rate for all tasks, increase proportional suction until sufficient tissue removal occurs, and finally decrease cutting rate only if the highest vacuum level does not produce adequate tissue removal. Continuous engage and advance technique is essential to safe, rapid, and sufficient vitreous removal.

INFUSION

Fluidic resistance is an advantage in cutter systems as discussed above but a significant disadvantage in infusion systems. Resistance to flow through the infusion cannula, stopcocks, and 84 inches of tubing results in a significant pressure drop between infusion pressure and intraocular pressure (IOP) during moderate to high flow rates. Air pressure or gravity is used in current systems to produce infusion pressure. Vented gas forced infusion systems (Alcon VGFI) produce a direct digital readout of infusion pressure (not IOP) and respond more rapidly to foot pedal commands to raise the pressure to stop or prevent bleeding than gravity-based systems. The infusion pressure must be raised when using higher resistance 25-gauge infusion ports and high vacuum levels, especially when using low resistance 20-gauge fragmenters or non-tapered extrusion cannulas. Unlike vitreous cutters, fragmenters and extrusion cannulas do not have coaxial needles or intermittent cutter closing of the port to interrupt flow.

Infusion pressure should be maintained at 35–45 mmHg with 20- to 23-gauge surgery and 45–60 mmHg with 25-gauge systems during flow scenarios. Low IOP results in miosis, bleeding, corneal striae, corneal deformation by the contact lens, and, ultimately, ocular collapse. Sustained high IOP results in retinal ischemia, especially with low systemic blood pressure seen with excessively deep levels of general anesthesia. High IOP can also cause corneal edema. 'Normal' IOP in the context of glaucoma is irrelevant during surgery.

SURFACE TENSION MANAGEMENT, EXCHANGES, AND DRAINAGE OF SUBRETINAL FLUID

Three-port vitrectomy systems are ideal for internal drainage of subretinal fluid (SRF) as well as exchanges of one intraocular fluid for another because the infusion port is physically separated from the egress port.[6–9]

Internal drainage of SRF can be performed using the vitreous cutter or preferably a variety of extrusion cannulas: rigid or soft tip, tapered or straight, straight or angulated, and blunt or sharp. Exchange nomenclature is often misstated; injecting air through the infusion port while removing fluid from the vitreous cavity is 'fluid–air' exchange, *not* gas–fluid exchange or air–fluid exchange (Fig. 21.1). Fluid–air exchange should only be started after internal drainage of SRF has been continued until the retina is no longer becoming more concave. This is because the interfacial tension of the air–retinal interface will 'seal' all retinal breaks as well as the gap between the internal drainage cannula outside diameter and the irregular retinal break or drainage retinotomy, preventing recirculation of infusion fluid through the breaks and subretinal space. An additional advantage of drain-before-exchange is that it stops peripheral SRF being shifted posteriorly, preventing it from being drained through peripheral retinal breaks. Internal drainage of SRF should

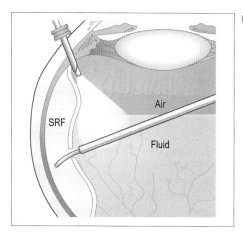

■ **FIGURE 21.1** Internal drainage of subretinal fluid and fluid–air exchange. (Adapted from Charles et al.[4] with permission from Lippincott, Williams & Wilkins.)

be continued while fluid–air exchange (FAX) is performed; often the extrusion cannula must be moved alternately between the subretinal and the preretinal space during this process. The view is often impaired as the air bubbles coalesce, necessitating a steady hand position so that the extrusion cannula remains immobile.

Drainage retinotomy can be very useful with very small peripheral breaks which are typical with post-cataract surgery retinal detachments. The 25-gauge cutter is ideal for drainage retinotomy because it produces a small hole matched to the 25-gauge extrusion cannula (soft tip or straight). Some surgeons mark the drainage retinotomy with endodia-thermy to facilitate locating it for laser retinopexy after internal drainage of SRF and FAX attach the retina. While there is no downside to endodiathermy marking, the author seldom finds it necessary to perform this additional step.

Air–gas exchange is performed as the last step before wound closure or cannula removal by connecting a syringe filled with an isoexpansive mixture of sulfur hexafluoride (SF_6) or perfluoropropane (C_3F_8) to the infusion port via the supplied three-way stopcock (Fig. 21.2). At least 30 cc of gas mixture must be injected to ensure complete exchange. Air is simul-taneously removed using an extrusion cannula with the tip positioned near the optic nerve. Injecting arbitrary amounts of gas into the unknown volume of an air-filled vitreous cavity is unwise and may produce very high postoperative IOP and ischemic damage, or a small, ineffective gas bubble.

Liquid perfluorocarbons such as perfluorooctane (PFO, Alcon Perfluoron) are absolutely necessary to repair giant retinal breaks but can be advantageous for removing SRF in rhegmatogenous retinal detachment surgery as well as stabilizing the retina during epireti-nal membrane dissection. As PFO is immiscible in water and has approximately twice the specific gravity of infusion fluid, it sinks in BSS, floating SRF anteriorly out through retinal breaks into the anterior vitreous cavity. PFO should be injected using a cannula connected via a short segment of tubing to a syringe operated by the assistant. The syringe is half filled with BSS to eliminate dead space and held with the BSS up until the needle is in the eye, and then inverted to inject when the cannula is over the optic nerve. Substantial amounts of SRF can be displaced anterior to retinal breaks, preventing retinopexy of the anterior breaks. The author recommends extending the most anterior retinal break to the ora serrata to allow egress of all SRF or making a small drainage retinotomy at the ora. FAX usually causes immediate fogging of the posterior surface of an intraocular lens if the posterior capsule is not intact. Although this problem is worse with silicone and poly-methyl methacrylate (PMMA) intraocular lenses (IOLs) than with acrylic IOLs because of their greater thermal mass, in reality it is the higher posterior capsular opacification (PCO)

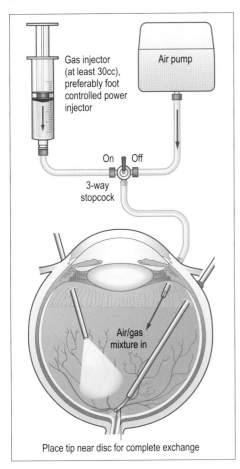

Place tip near disc for complete exchange

■ **FIGURE 21.2** Air–gas exchange. (Adapted from Charles et al.[4] with permission from Lippincott, Williams & Wilkins.)

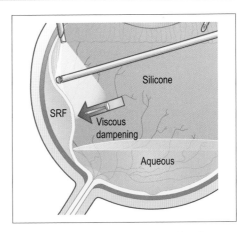

■ **FIGURE 21.3** Interface vitrectomy for silicone reoperation demonstrating viscous dampening.

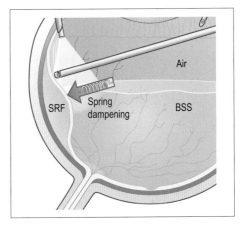

■ **FIGURE 21.4** Interface vitrectomy under PFO illustrating inertial dampening and gravitational force.

rates, and therefore excessive yttrium aluminum garnet (YAG) capsulotomy rates associated with silicone and PMMA lenses, that is the primary issue.

Interface vitrectomy is a term coined by the author to denote operating 'under' air, PFO, or silicone oil (Fig. 21.3). All three substances are immiscible in water—and therefore in the retina and SRF—and thus provide an interfacial tension 'barrier'. All three stabilize the retina against movement caused by the vitreous cutter or epiretinal membrane removal, as well as preventing increasing volume of SRF during the procedure. They differ in many ways: air and oil are less dense than retina and SRF, and therefore float anteriorly, displacing retina and SRF posteriorly. In contrast, PFO has greater density than the retina or SRF and sinks, displacing retina and SRF anteriorly. Air produces spring dampening of retinal motion (Fig. 21.4), silicone oil produces viscous dampening, and PFO produces inertial dampening as well as greater gravitational downforce because its mass is approximately twice as great as BSS (Fig. 21.5). It is crucial to keep the cutter port outside the interfacial tension agent and embedded in fluid or retina while removing residual vitreoretinal

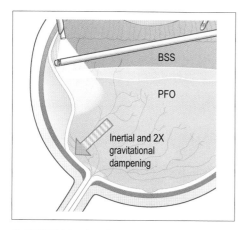

FIGURE 21.5 Interface vitrectomy under PFO illustrating inertial dampening and gravitational force.

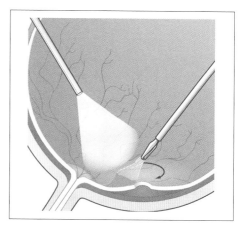

FIGURE 21.6 Internal limiting membrane peeling with conformal forceps. (Adapted from Charles et al.[4] with permission from Lippincott, Williams & Wilkins.)

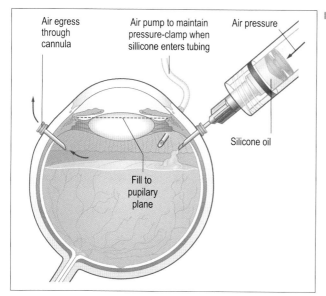

FIGURE 21.7 A 25-gauge air–silicone exchange with MedOne 25-gauge cannula. (Adapted from Charles et al.[4] with permission from Lippincott, Williams & Wilkins.)

traction, performing retinectomy possibly with simultaneous epiretinal membrane removal, or removing subretinal fluid, blood, or silicone oil. It is not necessary to remove silicone oil when reoperating for proliferative vitreoretinopathy (PVR) or epimacular membranes. Vitreous removal, retinectomy, forceps membrane peeling (Fig. 21.6), scissors segmentation and delamination, endodiathermy, drainage of SRF, and laser retinopexy can all be performed efficiently 'under' oil as well as PFO and air.

Air–silicone exchange is usually performed by continuing air infusion after FAX and internal drainage of SRF have been used to reattach the retina and perform laser retinopexy (Fig. 21.7). One 23- or 25-gauge cannula is left open to the atmosphere while infusing oil through the other cannula using a power injector such as the Alcon Accurus VFC (viscous fluid control) and cannula that fits in the 25-gauge cannula. Typically the patient's head is rotated somewhat away from the operative eye, placing the temporal cannula higher than the nasal cannula to facilitate air egress. The infusion line air pressure should be clamped with a hemostat when the fill is almost complete and the oil infusion terminated when all the air comes out the open cannula followed by oil. Care should be taken not to overpressurize the eye because oil is incompressible and more difficult to remove than gas.

MANAGEMENT OF EPIRETINAL MEMBRANES

A variety of methods have been developed to manage epiretinal membranes.[10] The strength of adherence determines whether membrane peeling or scissors methods are utilized. Peeling is used for low adherence epiretinal membranes (ERM)—typically epimacular membranes, internal limiting membrane (ILM), and the majority of PVR membranes. Scissors methods are required for diabetic traction retinal detachments and scar tissue secondary to trauma (Fig. 21.8).

Older outside-in membrane dissection techniques initially utilized bent needles, then bent MVR blades, and more recently picks or diamond-dusted membrane scrapers. These methods are dependent on finding an 'edge' and have not been used by the author for two decades. Membranes are thinner away from the epicenter, making edge finding problematic, potentially resulting in retinal breaks and bleeding. The author developed inside-out, forceps membrane peeling to address the retinal damage that often results from attempting to find an edge. Inserting any tool under the membrane is more likely to damage the retinal surface than grasping on the anterior surface of the membrane. Forceps membrane peeling was initially termed 'pinch peeling' to make the point that the membrane is grasped at the apparent epicenter using end-opening forceps rather than by passing one forceps blade under the membrane. The author developed diamond-coated forceps to prevent slippage of the ERM and conformal forceps so that the radius of curvature of the forceps tip conformed to the curvature of the retinal surface.

So-called 'bimanual' surgery is better termed 'forceps stabilization of epiretinal membrane'. Although many surgeons lift the membrane to visualize areas of adherence before severing them, this may result in tearing the retina which has approximately one-hundredth the tensile strength of the membrane. In general, 'bimanual' methods are used to offset dissection forces; however, the lower cutting forces associated with using disposable scissors such as the Alcon DSPs usually obviate the need for bimanual surgery.

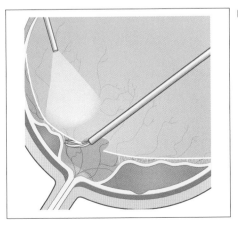

■ **FIGURE 21.8** Inside-out conformal delamination of diabetic traction retinal detachment prior to truncating posterior vitreous detachment (en bloc). (Adapted from Charles et al.[4] with permission from Lippincott, Williams & Wilkins.)

The author developed scissors segmentation three decades ago to eliminate tangential traction. Segmentation is used when the epiretinal membranes are too adherent for membrane peeling, typically for diabetic traction retinal detachments or late trauma. Segmentation means that the membrane is transected with one scissors blade under the ERM and the other blade on the anterior surface. The author developed scissors delamination a few years later which enabled complete removal of the ERM by placing both scissors blades under the ERM. The author prefers delamination because it results in lower glial recurrence rates and primarily uses segmentation as access segmentation to initiate the delamination process. Inside-out access segmentation and delamination are preferred to outside-in methods because the retina is stronger centrally, the 'edge' is often difficult to locate as described above for forceps techniques, and visualization is better centrally. An access segmentation cut is often made near the optic nerve to enable insertion of the second blade under the ERM to start inside-out delamination. Curved scissors are better than 'vertical scissors' for segmentation because the thickness of the blade is much less than the width of the blades which means that less space under the ERM is required for blade insertion so less force is applied to the retina at the ERM attachment points. Curved scissors are also better for delamination than so-called horizontal scissors (actually 135°) because the radius of curvature corresponds to the curvature of the eyeball, enabling conformal delamination, thereby reducing retinal penetration with the scissors tips (Fig. 21.9).

Conformal cutter delamination is dependent on port-based flow limiting and is best performed with the highest possible cutting rate and the compact tip of 25-gauge cutters (Fig. 21.10). The angle of attack is controlled by rotating the cutter port slightly away from the retina and feeding the ERM into the port as it is removed rather than pushing or aspirating the ERM into the port. The port can be placed over the membrane behind the cut margin to accomplish foldback delamination while protecting the retina from iatrogenic retinal breaks.

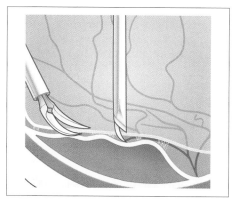

■ **FIGURE 21.9** Curved scissors are preferred for segmentation as well as delamination because the curve matches retinal curvature and blade thickness is less than blade width requiring less space under ERM. (Adapted from Charles et al.[4] with permission from Lippincott, Williams & Wilkins.)

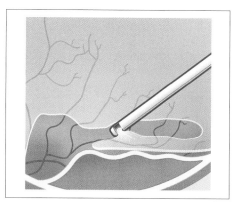

■ **FIGURE 21.10** Conformal cutter delamination of ERM. Angle of attack is continuously adjusted to reduce entry of retina into port and to feed ERM into port with minimal suction. (Adapted from Charles et al.[4] with permission from Lippincott, Williams & Wilkins.)

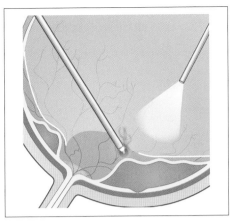

FIGURE 21.11 Laser coagulation of vascular attachment points severed during inside-out delamination of diabetic traction retinal detachment. (Adapted from Charles et al.[4] with permission from Lippincott, Williams & Wilkins.)

LASER COAGULATION AND RETINOPEXY

Endophotocoagulation was developed by the author[11] to replace cryopexy and perform focal and panretinal photocoagulation. Endophotocoagulation is preferred to use of the laser indirect ophthalmoscope during vitreoretinal surgery because it does not cause light scattering, cornea, lens or iris damage, or delay surgery. The Chang end-aspirating endolaser probe is ideal for 20-gauge surgery but is not available in 23- or 25-gauge. This tool enables removal of SRF or preretinal blood while performing retinopexy, laser coagulation of vascular attachment points, or panretinal photocoagulation (Fig. 21.11). The author developed the concept of using the laser for coagulation rather than endodiathermy because it is a non-contact method and not dependent on tool exchange.[12] Cryopexy is rarely used during vitrectomy because it damages the conjunctiva or requires a conjunctival incision, and, in contrast to laser retinopexy, it disperses viable retinal pigment epithelium (RPE) cells capable of causing PVR.

ENDODIATHERMY

Bipolar endodiathermy probes are available for 20-, 23-, and 25-gauge systems and can be used to coagulate elevated neovascularization, precoagulate vessels within diabetic ERM before segmentation, coagulate retinal vessels before retinectomy, or assist in making and marking drainage retinotomies. Elevated disc neovascularization must be treated very carefully with low energy and with a minimum of 0.75 mm offset from the surface of the optic nerve to prevent damage to the nerve fibers and vascular supply.

ILLUMINATION AND VISUALIZATION

Unlike transcorneal illumination, endoillumination eliminates light reflections and scattering from the contact lens, cornea, lens or intraocular lens which markedly improves visualization. Focal illumination with a moderate divergence light beam improves visualization of vitreous, relatively transparent ERMs, and ILM compared to diffuse illumination from a chandelier or Torpedo. All vitreoretinal surgeons instinctively and unconsciously use retroillumination to visualize transparent vitreous. The light can be reflected by the retina/RPE/choroid/sclera similar to the 'red reflex' essential for cataract surgery and lensectomy or, better yet, the vitreous probe, scissors, or forceps. Specular illumination is more difficult to explain but can be thought of as focal illumination of a nearly transparent object causing it to 'glow' when the light is directed at a critical angle. Clear vitreous is virtually impossible to see with diffuse illumination produced by chandeliers, dual-mode infusion cannulas, and Tornambe Torpedos.

Wide-angle illumination is ideal for viewing the periphery without bumping the lens or IOL. Since the endoilluminator is often used in the less dexterous hand, wide-angle illumination reduces the precision positioning requirement. Wide-angle illumination is essential for retinal detachment repair and is usually used with wide-angle visualization, scleral depression, or prism contact lenses to see the periphery. Wide-angle visualization enables visualization of retinal breaks, peripheral vitreoretinal traction, and other peripheral pathology. Contact-based wide-angle systems such as the Volk and AVI have a 10° greater field of view than non-contact systems such as the binocular indirect ophthalmomicroscope (BIOM) and eliminate corneal asphericity. Instrument flexion is an issue with 25-gauge systems, especially when used to repair retinal detachments. An additional advantage of contact-based systems over the BIOM is that they do not require large amplitude rotation of the eye to see the periphery which causes tool flexion with 25-gauge systems.

Wide-angle viewing systems significantly decrease axial resolution (depth) and lateral resolution, and therefore should not be used for macular surgery. A plano contact lens should be used for all macular surgery and most diabetic traction retinal detachments. Wide-angle illumination systems improve video images because of the limited dynamic range of charge-coupled device (CCD) video cameras but significantly reduce the ability to visualize epiretinal membranes, vitreous, and ILM. The decreased resolution of wide-angle viewing systems is a significant driver for use of triamcinolone acetonide (Kenalog) to see vitreous and indocyanine green (ICG) for ILM staining.

Brighter light sources such as the Alcon xenon illuminator are needed because of smaller 23- or 25-gauge fibers (especially first generation), high divergence large working distance tools (chandeliers, Tornambe Torpedos, dual-mode infusion cannulas), and illuminated tools with low light throughout. Care must be taken when using very bright light sources to avoid phototoxicity: the sources must conform to ISO standards, and the illumination level should start lower and be increased to just the level sufficient for the task, especially when performing macular surgery. ICG staining of the ILM has never been used by the author because of toxicity and phototoxicity issues and because it is unnecessary with end-gripping ILM forceps such as the Alcon DSP ILM forceps. ICG staining in combination with intense xenon or mercury vapor light sources is potentially a high-risk situation with respect to phototoxicity. White light is better than yellow or green light because it improves tissue identification: macular xanthophyll is yellow which would require blue light to improve contrast. As vitreous, ILM, ERM, and retina are colorless, green or yellow light will not improve contrast. Fundus cameras and all office examinations use white light although various color filters have been available for decades. Although blue light is more energetic than yellow or green light photon-by-photon, the action spectrum of light toxicity is 550 nm which is green.

Illuminated tools should never be used for macular surgery because of the risk of phototoxicity. The use of illuminated instruments for so-called 'bimanual' surgery is based on the problem of having two hands and therefore two tools but more than two functions. Forceps are used to stabilize ERM to offset forces created by scissors or picks. Illumination can be combined with scissors, forceps, or picks.

CCD cameras and liquid crystal display (LCD) and cathode ray tube (CRT) monitors have 10^2–10^3 dynamic range (2–3 log units or f-stops) while the human eye has 10^7 dynamic range. 3-CCD cameras split the light three ways using prisms and beam splitters, reducing the light that reaches each of the CCDs. They are therefore more than one-third less sensitive than 1-CCD cameras and need more illumination to achieve the same signal:noise ratio and contrast.

CONCLUSION

As techniques and technology continue to evolve as they have since the beginning of vitrectomy surgery, the constant drive to better understand physics and engineering principles will continue to enable us to more effectively address retinal and vitreous surgical diseases and pathology.

REFERENCES

1. Charles S. Vitreous microsurgery. Baltimore: Williams & Wilkins; 1981.
2. Charles S. Vitreous microsurgery, 2nd edn. Baltimore: Williams & Wilkins; 1987.
3. Charles S, Wood B, Katz A. Vitreous microsurgery, 3rd edn. Baltimore: Lippincott, Williams & Wilkins; 2002.
4. Charles S, Calzada J, Wood B. Vitreous microsurgery, 4th edn. Baltimore: Lippincott, Williams & Wilkins; 2006.
5. O'Malley C, Heintz RM. Vitrectomy via the pars plana—a new instrument system. Trans Pac Coast Otoophthalmol Soc Annu Meet 1972; 53:121–137.
6. Charles S (Developer, March 1976). Fluid–gas exchange in the vitreous cavity. Ocutome Newsletter 1977; 2:1.
7. Charles S (Developer, March 1974). Vacuum cleaning. Ocutome Newsletter 1977; 2(2):2.
8. O'Malley C (Developer). Extrusion method. Ocutome Fragmatome Newsletter 1978; 3:3.
9. McCuen BW, Bessler M, Hickingbotham D, Isbey E. Automated fluid–gas exchange. Am J Ophthalmol 1983; 95:717.
10. Charles S. Techniques and tools for dissection of epiretinal membranes. Graefes Arch Clin Exp Ophthalmol 2003; 241(5):347–352.
11. Charles S. Endophotocoagulation. Retina 1981; 1(2):117–120.
12. Chang S, McCuen B, Charles S. New techniques for hemostasis during diabetic vitrectomy. Retina 2003; 23(1):120–122.

Index

Please note that page references relating to non-textual content such as Boxes or Figures are in *italic* print. Numbers (e.g. 20) will be spelled out (e.g. twenty).